MW00579841

Heal Your Nervous System

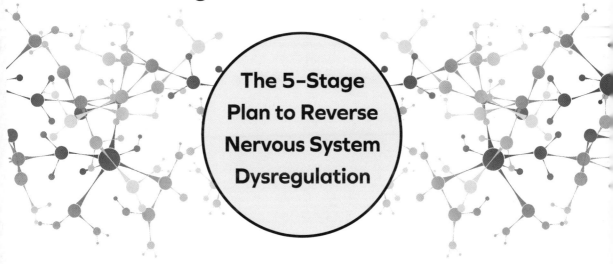

The 5-Stage Plan to Reverse Nervous System Dysregulation

Dr. Linnea Passaler

FAIR WINDS

Quarto.com

© 2024 Quarto Publishing Group USA Inc.
Text © 2024 Linnea Passaler

First Published in 2024 by Fair Winds Press,
an imprint of The Quarto Group,
100 Cummings Center, Suite 265-D,
Beverly, MA 01915, USA.
T (978) 282-9590 F (978) 283-2742

All rights reserved. No part of this book may be reproduced in any form without written permission of the copyright owners. All images in this book have been reproduced with the knowledge and prior consent of the artists concerned, and no responsibility is accepted by producer, publisher, or printer for any infringement of copyright or otherwise, arising from the contents of this publication. Every effort has been made to ensure that credits accurately comply with the information supplied. We apologize for any inaccuracies that may have occurred and will resolve inaccurate or missing information in a subsequent reprinting of the book.

Fair Winds Press titles are also available at discount for retail, wholesale, promotional, and bulk purchase. For details, contact the Special Sales Manager by email at specialsales@quarto.com or by mail at The Quarto Group, Attn: Special Sales Manager, 100 Cummings Center, Suite 265-D, Beverly, MA 01915, USA.

28 27 26 25 24 1 2 3 4 5

ISBN: 978-0-7603-8565-4

Digital edition published in 2024
eISBN: 978-0-7603-8566-1

Library of Congress Cataloging-in-Publication Data available.

Cover Design: The Quarto Group
Interior Design: *tabula rasa* graphic design
Illustration: Mattie Wells

Printed in China

The information in this book is for educational purposes only. It is not intended to replace the advice of a physician or medical practitioner. Please see your health-care provider before beginning any new health program.

To my children, Anais, Lelia, Amal, and Ariel—
May this work contribute to creating more regulated nervous systems and help shape a healthier world for you and all children everywhere.

Contents

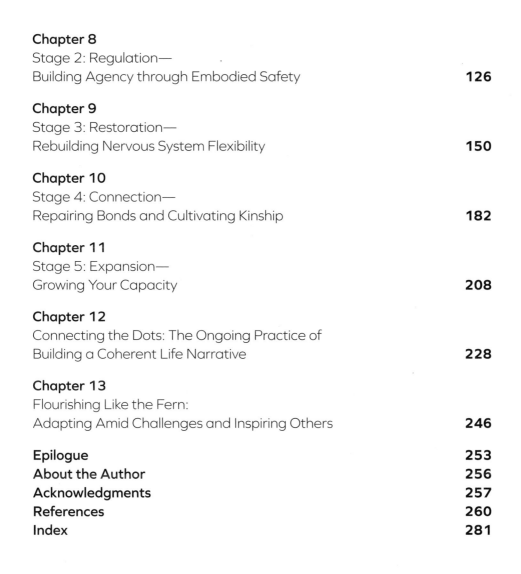

A Field Guide to Nervous System Regulation: How This Book Can Help You

DO YOU FEEL CONFUSED about what's happening in your body? Maybe you're caught in a loop of anxiety, fatigue, and strange symptoms, not knowing how to find relief. Clearly, your body isn't doing as well as it could. You don't know why this is happening, and nobody has given you a simple, complete explanation of what's really going on. What's worse, you haven't found solutions that truly work to help you feel better.

I was lost in the same chaos until, unexpectedly, an email popped into my inbox one day and turned everything around.

My life was spinning out of control, and I had no idea what to do. My physical health was declining. The first warning signs of rosacea, in the form of skin rashes, appeared, and I had constant gut pain that would later develop into a full-blown case of irritable bowel syndrome (IBS).

My emotional state was even worse—there were signs of high-functioning anxiety, stomach-churning sensations, chest tightness, constant dread . . . . As a busy oral surgeon and CEO of a digital health start-up, it was easy to brush off my feelings as nothing more than stress from work. But deep down, I knew there was more. On my way to a meeting, I emerged from the subway and crossed a desolate pedestrian bridge. It was a gray winter afternoon, about to rain. Everything, including my whole internal world, felt dull and lifeless. That's when I scrolled through my phone and saw that email waiting in my inbox that would change everything: a blog post by Jerry Colonna, cofounder of the coaching company Reboot, telling the story of Milarepa, a revered Buddhist master who learns to face his demons instead of chasing them away.

One day Milarepa returns to his cave on top of a mountain, after venturing outside to gather firewood, where he finds an unpleasant surprise: A troop of fierce and scary demons have taken over his home. Milarepa is filled with anger and fear. He immediately starts chasing them away, but they don't seem to care. In fact, they settle in his cave even more.

Milarepa decides to try something else—his current plan is not working! Since chasing them away doesn't work, perhaps they will listen to his spiritual teachings and leave. So he sits on a big rock and starts telling them about kindness, compassion, and life's ever-changing nature. After a while he stops and checks on the demons. Their eyes are fixed on him, but none will leave or yield.

This is when Milarepa realizes, if the demons won't disappear, perhaps there's something he must learn from them. He looks deep into the eyes of each demon and bows, saying, "It looks like we are going to be in here together. I am ready to learn anything you have to teach me."

Suddenly all the demons—except one, the biggest and most terrifying—vanish. Milarepa goes even further: He steps forward and gives himself over to the demon without reservations. "Eat me, if you wish," says Milarepa, putting his head in the demon's mouth. The terrifying beast immediately bows down before him and disappears.

Just like Milarepa, my life was full of inner demons. The more I fought against them, the stronger they seemed to get. Reading about Milarepa, I realized I needed to change my approach. Instead of trying to banish my inner demons, I had to learn to accept these parts of myself that I didn't really like or understand.

What if, I thought, instead of fighting my demons, I lowered my defenses and humbly acknowledged them? Could these demons help me understand my anxiety, burnout, and physical symptoms? So I made a commitment. I decided to stop running, stop trying to fix everything, and, instead, started to acknowledge and accept the parts of myself I had feared. Instead of trying to eliminate my demons, I started stepping toward them and saying, "Eat me, if you wish." This change in perspective, this act of courage and acceptance, was the first step I took toward healing my dysregulated nervous system.

This was just one initial step, of many, on a journey that would turn out to be long and challenging. Over time, that journey led me to a place of better health, a calm mind, and eventually, a mission to help others going through similar struggles. Eventually, this new mission led me to start a community for people going through a similar journey. Based on the comprehensive nervous system approach I and many others found successful in our healing journeys, I called this community Heal Your Nervous System.

Inside our community today, many people all over the world are bravely facing their personal demons and healing nervous system dysregulation. They're discovering how this approach doesn't just help relieve the symptoms that trouble them, but also opens a path to a more fulfilling life.

Now, after years of working with nervous system dysregulation, I've seen thousands of people in the Heal Your Nervous System community go from feeling chronically anxious, exhausted, burned out, and overwhelmed to feeling reliably calm, confident, resilient, and energetic. As their nervous system starts to regulate better, they gradually feel more at peace with themselves and those around them. They typically feel more confident and capable of handling the inherent stressors of life. Often they even start to spontaneously feel motivated to help others. Additionally, people who have reversed nervous system dysregulation have found that many of their physical health symptoms, such as autoimmune conditions, irritable bowels, rosacea, and chronic fatigue, have eased and no longer cause significant disruption to their lives.

Many of the people who have found our community have a long list of painful symptoms that are poorly addressed by the traditional medical system. Some are chronically stuck in a high state of activation, feeling a background sense of anxiety and worry, and have difficulty settling their mind on anything. Others are stuck in a chronic state of low energy, where they may regularly feel disengaged, like life is passing them by without much sense of purpose or meaning. Still others find us after physical health diagnoses like autoimmune conditions, IBS, postural orthostatic tachycardia syndrome (POTS), and rosacea.

Although the specific list of issues and diagnoses that may have led someone to connect with us is different for everyone, they all have something important in common. At the root of all these different symptoms is one underlying cause: a dysregulated nervous system that has lost its ability to respond flexibly to stressors.

I have designed this book to provide effective, practical guidance you can use to heal your nervous system, relieve your symptoms, and reclaim a sense of agency, resilience, and vitality.

In this book, I offer solutions rooted in science and that are designed to work in synergy with regular medical treatment—not replace it. I share the considerable wealth of experience that our team of practitioners at Heal Your Nervous System has gathered by guiding thousands of people to effectively heal and reverse the symptoms associated with a dysregulated nervous system.

In chapters 1 through 4, I orient you to the territory we will cover together, explaining what nervous system dysregulation means and how to assess the state of your nervous system. The approach to healing I offer in this book is significantly different and more expansive than what you might have encountered before. So I explain why such a broad and in-depth strategy is necessary for healing nervous system dysregulation, and then introduce a framework for the comprehensive approach called the 4 Pillars of Nervous System Health. Wrapping up your orientation, you'll learn about the main factors that may have contributed to your dysregulation and how you can leverage them to reverse it. You will explore the unique sensitivity of your nervous system, your innate stress response, and your fear system. You might feel the urge to jump directly to the solutions, but having a clear understanding of your nervous system is crucial before moving forward. Grasping the basics of your nervous system allows you to understand each stage of the healing process more thoroughly, paving the way for a smoother, more effective progression.

Then, in chapters 5 through 11, I'll show you a straightforward path to healing a dysregulated nervous system called the 5-Stage Plan. There are many practices that can help your nervous system, but without the right timing, these can be ineffective, inefficient, or even harmful. I've found that following a specific sequence helps people get more effective results in less time.

1. In stage 1, Awareness, you'll use what you've learned to recognize what's happening inside your nervous system, moment by moment.
2. In stage 2, Regulation, you'll learn short body-based interventions to change how you're feeling in the moment, shifting to a more relaxed state. Many people find this stage gives them a new sense of control over their body and feelings, which can be relieving and freeing.
3. In stage 3, Restoration, you'll focus on understanding and tackling the root causes behind your dysregulation. I'll show you how to shift the most fundamental patterns that keep throwing your nervous system out of a regulated state.
4. In stage 4, Connection, with a more regulated nervous system, it's time to help it thrive. Thriving nervous systems form deep connections with other people, nature, beauty, and a sense of purpose. During this stage, I'll guide you toward fostering a profound sense of interconnectedness with the people and the world around you.
5. In the fifth and final stage, Expansion, I'll guide you to harness the capabilities of your regulated nervous system. I'll show you how to use stress intentionally, along with experiences of awe, to expand your capacity for intensity and vitality.

Finally, chapters 12 and 13 will pull everything together. I've done my best to make this book helpful and easy to use: It's my attempt to offer the kind of clear, specific guidance I wish had been available during my own healing journey—guidance that countless people in our community, and beyond, rely upon daily. My sincere hope is that this book can provide that same valuable support for you too.

1

The Missing Piece of Your Healing Journey: A Dysregulated Nervous System

MOST OF THE WAYS WE'RE TOLD to go about healing our symptoms—whether from our favorite Instagram influencer or a specialized doctor—lack a comprehensive approach to the underlying issues that lead to suffering. If you've spent time in the modern medical system, you've probably experienced how siloed it is: one medical professional for your ears, nose, and throat; another for your mouth; another for your digestion; and another for your mind. Although this specialized approach to healing has certain advantages, it leaves little room for understanding that many symptoms, whether they show up in your feelings and behaviors or in certain parts of your body, have a common cause. This approach can leave you addressing each symptom individually and missing the bigger issue, like pulling the leaves off weeds in your garden without pulling out the roots, only to see the weeds grow back just as fast.

For example, you may be struggling with:

- Anxiety (health anxiety, high-functioning anxiety, social anxiety, and more)
- Autoimmune conditions
- Burnout
- Chronic fatigue syndrome and fibromyalgia
- Chronic pain
- Depersonalization, derealization, and dissociation
- Extreme sensitivities and sensory overload
- Functional neurological disorder

- Insomnia and sleep anxiety
- Irritable bowel syndrome (IBS)
- Multiple, unexplained food or chemical sensitivities
- Neck and shoulder tension
- Panic attacks, phobias
- Postural orthostatic tachycardia syndrome (POTS)
- Post-viral syndromes, such as long COVID
- Rosacea, eczema, hives, and other stress-related skin conditions
- Stress- and anxiety-related gut issues (nausea, vomiting, constipation)
- Stress-related hair loss
- Temporomandibular joint (TMJ) pain and jaw clenching
- Other chronic mind-body conditions

For a wide variety of symptoms, from generally feeling unwell and unmotivated day after day to irritable bowel syndrome and chronic fatigue, the underlying issue that led to developing your particular set of symptoms is that your nervous system is dysregulated.

THE DIFFERENCE BETWEEN REGULATION AND DYSREGULATION

Your nervous system is an intricate network of nerves and cells responsible for communicating with all the other systems in your body and telling them how to respond to different situations. Imagine that you just woke up, you check your phone, and you suddenly realize your alarm didn't go off. You have a sinking feeling in your gut as you realize that you need to rush to work right now or you're going to be late. Your nervous system integrates all this information almost instantly and tells your body systems how to respond. It sends stress hormones to your gut and immune system telling them to stop what they're doing because you need all your energy to get out the door. It signals your heart to beat faster, and your liver and muscles to take up more fuel, preparing your cells to make more energy available so you can move quickly. It signals your thought processes to focus on getting ready quickly, and, perhaps, fixing the problem with your alarm so it doesn't happen again. And it might change your mood to make you feel a sense of urgency so you don't suddenly forget you're in a rush and start scrolling on Instagram or call your mother for a chat.

Whether you're rushing to work, relaxing with a partner, or deep in sleep, your nervous system is constantly taking in information from your surrounding environment and communicating with all the other systems in your body. All of your body systems, such as your digestion, hormone regulation, and immune system, rely on the nervous system, so if your nervous system gets out of balance, many different aspects of your health can be affected all at once.

Because your nervous system plays such an important role in your overall health, you might imagine that stressful situations would be bad for it. But stressful situations are not a problem, and can even be good for your health. When your nervous system is in a regulated state, it responds to stress easily without the stressful circumstances becoming a problem for your health.

It's like a fern that bends under stressors—it is flexible. Just as a fern can quickly recover from being bent, a regulated nervous system can come back to a calm baseline state relatively quickly after being stressed. This flexibility allows your nervous system to cope with stressors without becoming overwhelmed or dysregulated, maintaining an environment in the body that allows all the other systems to function smoothly.

A regulated nervous system can respond to everything from a small, acute stressor, like a sudden loud noise, to a longer-term stressor, like being given too much work by your boss. It can also respond to both emotional stressors, like a difficult breakup, and physical stressors, like a virus, with the same flexibility, increasing the intensity of the stress response until the stressor has passed, and then turning down the intensity of the stress response to a baseline state of natural, easy relaxation.

A *dysregulated* nervous system, on the other hand, has lost its natural flexible response to stressors. It is stuck. If your nervous system is dysregulated, it may spend too much time stuck in a chronically activated state and not enough time in a rest-and-recovery state. You may feel anxious all the time, like there's always something wrong and you can never fully relax. It may also get stuck in a state of burnout or shutdown, where you feel exhausted, depressed, or like nothing really matters. Often, a dysregulated nervous system will cycle between these states, and you'll feel like you're caught in a loop of anxiety and fatigue.

Over time, a dysregulated nervous system can cause other systems in your body to accumulate damage. Although a regulated nervous system spends time in higher-stress states and then comes back to a baseline of lower-stress states, a dysregulated nervous system gets stuck in the higher-stress states and can't come back to the lower-stress states as a baseline. Many important processes that maintain your health in all parts of the body happen when you're back in a lower-stress state. For example, in very low-stress states, like deep sleep, your damaged cells get repaired or replaced with new cells, your brain flushes out waste material, and your immune system hunts down bacteria. If your nervous system is dysregulated and stuck in a high-stress response state, your body does not have enough time to do these important repair processes.

The damage your nervous system accumulates is a lot like if you never have time to take care of house chores and maintenance. Sometimes you're just too busy to take out the trash, clean, and call the plumber to replace that leaking pipe. That's okay—taking out the trash is most urgent, so do that now, and you can put off calling the plumber until next weekend. But if this pattern happens every week, the leaking pipe will become a major problem. The leak will get worse and, eventually, the puddle on the floor from the water leak will cause your floors to rot and mold will start growing. Similarly, when your nervous system is dysregulated, your body doesn't have time to do all the maintenance and repairs it needs, which will eventually lead to disease and illness.

Your body is naturally resilient and does not need to function perfectly all the time to maintain good health, but if your nervous system dysregulation goes on too long, the accumulated damage, eventually, results in symptoms like anxiety, depression, burnout, and chronic health conditions.

In this book, I'll guide you through exactly how to heal dysregulation and re-regulate your nervous system using a structured, 5-Stage Plan. Following this plan, you'll restore flexibility to your nervous system responses, which will allow you to respond much more easily and gracefully to stressors. Moreover, by reestablishing nervous system regulation, your body will finally have the time it needs in restful states to repair any damage that's accumulated in all of your bodily systems. This can significantly ease chronic conditions and restore your mood and energy. You will finally be able to return to a state of regulation.

Healing dysregulation is not a replacement for working with your doctor to treat any diseases or clinical diagnoses. When my nervous system was dysregulated, one of my primary physical symptoms was a skin condition called rosacea. The rosacea had developed because my nervous system was dysregulated, but it was absolutely essential for me to find a good doctor to treat me. And the treatments my doctor gave me were critical for getting the rosacea flares under control. But if I hadn't also healed my dysregulated nervous system, the rosacea would have come back, or a new symptom would have cropped up. If dysregulation is the root cause of your symptoms, then simply treating the symptoms without addressing the root cause won't provide long-term relief.

The next step is for you to start to understand how much nervous system dysregulation may be impacting your health and your symptoms. You may be surprised to discover that many things you thought were just a part of you, are, in fact, symptoms of nervous system dysregulation and no longer have to cause you distress.

IS YOUR NERVOUS SYSTEM DYSREGULATED?

To date, there are not yet any good comprehensive assessments of dysregulation that have been validated by scientific researchers. Also, no test or self-assessment can truly capture your full personality or perfectly depict your current situation. However, a good assessment can help you understand a little more about what is happening inside. Although it can't show you everything, and you might be different tomorrow, an assessment can be extremely useful for getting a general sense of what's happening to you right now.

To help you assess your level of nervous system dysregulation, I've created a self-assessment tool (see page 16) that will help you understand how much nervous system dysregulation is affecting your life. My self-assessment tool combines aspects of other validated assessments to give you a general sense of how much nervous system dysregulation might be showing up in your health. Treat this like a photograph, a point in time, marking where your nervous system dysregulation is right now, at the beginning of your healing journey.

For an online version of this assessment, as well as other self-assessment tools that will give you a more complete picture of the state of your nervous system, go to the online resource section for this book: healyournervoussystem.com/book.

>> DO THIS

ASSESSING YOUR NERVOUS SYSTEM

To take this assessment now, grab a pen and some paper, or open a note on your phone. For each of the following six items, rate **how much each affects your life** on a scale of 1 to 5, with 1 meaning it does not affect your life at all, 3 meaning it affects your life a moderate amount, and 5 meaning it affects your life a great deal.

1. Feeling overwhelmed ________
2. Feeling irritable, angry, easily frustrated ________
3. Experiencing sleep problems: falling asleep, waking up during the night, sleeping too little, sleeping too much ________
4. Feeling increased alertness, anxiety ________
5. Feeling dissociated or emotionally disconnected ________
6. Having difficulty maintaining lasting and satisfying relationships ________

For each of the following eight items, rate each based on **how much stress it causes you due to your sensitivity to it**. Use the same 1 to 5 scale, with 1 meaning it does not affect your life at all, 3 meaning it affects your life a moderate amount, and 5 meaning it affects your life a great deal.

7. Sounds ________
8. Smells ________
9. Feeling hot or cold easily ________
10. Certain food textures ________
11. Creams or lotions when they're on your skin ________
12. Lights, contrasts, reflections ________
13. Touching dirt, glue, or paint ________
14. Turtleneck tops, tight-fitting clothes or belts, elastic waistbands, materials and tags in clothes ________

For each of the following seven items, using the same 1 to 5 scale, rate **how much this condition applies to you**.

15. Sore muscles in the neck and shoulders area ________
16. Back pain ________
17. Headaches ________
18. Tense jaws, clenched teeth ________
19. Chronic pain ________
20. Skin conditions ________
21. Irritable bowels, stomach problems ________

Now, total your scores. ________

Interpreting Your Scores

Mild Dysregulation: Less than 34

If your score is less than 34, your nervous system may be regulated or you may have only mild dysregulation. If it's mildly dysregulated, you may notice that your energy levels don't stay balanced throughout the day, or you may have trouble sleeping fully through the night and, especially, getting enough deep sleep. Although mild dysregulation will show up differently for everybody, you may experience common physical symptoms like on-and-off difficulty with your digestion and a clenched jaw or teeth grinding at night. You might have a hyperactive mind even when you're trying to relax, and get easily frustrated or feel disconnected. Overall, you are likely still keeping it together quite well. You may even feel fairly typical compared to the other people around you because mild dysregulation is extremely common in our modern society.

Short periods of stress aren't dysregulation. It's completely natural for a regulated nervous system to experience periods of stress. So if your symptoms have only lasted for the past few days or weeks, or in rare cases the past few months, and they aren't causing you major suffering, your nervous system may just be in a temporary high-stress state, but not dysregulated. Once this intense period passes, your nervous system will naturally come back to a more relaxed state, and your body will be able to clean up any short-term damage caused by this intense period.

However, if your symptoms have lasted for more than a few weeks or months, your nervous system is likely mildly dysregulated. Even if you feel like your symptoms are relatively manageable right now, without intervention to re-regulate your nervous system, your dysregulation will worsen over time. Right now is the perfect time to use this book and start the 5-Stage Plan to Reverse Nervous System Dysregulation, relieve your current symptoms, begin to heal the damage it may be causing, and prevent any further damage from accumulating.

Moderate Dysregulation: 34 to 67

If your score is between 34 and 67, you likely have a moderately dysregulated nervous system. The symptoms of nervous system dysregulation show up differently for everyone, but it's very common for people with moderate dysregulation to have difficulty falling asleep or staying asleep, and then to feel both tired and anxious during the day. Your emotional landscape may be challenging to navigate, often feeling like it's just too much. You may become overwhelmed by life's stressors often and need a lot of time by yourself or with people who help you feel safe just to get through each day.

Notable physical symptoms are common for people with moderate dysregulation, which can show up in the body as inflammation and constriction. You may have chronic pain in parts of your body that hold tension, such as your shoulders or back.

And, at this level of dysregulation, inflammation may have contributed to one or more diagnosable conditions, such as rheumatoid arthritis, IBS, or depression. Additionally, you might notice that certain sensory stimuli, such as loud noises or fluorescent lights, are especially stressful or uncomfortable for you.

If you have moderate nervous system dysregulation, this book will help you. You'll learn how you got here and how you can work with your sensitivity to make it a source of joy and purpose rather than a vulnerability. The 5-Stage Plan to Reverse Nervous System Dysregulation will help you find a new baseline where you can finally heal and relax.

Significant Dysregulation: Above 67

If your score is above 67, you may have a significantly dysregulated nervous system. You are likely really struggling to get through each day and just going about your daily tasks can often seem insurmountable. You may have one or more clinical diagnoses and you might be working with a doctor or therapist to address various aspects of your health. You may have been struggling for many years or even most of your life just to feel all right.

Getting a good night's sleep may be rare or nonexistent. You may often feel overwhelmed by things that other people don't seem to struggle with, and when you're not overwhelmed, you can often fall into a low mood or feel numb or dissociated. On top of all this, your nervous system may have shifted into a mode of sensory defensiveness and many different sensory stimuli can increase your sense of feeling stressed or unsafe. Things like certain lights, loud or annoying sounds, and certain textures put an additional burden on your nervous system and make you feel even worse.

If you have significant dysregulation, you may be suffering seriously. I wrote this book to help you. It may feel particularly easy for you to become overwhelmed on your healing journey, so take it slowly, one step at a time. In the next few chapters, I'll help you understand how your sensitivity works so it can become an ally on your healing journey and in life. You'll discover the science behind how you got here and why attempts to heal in the past didn't work. Most importantly, I'll walk you through the 5-Stage Plan to Reverse Nervous System Dysregulation so your suffering can be a thing of the past. You'll be able to feel confident in your body, your health, and the natural gifts you have to offer others.

HOW DYSREGULATION SHOWS UP FOR YOU

The self-assessment of nervous system dysregulation you just took is divided into three components, or areas, of life where you're most likely to notice symptoms of dysregulation: *emotional, sensory, and physical.* Because the symptoms of dysregulation show up differently for everybody, noticing the trend of your scores in each section can give you a glimpse into how your body processes dysregulation and where the symptoms tend to manifest. Some people have higher scores in just one or two areas, whereas others have higher scores in all three.

The way your symptoms can show up in the *emotional component* includes feeling regularly overwhelmed, dissociated, and like your mind is racing and won't shut off when you're trying to relax. The emotional component is associated with an aspect of your sensitivity called "high reactivity." Your dysregulation is likely to show up here if you have an innate tendency to feel emotions more intensely than others.

The *sensory component*, including stress reactions to sensory stimuli, like certain sounds, smells, heat and cold, lights, and textures, is associated with sensory defensiveness. In chapter 3, I'll show you how you may be naturally more sensitive than other people, and how this can be a benefit if your nervous system is regulated. But if your nervous system is dysregulated, your natural sensitivities can cause your nervous system to go into a defensive mode and react negatively to a wide range of stimuli.

The *physical component*, including things like chronic pain, shoulder and neck tension, irritable bowels, and frequent headaches, is often associated with inflammation or your body holding tension. You might notice dysregulation showing up here if you have painfully tense shoulders or a clenching jaw. Alternatively, dysregulation in your body can show up as inflammation, which can lead to symptoms like digestion issues and skin conditions. It may even lead to autoimmune conditions or a whole range of other physical manifestations.

Everybody's journey will be different based on how your particular symptoms show up and which aspects of your dysregulation are most in need of relief, but you *can* find relief from all your symptoms. As you read the next few chapters, keep in mind how dysregulation shows up for you.

THE BIOLOGY OF DYSREGULATION

Inside your body, there are many things that contribute to nervous system dysregulation. Although scientific research is far from understanding the full picture of dysregulation, a few of the most significant factors in play are:

- How efficiently your cells produce and utilize energy
- How sensitive your nervous system is to different types of input
- How your brain has stored past information about difficult or disturbing experiences you've gone through

Mitochondria: The Energy Producers in Your Cells

Emerging scientific research is showing that energy production within each cell plays an important part in maintaining a regulated nervous system. The parts of each cell that are responsible for producing energy are called "mitochondria." So when your mitochondria are functioning smoothly, your cells are getting all the energy they need at the right time. However, when your mitochondrial function becomes disrupted, such as when too many waste products, or "free radicals," accumulate in your cells, it can stop producing enough energy for the cell. Not having enough energy in your cells can affect all aspects of health, from your mood to your hormones to your immune system.

Nervous System Sensitivity: How Your Body Responds to Stimuli

Sensitivity is another important factor that can affect both how your nervous system gets dysregulated and how dysregulation leads to your specific symptoms. Scientific research into nervous system sensitivity has shown that sensitivity is a spectrum, meaning we all have different levels of sensitivity to different stimuli and sensations. Like any other aspect of your personality, there are both advantages and disadvantages to being more sensitive. If you are a highly sensitive person, you may be better at things like attuning to others' feelings and sensing subtle aesthetic differences in art, music, or writing. These advantages can, among many other things, make you an especially good friend, and even lead you to work in the arts or other creative fields. But one disadvantage of being higher on the sensitivity spectrum is that you are more susceptible to nervous system dysregulation.

Simply learning about your sensitivity is an important first step to increasing the advantages of being more sensitive, while decreasing the disadvantages. In chapter 3, I dive deeply into understanding your sensitivity.

How Your Brain Is Wired to Process Stress

Another critical factor in nervous system dysregulation is how your nervous system is wired to process stressful situations. You may have gone through some extremely distressing experiences in your life, which could have left your nervous system less capable of responding to stress with flexibility. As a child, your nervous system may not have received comprehensive training about how to respond flexibly to stressful situations and then come back to a relaxed baseline easily. Both of these situations can lead to dysregulation.

However, your nervous system has a remarkable power to reshape and heal itself from damage caused by stressors. In fact, your nervous system is constantly in the process of forming and reorganizing connections between different neurons, the cells that make up the nervous system. This process is called "neuroplasticity," and although neurocientists used to think that only children's brains had neuroplasticity, they now agree that the brain remains neuroplastic throughout one's life-span. That means that no matter what experiences you had during childhood, or what traumatic stressors are contributing to dysregulation as an adult, you can rewire your nervous system to become regulated.

To picture this, think of your nervous system like a piece of play-dough. You have the power to mold and reshape it, directing its rewiring. Of course, your ability to shape your nervous system has limitations: Lost neurons from brain damage, such as traumatic brain injuries or stroke, cannot be replaced. But your nervous system is fully equipped for you to rewire the neural pathways that lead to dysregulation and restore a flexible stress response. The 5-Stage Plan to Reverse Nervous System Dysregulation will give you all the tools you need to shape your nervous system and restore its flexibility and regulation.

THE PINBALL EFFECT

Now that you understand the nervous system and have assessed your system's state of functioning, the next step is to figure out how it got this way so you can begin to heal it. If nervous system dysregulation were like a bacterial infection, you could just take a course of antibiotics and feel better. Unfortunately, it's not that simple.

Mitochondria, brain wiring, and sensitivity operate through complex networks of feedback loops. This means that a cause can lead to a consequence, but the consequence can lead to another cause.

You can think of this complicated system as like a pinball machine. Mitochondria and brain wiring act as the "flippers" that guide signals around our bodies. When they work together in harmony, they create a feedback loop that helps keep the brain and body functioning optimally, like when a pinball expert uses the flippers just right to keep the ball bouncing around the machine and racking up points.

But when something malfunctions in the machine—for example, one of the flippers slows down or a bumper loses some of its bounce—the pinball expert's strikes miss the target. Even a small difference from a faulty flipper can cause the ball to careen into an entirely different sequence and end up in the gutter.

When things go wrong with one component of the system, sooner or later, that affects the other components—the immune system, gut, skin, and more—leading to dysregulation and a cascade of symptoms, like inflammation or poor regulation of emotions and bodily functions, which can feel overwhelming to diagnose and treat.

This is what I call the "pinball effect": Causality is often complicated, with a cause generating a consequence that becomes another cause in turn, creating a cycle of events, just like when playing pinball. This is the reason many people struggle to identify what's going on in their body and how to heal it. Cause and effect become so intertwined that it's hard to know where to start and how to untangle it all.

Despite the mystery surrounding the exact mechanisms of cause and effect in bodily systems, one thing is clear: It is possible to break the dysregulation loop with small, consistent interventions that are known to improve the function of mitochondria, offset the challenging aspects of high sensitivity, and modify brain wiring to respond better to stressors.

Sometimes it's possible to link symptoms to a specific problem and solve them with simple, effective interventions. For example, if your doctor finds there's a lack of a specific vitamin in your body, replenishing that vitamin can help heal your symptoms and restore regulation to your nervous system.

But most of the time, identifying the issue and resolving it are more complicated. Many of the practices in this book aim to specifically address the biological factors that may be playing an important role in your dysregulation, such as mitochondrial dysfunction, sensitivity, and brain wiring. However, healing from a dysregulated nervous system and rediscovering your innate resilience and ability to thrive require a comprehensive solution.

In the next chapter, I introduce you to a new comprehensive framework, the 4 Pillars of Nervous System Health, which includes all four essential elements of mind-body health your nervous system needs to thrive.

2

Transitioning from Quick Fix to Long-Term Solution: The 4 Pillars of Nervous System Health

IN THIS CHAPTER, WE'LL LEARN TO RECOGNIZE the "quick-fix cycle" and why it keeps you stuck in a loop of pain—as well as how it can be broken using a new model called the 4 Pillars of Nervous System Health—body, mind, connection, and spirituality. Unlike the "quick-fix cycle," this new model provides real, long-lasting relief to symptoms and progressively reverses the damage you have accumulated over years of having a dysregulated nervous system managed with quick-fix trial and error.

THE "QUICK-FIX CYCLE"

Sometimes it can feel as though you're caught in a vicious cycle when trying to manage your current symptoms. You look for a quick fix to help relieve your most urgent symptoms, but the relief doesn't last long. These solutions are only temporary and make you feel frustrated and disappointed in the end.

You will likely recognize some aspects of this vicious cycle in your own story. Here's how this cycle can play out: You've spent years in a highly stressful environment, such as a high-stakes job, raising a family, patching together gigs to make ends meet, or as a caregiver for a loved one. Perhaps you've gone through some especially difficult periods, such as a challenging childhood, a complicated relationship, a debilitating illness, or a devastating breakup. Maybe you had a very difficult childhood where you didn't feel safe or your emotional needs weren't met. And now, you're struggling with symptoms such as overwhelming fatigue, body aches, digestive issues, and general anxiety as a result of the damage your body has accumulated.

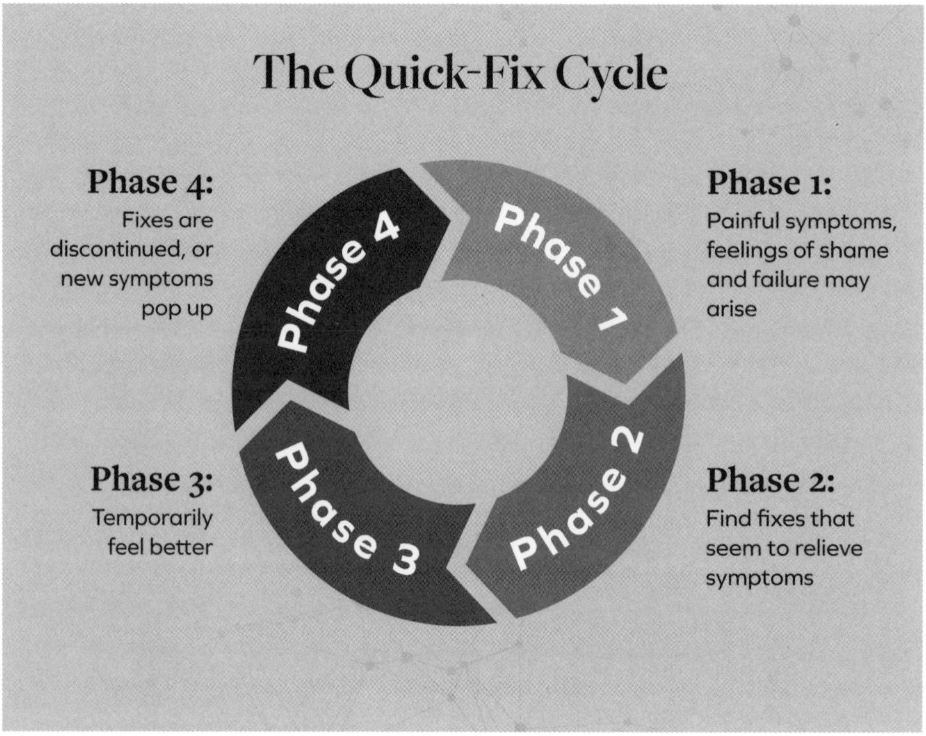

After everything you've been through it might feel especially unfair, or even cruel, that you're now struggling with these symptoms. But you do your best to address them: you research the latest treatments and scour the internet for a solution. For example, you try a new diet to increase your energy, and you implement various lifestyle modifications that you've heard can ease the growing burden of anxiety and fatigue. You might have talked to your doctor about the fatigue, a gastroenterologist about the bloating, and a psychiatrist about the anxiety. You might have done years of talk therapy or seen a host of alternative health-care providers such as acupuncturists or alternative medicine specialists. You are desperate to find an answer that will give you some relief.

Although many of the solutions you've found provide some relief, and some of your symptoms might even completely go away, it never seems to last no matter how much progress you make. Your symptoms return with a vengeance, or new ones pop up. Over months and years of this cycle, you might start doubting yourself. Your confidence in healing yourself diminishes with each new attempt and failure. At this stage, many people start thinking that something must be wrong with them. Something inside feels broken.

On the outside, it may still look like you have everything under control. Inside, however, you feel lost.

When your symptoms get bad enough, you start to have trouble relaxing even when you're home from work, sleep feels impossible, and you have frequent meltdowns. You snap at people easily and withdraw from connections more so you don't have to deal with the stress that others can cause. You're impatient to feel better, and this never-ending delay fuels your anger, frustration, or despair. You feel at the end of your rope.

When looking for lasting relief from anxiety, burnout, and overwhelm, many people face challenges that follow a predictable and frustrating pattern. I call it the "quick-fix cycle" and it looks like this:

1. You experience mind or body symptoms that cannot be attributed to a well-defined and treatable disorder.
2. You start searching for a fix, which often leads to trying a wide variety of practices and treatment modalities. However, you don't really understand the root causes of your symptoms and how to address them.
3. You feel better, and symptoms subside.
4. Because you have not addressed the root cause, when you inevitably become less diligent about implementing the fix or you discontinue it altogether, symptoms come back with a vengeance. Alternatively, another symptom pops up to replace the old one you've worked so hard to fix. You are back to square one, maybe feeling even more discouraged than before. You might even notice yourself feeling embarrassed or ashamed in front of your loved ones who supported implementing this fix and thought you had healed.

Over time, rather than healing your symptoms, the repetition of this cycle adds to the toll on your nervous system, making the problem even worse.

Your increasing number of symptoms and the painfulness of each can make your body a scary and uncomfortable place. The "quick-fix cycle" can reinforce the awful feeling that you have lost control and nothing that you do will help you heal.

When this happens, your mind may try to protect you by pushing you even harder to try to fix the problem, obsessively jumping from one fix to the next in search of relief. Another way it may try to protect you is to simply shut down into a state of despair, where you start to believe that you are beyond any hope of healing. After enough repetitions of the "quick-fix cycle," you may find yourself deeply disconnected from your body. You may have completely lost trust in your body's ability to heal, and embarking on (yet another) healing journey may seem almost hopeless.

These feelings of suffering and helplessness, reinforced by the "quick-fix cycle," can lead to the emergence of a protective part of yourself that I call the "disconnected part." In response to your dysregulated nervous system and the failures of the "quick-fix cycle" to heal, your disconnected part learns to protect you by disconnecting you from your body.

In my experience, the disconnected part is one of the biggest obstacles in the journey to healing the underlying causes of anxiety, burnout, and overwhelm. This disconnected part doesn't mean to harm you; on the contrary, it disconnects *because* you have been wounded deeply by previous experiences and feelings of failure. But its strategy to protect you can end up blocking real healing. It tries to protect you in a few ways:

- It's suspicious, always looking for things to go wrong. Its way of protecting you is to give you reasons to pull away and to second-guess your choices when it comes to healing.
- It relies heavily on cognition, overanalyzing and overplanning, trying to make sense of everything at the cost of sacrificing your healing progress, body, and intuition.
- It's very critical; from its point of view, if things are not perfect, they are not worth doing. For example, if you don't have hours to meditate or do yoga, or if you must take breaks for whatever reason, this disconnected part will say, "This will not work."
- It's impatient and always in a hurry. It won't let you slow down; if results don't come quickly, it convinces you that you don't have time for this and you should just try something else.

To heal the underlying causes of your symptoms, you need a new plan to reassure the disconnected part that you're safe, while still allowing your healing journey to progress. Many of the practices you'll find later in this book will help calm and reassure your disconnected part and allow it to let go a little bit so you can continue your healing journey.

You can start working with the disconnected part if you notice it coming up. Here's a simple practice to get started (see page 29).

The disconnected part is also a reflection of our culture's narrative around healing—distorted by skewed and inaccurate lenses. We are taught to consume the newest

>> DO THIS

REASSURING YOUR DISCONNECTED PART

First and foremost, set the intention to notice the disconnected part when it becomes activated. When you become aware that the disconnected part is active and trying to protect you, stop and take a deep breath. Instead of trying to reason with it or follow its train of thought, simply switch your attention to noticing bodily sensations that arise when this part comes online. You can use a journal to describe body sensations such as tension, tingling, tightness, or pressure and where those sensations are located in your body. It can be useful to describe what they would look like if you could see them. What size would they be? What shape? What color?

Next, offer warm, compassionate reassurance to this disconnected part. You can tell the part that you are going to take good care of yourself now and you will not let your guard down. Thank the part for its hard work at keeping you safe.

trend or supplement, practice the latest meditation technique, or try the hottest diet craze to become healthier, happier, and more successful. Real healing requires patience and deep acceptance of our imperfect humanity. When we follow the misguided healing narratives our culture espouses, we find ourselves seeking:

Immediate gratification, with the expectation that healing should be fast and convenient. This encourages people to take shortcuts when addressing their health concerns and to focus on symptomatic relief instead of healing the underlying causes of those symptoms.

Performance increases, because the idea is that healing should make you faster, more productive, stronger—rather than being a way to restore the integrity of the individual. This strong emphasis on performance can create a feeling of urgency, to hustle and produce more, eventually leading to an even greater sense of powerlessness and burnout.

Healing as a way to become an improved version of yourself, which can further disempower you by creating the expectation that you should always be striving to reach some level of perfection. This type of thinking assumes that your current state is not good enough or there is something wrong with you, which can result in feelings of guilt and shame. It also sets up an unhealthy comparison loop in which you compare yourself to those who seem more successful or "better" than you, resulting in self-doubt and a lack of confidence. This just perpetuates the "quick-fix cycle" and makes it difficult for you to break the pattern.

Becoming an enlightened version of yourself, which can encourage you to bypass your own sense of self and your body's natural healing process in order to feel better. A view that healing should result in some kind of "enlightenment" is disempowering and reinforces the belief that your body is not capable of healing itself. It also perpetuates the idea that healing should be a mystical experience, which can result in confusion and frustration as you try to make sense of what this means for you. This is sometimes called "spiritual bypassing," and it's a form of avoidance that can, ultimately, lead to further dysregulation.

Given the dysfunctional nature of our culture's narrative around healing, we need to stop relying on it to heal. It's completely normal to want relief from physical and emotional pain, and even to want to expand your capacity to be human. I dedicate a whole chapter (chapter 11) to expanding your capacity to be human once your nervous system is regulated. But problems arise if your healing is centered on the need to feel validated by society, with its impossible standards. This fuels anxiety and self-doubt and bolsters your "disconnected part," making it even harder to break the "quick-fix cycle" and find lasting relief. Our society's misguided narratives around healing do not lead to real nervous system regulation and lasting relief from your symptoms.

HOW THE HEALTH-CARE SYSTEM FUELS THE "QUICK-FIX CYCLE"

Is modern medicine inadvertently reinforcing the "quick-fix cycle"? I believe so.

Modern medical training has made it difficult for clinicians to navigate the complex terrain of illnesses that don't fit a clear diagnosis. Every doctor specializes in a particular area of health care, such as an organ or a surgical treatment. The dermatologist focuses on skin diseases and conditions, the gastroenterologist treats the digestive system, and the ophthalmologist specializes in the eyes.

One advantage of this specialization system is that it ensures doctors can provide the highest quality care for patients experiencing symptoms in their area of expertise. It also gives them the confidence to make diagnoses quickly and prescribe effective treatments for a large number of diseases. Additionally, as a result of this siloed approach to medicine, doctors become more efficient, stay informed about cutting-edge advancements in their field, and are able to conduct specialized research that may lead to the development of innovative technologies and treatments.

However, this comes at a high cost for those of us whose symptoms don't fit neatly into one focused area of the body. This fragmented approach to health care fails to recognize the interconnectedness of the human body and mind. It isn't equipped to handle illnesses or conditions that don't originate from a localized physical problem or other obvious cause.

Clinicians are limited in their approach to healing because of their strict adherence to the practice of identifying symptoms, diagnosing diseases, and prescribing medications or treatments.

Illnesses such as chronic pain, autoimmune disease, depression, and anxiety are multifaceted and often can't be lumped under one diagnosis or treatment plan. Even worse, clinicians become accustomed to viewing individuals as a compilation of their parts, and they often feel inadequately trained to provide more comprehensive care. The consequence is that you, as the patient, receive disjointed care that leaves little room for exploring the root causes of your physical and emotional suffering. It also leads clinicians to prescribe medications that, at best, provide temporary symptomatic relief but do nothing to address the underlying causes of illness.

An additional problem is that, in the current medical model, we are encouraged to feel our suffering is valid only if it fits into an official medical diagnosis. It is natural to feel validated and relieved when we receive an official diagnosis, something that tells us why we feel the way we do. However, it is important to recognize that although diagnoses are indispensable for the health-care system and for scientific research, *they do not define us as human beings.*

Relying on a diagnosis to make sense of our suffering is not good for us. We need to stop giving diagnoses the power to validate our pain. Your physical and emotional experiences are valid whether or not they're measured against an external system designed by medical institutions. Luckily, over the last fifty years, numerous scientists, physicians, and medical researchers have started a paradigm shift toward acknowledging that modern medicine is not an all-encompassing solution for treating illness and understanding the human experience.

In the 1970s, Dr. Marshall Marinker—a brilliant British general practitioner who was also a sensitive poet and writer—laid the groundwork to redefine what constitutes being a primary care physician. In the famous paper, "Why Make People Patients?" published in the *Journal of Medical Ethics* in 1975, he redefined the role of diagnoses in a way that can reframe your experience of feeling unhealthy.

According to Marinker, there are three different modes, or perspectives, of being and feeling unhealthy. One has to do with measurable biology, another with your internal experience, and the third with how your health challenge is labeled by society. None of these modes is better than the others, but instead they are each valid and serve different purposes. Marinker's model can help us disentangle the different aspects of being unwell and see them more clearly.

The Three Modes of Unhealthy

Disease: Disease is the realm of doctors. Disease happens when the structure or function of the human body differs from the biological norm. Doctors use objective measures, such as laboratory tests, to detect disease, which then allows them to prescribe treatments and medications. In the medical view, diseases are seen as central—to restore the biological norm, the disease needs to be resolved.

Illness: Being ill is a personal feeling, different for each person. It is the realm of patients: an experience that comes from inside of them. It's important to understand that illness and disease don't always go together. Sometimes, for example in the early stages of cancer or diabetes, the doctor can detect a disease by running some lab tests, but the patient is not experiencing any illness. Other times, the patient experiences illness, but the doctor can't find any disease.

Clinical diagnosis: Clinical diagnoses, or what Marinker defines as "sickness," is the realm of society. It is an identity co-created between you and society that you are a "sick" person and need to be regarded differently than if you were well. Marinker wrote that having a clinical diagnosis "is a social role, a status, a negotiated position in the world, a bargain struck between the person henceforward called 'sick,' and a society which is prepared to recognize and sustain him." Having a clinical diagnosis can help you feel seen and validated in your illness. It can also get you access to the support needed to function in society with your illness or disease, as well as to navigate the journey back to health.

If you have a clearly defined clinical diagnosis, people are more likely to acknowledge that you are sick and help you get well again. Your family might bring you soup or let you skip out on chores. Your doctor might write you a prescription for medication to help manage or cure your condition. A diagnosis might make you eligible for financial assistance, such as insurance payouts or disability support. You may also get some accommodations at work or school, like extra breaks, reduced hours, or a more comfortable workspace. Additionally, an official diagnosis can help you find social support and get you access to people living with a similar illness or disease. Support groups, whether online or in person, often welcome only those who have been officially diagnosed.

UNTANGLING DISEASE, ILLNESS, AND DIAGNOSIS

The mainstream medical model says that diseases, the objectively measurable "hard facts" of our biology, are all that matter for health. The medical model views clinical diagnosis as the way to talk about and bill for treatment of what really matters—the disease. It rarely acknowledges that illness, your subjective experience of being unhealthy, exists at all. On the other hand, our social institutions, such as schools, workplaces, insurance companies, and governments, treat clinical diagnosis as the most important "hard fact" and assume that disease doesn't exist until it is clinically diagnosed. Like the medical model, these institutions also completely ignore your experience of illness.

But your health is not reduceable to any one of these perspectives. Your well-being includes objectively measurable biology (disease), society naming and accommodating your needs (clinical diagnosis), and your individual experience of being unwell (illness). In fact, all three of these perspectives are valid and important in understanding the state of being unhealthy and the journey back to health.

When you understand that these are equally valid but separate aspects of being healthy, you can see that we often get confused between them, and our confusion leads to unnecessary suffering. The truth is that not all diseases lead to the feeling of being ill. And sometimes, we feel ill without any identifiable disease. Confusing *illness* and *disease* can be frustrating for both the patient and the doctor. Illness is deeply personal. It's about how you feel, and not all illnesses show up on a lab test or a doctor's examination.

But your feelings are important, even if there's no disease or clinical diagnosis to pin them on. Additionally, not all clinical diagnoses are associated with an illness or a disease. For example, a person with dyslexia might find a clinical diagnosis helps them get their needs met in school, yet they don't feel ill and they have no disease. By valuing all three modes of unhealthy, you can bring more clarity and understanding to your health experiences and needs.

WHAT IS HEALING?

Now that you understand there is a better way to talk about what it means to be unhealthy, you need a clear working definition of healing. *Healing is the process of resolving illness and restoring physical, emotional, relational, and spiritual well-being.* The process of healing *may involve* curing a disease, but it is not limited to that. When it does involve curing a disease, the person receives a clinical diagnosis and enters a patient-doctor relationship to treat the disease, or at least manage it.

Importantly, *the lack of a clinical diagnosis does not invalidate an individual's experience of illness*, nor does it diminish their need for healing. To bring about genuine healing, it's crucial to address the illness, alongside curing any diseases and navigating clinical diagnoses with health-care professionals.

As you have seen, the "quick-fix cycle" is a failed model of healing. It doesn't address the underlying causes of illness. Similarly flawed is the cultural narrative that promotes perpetual self-improvement until you reach an ideal, enlightened version of yourself. Even our modern medical system and societal institutions, which are primarily equipped to recognize disease and clinical diagnosis, typically overlook many critical components of healing and health. To become truly healthy again, you need a new model of healing.

A NEW MODEL OF HEALING: THE 4 PILLARS OF NERVOUS SYSTEM HEALTH

Now that we have clearly identified the problems that keep us stuck in the ineffective "quick-fix cycle," and have a definition of healing we can work with, and toward, let's discuss an alternative model of healing to replace this flawed system: the 4 Pillars of Nervous System Health.

In 1977, the highly esteemed journal *Science* featured a paper written by American psychiatrist and internist George Engel. In the article, titled "The Need for a New Medical Model: A Challenge for Biomedicine," Engel suggested that doctors were too focused on the biological and physical causes of diseases and not enough on how people's thoughts, feelings, and social environment could play a role in making them sick.

Engel expanded on previous ideas that had been circulating in the medical community, and proposed the "biopsychosocial model" of health. It involves looking at all the different factors that can cause illness and figuring out which ones are most important for each patient.

Engel said that doctors should use information from a person's body, mind, and social life to create a complete picture of their health. He understood that it's essential to look at all these systems together to understand the patient's story of illness. This means that doctors and patients need to talk to each other a lot to understand what's going on. Engel argued that if doctors used this approach, it would make health care both more caring *and* more scientific.

Over the past forty years, the biopsychosocial model has become one of the most popular alternatives to the traditional biomedical model in health education and clinical settings.

Based on Engel's biopsychosocial model, I've created a simplified comprehensive approach that includes all the essential aspects of maintaining a regulated nervous system: I call it the 4 Pillars of Nervous System Health.

Pillar 1, body: This pillar includes all the biological components that influence regulation and health, from the genetic and cellular level to organs and systems. If we don't include healing at the body level, our journey toward a regulated nervous system is almost guaranteed to fail.

Pillar 2, mind: This pillar addresses the psychological factors that contribute to dysregulation and includes our thoughts, emotions, coping strategies, internal working models, and how we see ourselves and the reality around us.

Pillar 3, connection: We heal and grow in connection with others, and this includes how we relate in the context of close relationships, within our community, and society at large. Relationships are an essential source of support, comfort, and joy and can provide a sense of belonging that is crucial for healing. This pillar involves not only how we

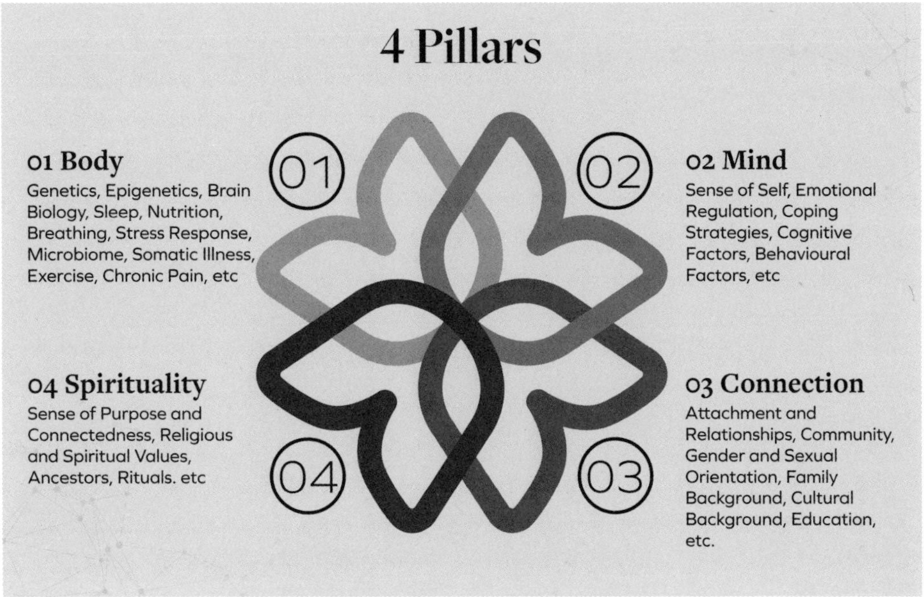

regulate in the presence of other people, for example, when there is conflict, but also our ability to help others when they are dysregulated.

Pillar 4, spirituality: We need to feel part of something larger than ourselves to have a thriving nervous system. And spirituality, at its core, is the fulfillment of this need. For some people, it's religion, and for others, it's a connection with nature or with a big purpose like creating more justice and equity in the world or raising emotionally competent children who are confident, empathetic, and adaptable in the face of life's challenges. This pillar recognizes the importance of understanding our place in the world and cultivating a sense of connectedness and meaning that goes beyond relationships with other people.

These 4 Pillars are interconnected and mutually influence and support one another, creating a feedback loop. Therefore, you can't just focus on one pillar and expect to heal your symptoms; you must work on all four to achieve lasting relief. By restoring health in each pillar, you can create a regulated nervous system—one able to withstand stressors without tumbling into chronic dysregulation. Additionally, the more you strengthen each pillar, the more your nervous system will have the support it needs to reverse or ease the symptoms of dysregulation that have caused you so much suffering. In this book, I take you through the journey of comprehensively addressing each pillar, putting the power to regulate your nervous system back in your control.

Although the pillars can never be fully separated, each stage in the journey to reversing nervous system dysregulation focuses more on some pillars than on others. Your journey will start by focusing on the body to establish a structure to support the biological aspects of nervous system regulation, including resetting your circadian rhythm and creating a routine to provide the right amount of physical stimulation to different parts of your nervous system. This underlying structure will support your nervous system throughout the rest of the journey.

In the first stage of the 5-Stage Plan, Awareness, you'll emphasize the mind pillar, learning to open the mind to clearly understand what is happening throughout the nervous system. The second stage, Regulation, moves back to the body, but this time emphasizing how you can use physical activities, such as breathing and muscles, to shift to a more calm and relaxed state. In the third stage, Restoration, you'll bring these two pillars together, emphasizing both mind and body as you address the root causes of your dysregulation. The fourth stage, Connection, moves to focus on the connection pillar, emphasizing connection to others, to nature, to beauty, and to purpose. And the fifth stage, Expansion, focuses on all 4 Pillars at once, building your nervous system's capacity once it's regulated. Ultimately, a thriving nervous system is supported by all 4 Pillars being strong and healthy. No matter which pillars are stronger or weaker right now for you, the 5-Stage Plan will show you how to make each pillar a robust support for your nervous system.

RETAKING CONTROL OF YOUR HEALING JOURNEY

Although Engel's biopsychosocial model has become an increasingly popular alternative to the mainstream reductionist models of healing, it can't be plugged into our modern medical system easily. Clinicians are limited in their ability to work from this more comprehensive framework in several ways, including:

- It takes a lot of time to do a full evaluation and provide care for a patient. The way our health-care system is set up, clinicians are not compensated for spending time doing this level of in-depth biological, psychological, and social evaluation.
- Health-care providers need to learn about the biological, psychological, and social aspects of their practice. Achieving this level of comprehensive and in-depth understanding can be difficult.
- It can be challenging to figure out how the biopsychosocial model applies to an individual patient. There are many psychological, social, and spiritual components to consider.
- Physicians focus on medical tests and labs that will be paid for by insurance companies. They spend less time on care that is not paid for, such as social and emotional care.

These are valid concerns and help explain why, to this day, the traditional model of care still dominates medical practice. Although improving our health-care system is a worthy goal, it may take many decades, and improvements will likely be incremental. But you need a solution now that will allow you to get the care you need, address all 4 Pillars, and regulate your nervous system.

The solution is for you to take the lead in your healing journey. It's your body; what you say goes. You know when something doesn't feel right, even if you can't put your finger on it. You know your triggers and what makes you feel good. So it makes sense that you are the best person to lead your healing journey. When you take control of your healing journey, you regain a sense of agency and autonomy.

Taking responsibility for your healing journey and finding the strength to advocate for yourself is empowering, but it can also be daunting: All humans have an innate need to be cared for and to trust others to help them. But this isn't about rejecting help; it's about working hand-in-hand with your care team to create a comprehensive health plan that suits you. This could mean finding comfort in the reassuring care of a physician or nurse, developing an understanding with a therapist, or taking small steps toward growth with a coach by your side. As you embark on this journey, you can find a new sense of security in knowing that you are in control of your health and you are, ultimately, the one responsible for it. Using the 4 Pillars of Nervous System Health is the most effective way to break the "quick-fix cycle"; achieve lasting relief from anxiety, burnout, and overwhelm; and reverse the accumulated damage.

Healing your nervous system is a big undertaking, requiring strategy, dedication, and hard work. But with the right plan and support, it is absolutely possible. You'll be able to achieve lasting relief from your symptoms, restore flexible and appropriate reactions to stressors, gain a deep sense of self-trust, and develop a meaningful connection to life. This systematic approach is exactly what I cover in the chapters throughout the rest of this book.

However, before we get there, we need to address another piece of the puzzle to understanding your unique nervous system: your sensitivity. Recent research is revealing that some people have more sensitive nervous systems than others. Higher sensitivity can be a double-edged sword. On one hand, it can amplify your awareness of your surroundings, deepen your understanding, and enable you to perceive subtleties that others might overlook. However, it can also intensify your feelings of stress and fear, along with other sensations, potentially making you more susceptible to nervous system dysregulation. In the next chapter, we'll delve into the emerging science of nervous system sensitivity and explore its implications for your personal healing journey.

3

The Sensitive Nervous System: Its Role in Your Path to Healing

SOME PEOPLE CAN ADAPT MORE EASILY to stressors, whereas others become overwhelmed and depleted more quickly, which can eventually contribute to a dysregulated nervous system. A significant factor influencing your susceptibility to stressors is the depth at which your nervous system processes experiences. If it processes experiences more deeply, it can be more sensitive to external stimuli like touch, smell, and light, as well as internal sensations and bodily feelings. Understanding the components of your unique sensitivity is extremely useful as you begin the process of healing a dysregulated nervous system. With this understanding, you can implement a customized approach to regulate stressors, making them more manageable and less overwhelming.

In this chapter, we will discuss what sensitivity is and why it plays a significant role in healing dysregulation. We will also break down different components of your sensitivity in your sensitivity profile, so you can start to understand how they show up in your life. Learning about your sensitivity components will make it much easier to regulate your nervous system.

Studies have shown that when highly sensitive people educate themselves about this trait, they don't just learn—they evolve. When you learn to navigate your particular sensitivities more effectively—in your feelings and physical sensations—you will have less anxiety, an increased belief in your own capabilities, and a heightened resilience to challenges. By understanding sensory processing sensitivity and how best to support this trait, you're not just acquiring knowledge, you're actively empowering yourself.

To get started, I need to clear up a common misunderstanding about sensitivity and how to approach healing if you're a highly sensitive person.

BREAKING STEREOTYPES ON SENSITIVITY

There's a widespread misunderstanding about sensitivity in our culture. Just like any aspect of your personality, increased sensory processing sensitivity can be challenging in certain circumstances, and it can also be a gift in others. Yet often in our culture we get the message that sensitivity is a problem, and you need to deal with your sensitivity by numbing yourself and "toughening up."

Perhaps you can trace back this belief to some particular experiences you had in your life. Maybe you were told to "stop being so sensitive" or to "just get over it." Or maybe you feel overwhelmed by the fast-paced nature of our modern always-connected culture and yet feel that, somehow, other people seem to manage it without any problems. Over time, you might start to feel as though if everyone else can manage it, there must be something wrong with you.

For example, imagine yourself at a family gathering, where you feel anxious due to the number of people there, the loud conversations, and the chaos of it all. When you look around, your siblings or cousins seem to be enjoying themselves without any trouble. You might start to question why you're reacting differently—why you can't just "keep your chin up" and enjoy the event like everyone else.

Or consider a scenario at work where you're under significant pressure to meet a deadline. Your heart races, your palms sweat, and you can barely focus due to the stress. Meanwhile, your colleagues seem to manage the same pressure without any visible distress. In such a situation, you may have been told to just "deal with it" or "push through"—essentially, to numb your sensitivity and react as others do.

Modern work environments can be especially challenging for highly sensitive people. You may find the constant availability demanded by today's digital culture to be exhausting. But if you struggle to keep up, that's often mistaken for lack of commitment, rather than seen clearly as a need for boundaries. The modern work environment's obsession with productivity doesn't help either. You may be especially sensitive to the deeper meaning and purpose of the work you're doing, which can be misinterpreted as a lack of drive to succeed. And if you need a quieter, slower-paced environment to perform your best, you may be unfairly seen as lazy or ineffective.

You might also recall a difficult breakup where you felt immense pain while your ex-partner seemed to move on easily. You might have been advised by well-meaning friends to "get over it" or "stop being so sensitive," reinforcing the idea that showing less sensitivity or emotion is the way to heal. Each of these instances can make you feel as though your natural reactions and feelings are incorrect or exaggerated. They can plant the idea that to fit in or to be okay, you need to stifle your feelings and responses—to become less sensitive.

Over time, these messages can lead you to accept a distorted view of your sensitivity—that it's a fault rather than a natural part of your identity. You might start to feel like you're fundamentally different from everyone else, like you just don't fit in, or are even "broken." You might even think "sensitivity" is merely a polite way of denoting weakness.

Many people with a sensitive nervous system, perhaps without even realizing it, have learned to dull or numb their sensitivity as a way of managing it. If you internalized a belief that there's something wrong with your sensitivity, you may have learned ways of coping that seem to temporarily get rid of it or reduce its impact. Perhaps you avoid social gatherings because they are overwhelming. Maybe you constantly suppress emotions for fear of being judged for your strong reactions. You might have even started using alcohol or other substances to numb your feelings and temporarily become less impacted by your surroundings. Although these strategies might offer momentary relief, in reality, they are like putting a bandage on a wound that needs attention.

Numbing out doesn't solve the underlying issue; it just makes your discomfort temporarily less noticeable. Moreover, it ignores the rich insights your sensitivity can offer about your needs and limits. In fact, continually numbing sensitivity can keep your nervous system stuck in a state of high alert and prevent you from addressing the root causes of your discomfort.

So instead of trying to dull your sensitivity, understand and embrace it. Your sensitivity isn't a flaw. It's a signal, a way for your nervous system to communicate with you. By tuning in to this communication, instead of turning away, you can better understand your unique needs and how to support your nervous system in a healthier, more sustainable way.

WHAT IS SENSITIVITY?

All living organisms have the ability to sense and respond to changes in their environment. Some are more sensitive than others. The more sensitive ones are better equipped to identify potential opportunities and threats with accuracy and speed, often giving them a leg up over their less sensitive counterparts when finding food, making connections, or defending themselves from predators.

Imagine a gazelle on the African savanna who is a little more sensitive than her sisters. She is a little bit more attuned to slight differences in the color of grass and has an easier time spotting the most nutritious tufts of grass than her less sensitive herd mates. She is also a little more sensitive to the sound of rustles in the grass and might respond a few milliseconds sooner than her sisters to a lion attack, which could be the difference between life and death.

On the flip side, having increased sensitivity means increased metabolic demand—greater effort is needed to process incoming information, and more energy must be expended as a consequence of this greater sensitivity. For example, sometimes when our sensitive gazelle friend hears a rustle in the grass, she takes off running for a few seconds only to discover that it was just the wind and not a lion. Compared to her less sensitive sisters, our gazelle has wasted precious energy and time that could have been spent grazing.

From an evolutionary point of view, if just one level of sensitivity were most optimal for survival and reproduction, then scientists would observe only that one optimal level of sensitivity among all individuals of a species. But in fact, scientists have found variations in individual sensitivity in more than one hundred species. This means that, just like other well-studied personality traits, such as introversion versus extroversion, having higher sensitivity is likely more advantageous for survival and reproduction in certain situations whereas lower sensitivity is better in others.

Unlike other personality traits, researchers have only recently started investigating differences in sensitivity. The term "highly sensitive people" was introduced in the 1990s by Dr. Elaine Aron's research. She set out to explore sensitivity through the perspective of personality psychology and coined the term to define people who had increased nervous system sensitivity. Aron's work opened avenues for further research and raised important questions about how sensory processing sensitivity affects different aspects of our lives.

Initially, scientific researchers thought that just a small percentage of the population was highly sensitive, suggesting a simple division of people into two groups: those who were highly sensitive and those who were not. However, most researchers now see sensitivity as a spectrum. Instead of being a trait you either possess or don't, like blue eyes, sensitivity varies in degrees among individuals, like height. So we all fall somewhere on the sensitivity spectrum.

In the early days of studying sensitivity, scientific researchers framed high sensitivity as a form of *vulnerability*. However, recent research is showing that vulnerability is only one side of the coin. The study of sensitivity is complex and still maturing. Researchers are just starting to scratch the surface in understanding how sensitivity affects various aspects of our lives, such as our personality traits, behaviors, and physiological responses. And the more they explore, the more they see that, with the right care and nurturing, higher sensitivity can be a great benefit for the individual and their community. For instance, highly sensitive people are often more creative, generate insightful ideas more easily, have deeper connections with loved ones, and are especially good at appreciating beauty.

If you're highly sensitive, you may have the ability to notice subtle details that other people miss. This can give you a natural predisposition to become a talented creative, such as an artist, a musician, or a writer. Likewise, you can pick up the finer details or emotional nuances in your environment, leading to unique and profound insights and ideas. In social situations, you may be more attuned to others' feelings and needs, making you an empathetic friend, considerate partner, and insightful leader. You might be the first to notice if a friend is upset or if a team member is feeling left out. Moreover, sensitivity can allow a deep appreciation for beauty. Highly sensitive people might find immense joy in a beautiful sunset, a piece of music, or a well-written sentence, which can significantly enrich their life experience.

Your sensitivity can be a great gift when you're in a nurturing environment, or when you learn how to nurture it yourself, but people with higher sensitivity are also more prone to becoming stressed. And if you're stressed for too long without adequate periods of recovery, your nervous system can become dysregulated.

Sensitivity versus Dysregulation

Nervous system dysregulation and high sensitivity are two different things. Dysregulation happens when your nervous system gets stuck in high states of activation and loses its flexibility to respond appropriately to stressors. Sensitivity, on the other hand, describes the way your nervous system responds to stimuli.

Dysregulation can affect anyone, regardless of their sensitivity level, but is more common among those who are more sensitive. In other words, people who are highly sensitive tend to be more susceptible to dysregulation and often experience symptoms more intensely. So although anyone's nervous system can become dysregulated, if you are highly sensitive, your nervous system is more likely to become dysregulated. And when your nervous system does become dysregulated, you are more likely to experience painful symptoms of dysregulation, such as anxiety, burnout, and a wide range of other mind-body conditions.

Research shows that simply understanding your sensitivity can help you increase the benefits of being sensitive while mitigating the downside. To help you do that, I'll introduce you to your personal sensitivity profile, a breakdown of your particular types of sensitivity. Understanding your profile is an important step toward effectively supporting your nervous system, regardless of whether you are on the lower or higher end of the sensitivity spectrum. In the next section, I break down the components of sensitivity, examine their role in your daily life, and provide practical advice on how to support them.

ASSESSING YOUR SENSITIVITY PROFILE

Sensitivity is a complex aspect of the human nervous system, a trait that has captivated researchers across various fields. In the last thirty years, sensitivity has been explored from multiple perspectives: psychological, behavioral, physical, and more. Each perspective brings unique findings, contributing to our understanding of sensitivity, and along with this, each field has created assessments to determine where you might stand on the sensitivity spectrum.

However, as insightful as these diverse assessments are, researchers have not yet developed a unified method to assess all different components of sensitivity. Each year, new assessments emerge that get closer to comprehensively assessing all the different aspects of sensitivity, but new assessments often raise new questions. Because there is not yet one validated sensitivity assessment that is widely recognized as being comprehensive, the best way to measure your sensitivity is by using a combination of the latest assessments. I have set up an online resource section for this book where you can find the most recent and comprehensive sensitivity assessments.

Your sensitivity profile is unique to you. It helps you understand how your nervous system experiences and interacts with the world around you. It's like a personalized set of eyeglasses that influences how you react to different stressors, how you process information, and how you respond to various emotional and physical stimuli. Using these assessments, you can get a good picture of where you fall on the sensitivity spectrum, so that you can better understand and appreciate your sensitivity. I highly encourage you to take a self-assessment before you continue with the next sections. You can find the most up-to-date assessments for understanding your sensitivity at healyournervoussystem.com/book.

UNDERSTANDING YOUR SENSITIVITY COMPONENTS

One of the most useful ways of understanding where you land on the sensitivity spectrum is by using the flower metaphor. In 2005, Professors Thomas Boyce and Bruce Ellis introduced orchids and dandelions to explain sensitivity. They likened highly sensitive people to orchids, flowers that require a caring and nurturing environment to bloom. Just like the orchid, highly sensitive individuals can flourish beautifully when they receive special nurturing and care. But in the absence of a supportive environment, both orchids and highly sensitive people may not bloom at all.

On the other hand, dandelions symbolize individuals who are less sensitive but more resilient and robust. Dandelions can grow and blossom in a wide range of conditions, even harsh ones, which parallels the ability of less sensitive people to thrive in less nurturing environments.

Adding to this metaphor, developmental psychologist Michael Pluess and his research team proposed a third category of sensitivity—the tulips. This category represents people who exhibit moderate sensitivity levels, just as the common tulip flower displays a medium sensitivity to its surroundings.

Current data suggest that 25 to 30 percent of people are orchids, exhibiting the highest levels of sensitivity. Dandelions make up another 30 percent of the population, whereas the largest group, around 40 percent, are tulips, displaying a medium level of sensitivity.

Although it can be useful to understand where you land on a general sensitivity spectrum, sensitivity shows up differently for each person. Your sensitivity profile is a rich tapestry woven with various threads, each representing a unique component that contributes to your overall profile. These components blend in unique ways in each person, crafting a sensory profile as distinctive as a fingerprint.

While each sensitive individual possesses a unique mix of components that make up their sensitivity, researchers across various fields have pinpointed five key elements of sensitivity that distinguish people with higher sensitivity from those with lower sensitivity: strong sensory preferences, sensitivity to subtle internal and external stimuli, emotional and physiological reactivity, social and affective sensitivity, and aesthetic sensitivity.

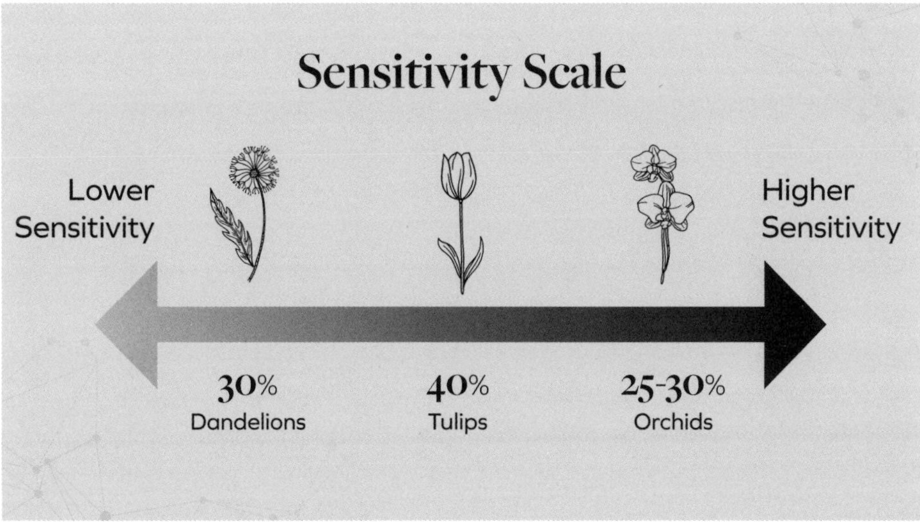

Strong Sensory Preferences

Researchers have found that more sensitive people tend to have stronger sensory preferences. If you are more sensitive, you may seek out or try to avoid certain sensory experiences to help your nervous system find the right amount of stimulation. Going out of your way to get certain types of stimulation, such as feeling the texture of certain foods or the slight pain of pulling out a hair, is called "sensory seeking." Avoiding certain types of stimulation that stress you out more than others, such as loud noises or certain textures, is called "sensory avoidance."

Navigating these preferences so you're no longer controlled by them requires a structured approach that supports your nervous system in handling sensory input. In chapter 6, I will show you how you can build such a structure and discuss the importance of establishing routines, creating sensory-friendly environments, and employing techniques to manage sensory overload.

Sensitivity to Subtle Internal and External Stimuli

This component of your sensitivity involves being highly attuned to subtle details or changes in the surrounding environment and within yourself. If this component of your sensitivity profile is strong, you might, for instance, notice the faintest scent of a flower in a garden, hear the quietest rustle of leaves in a forest, or feel the smallest change in room temperature. Internally, you might be attuned to minute shifts in your body's state: You could notice a slight increase in your heart rate when feeling anxious or minor discomfort in your stomach when something is off.

Like all components of sensitivity, research shows that simply understanding how your sensitive nervous system responds to these subtle stimuli can help this extra attentiveness to details become more of a strength and less problematic. However, understanding is just the tip of the iceberg in making this aspect of your sensitivity an ally. Later in this book, in chapters 7, 8, and 9, you'll learn awareness, regulation, and restoration techniques so your high level of attentiveness stops throwing you off balance.

Emotional and Physiological Reactivity

If this component resonates with you, your emotional responses are likely more intense than those around you. It's as if your emotional world is painted with vibrant, bold colors whereas others may experience more pastel shades. Simultaneously, your body responds to these emotions and various other stimuli with a heightened physical reaction. Perhaps your heart pounds a bit faster when you're anxious, or you might feel a rush of adrenaline during a suspenseful movie. You could also find more pleasure in comforting experiences, like the warmth of your favorite blanket or the rich flavor of a well-made coffee. The upside of such intense emotional and physiological reactivity is the richness and depth of experience it brings to your life. You feel life in its full intensity. However, the downside is that without proper understanding and management, this intensity can lead to emotional exhaustion or chronic stress. Therefore, recognizing and learning to navigate this intensity will be an essential part of your journey.

Like high sensitivity to the subtle aspects of your body and your environment, for high emotional and physical reactivity to be a benefit, your nervous system must remain regulated. The practices in chapters 7, 8, and 9 will help you shift your nervous system back to a regulated state and allow this aspect of your sensitivity to flourish.

Social and Affective Sensitivity

This sensitivity reflects your ability to tune in to the emotions of others and understand social situations on a deeper level. You might notice when your friend is feeling down, even if they haven't said anything. Or you might walk into a room and immediately pick up on a tense vibe. On the positive side, this can make you a great friend, partner, or colleague because you're always aware of what's happening emotionally around you. You're the one people turn to when they need someone who truly understands them. This ability can also be great in teamwork situations because you can sense and navigate group dynamics effectively.

But this sensitivity can also be challenging. For example, you might find yourself taking on other people's emotions as if they were your own, which can be draining. You might also find yourself habitually putting other people's needs before your own, which can lead to burnout if you're not careful.

In chapter 10, I show you how to effectively manage increased social and affective sensitivity and share strategies for cultivating healthy connections, setting boundaries, and managing emotional regulation. Additionally, I discuss how to use your sensitivity as a strength in various contexts, such as personal relationships and professional environments, without compromising your well-being.

Aesthetic Sensitivity

If you have high aesthetic sensitivity, you have a unique ability to appreciate beauty in its many forms, such as art, music, literature, and nature. You might find yourself greatly moved by a captivating melody or spend hours absorbed in an art gallery. You may also have a talent for designing beautiful environments or find yourself naturally drawn to creative professions. People with aesthetic sensitivity often utilize their strengths by becoming artists, musicians, writers, or architects, using their gift in ways that resonate deeply with others.

High levels of aesthetic sensitivity are also associated with a personality trait called "openness to experience." This means you're likely to seek out new experiences and have a deep connection with art or nature. This openness can inspire self-compassion, acceptance, and a broader appreciation for life. Your aesthetic sensitivity can be a tool to navigate the world, mitigating anxiety and encouraging meaningful connections. In chapter 11, I show you how you can leverage aesthetic sensitivity to expand your nervous system's capacity.

Making sense of the different facets of sensitivity can be a challenge, especially given that it's a relatively new area of study. I use these facets as tools to help you understand yourself better, not as fixed boxes to define and confine you. Remember, you're much more than any label could ever capture.

SENSORY SEEKING VERSUS SENSORY AVOIDING

Some people tend to be more of a "sensory seeker," meaning they actively seek out sensory stimulation. Others may be more of a "sensory avoider" or hypersensitive, meaning they are overwhelmed by sensory input and try to avoid it altogether. Most people don't fit into these two categories exclusively but, rather, combine both tendencies. Recognizing and understanding your combination of sensory-seeking and sensory-avoiding tendencies can be one of the most important steps in supporting heightened sensitivity.

Counterintuitively, if you are highly sensitive you may under-register certain types of stimuli and seek more stimulation to allow your nervous system to process and organize the input. This could mean you love the thrill of physical activity, or are drawn to the melodic pulse of loud music, yet you may still find the intensity of bright lights overwhelming or the feeling of certain textures unbearable.

Sensory seeking occurs when you are not fully aware of all the incoming sensory information, but actively try to increase sensory input to find the right amount of stimulation. This may lead to hyperactivity, as you seek more intense experiences both physically and emotionally to fulfill your sensory needs. When you're in a sensation-seeking state, you may engage in riskier behaviors or activities that provide some level of stimulation or thrills, such as jumping from heights, listening to loud music at volumes that can damage hearing, engaging in risky sexual behaviors, or taking part in other dangerous pursuits.

Sensory avoiding is a pattern where you actively try to avoid certain sensory information that feels overwhelming. This means you may avoid loud or busy environments or cover your ears when overstimulated by noise. You may also feel the need to wear gloves or other protective items when faced with tactile sensations such as paint textures, fabrics, and more. In some cases, avoidance behaviors extend

>> DO THIS

UNDERSTANDING YOUR SENSORY NEEDS

This exercise will help you better understand your sensory needs.

1. Create two lists, one with the types of sensory input that are comforting to your nervous system, and the other with the types of input that bother it. Be as specific as possible, noting the type and intensity of sensations that both provide relief and cause distress.
2. Look closely at the lists you've created. Consider whether your preferences and aversions are specific to certain sensory systems, such as vision, touch, sound, taste, or smell.
3. Take note of any patterns that emerge. What do you need more or less of? Are there specific activities or situations you regularly engage in that increase your level of comfort or lead to heightened sensitivity?
4. Keep adding to this list over time as you notice new sensory experiences that feel comforting or bothersome. Writing a comprehensive list of your sensitivity preferences can be extremely beneficial in creating an organized and effective structure to help support your nervous system. You may have been shamed in the past for some of your sensory preferences, and writing a list like this can be distressing as your body remembers those feelings of shame. I encourage you to be as honest with yourself as possible. Making your list as comprehensive as possible will help you understand yourself and prepare you to regulate your unique nervous system. Besides, no one needs to read this list except for you.

You may feel alone in dealing with your unique sensory sensitivities, but you're not. Here are a few examples I have heard from members of our community:

Intolerances: Hand sanitizer texture and smell, difficulties opening cardboard boxes, chalkboards, mouth noises, sensation of having dry hands or feet, touch and other forms of physical contact (which can pose unique challenges to intimate relationships), fluorescent lights, the smell of some perfumes or scented candles, food textures like cooked onions, mashed potatoes, or the pulp in orange juice, being in large crowds

Cravings: Need to stay moving, jumping from heights, spinning, intense exercise, loud music where you can feel the bass, multitasking like talking on the phone while doing household chores, desire to touch everything, eating strong-tasting or extra-spicy foods, hair pulling, nail biting, fidgeting

beyond physical sensations and into social situations where your nervous system will avoid certain types of social stimulation to remain comfortable and unstimulated.

Your sensory preferences can also change over time, making navigating them even more complex. For example, during pregnancy and menopause, you may experience heightened levels of sensory avoidance as hormone levels fluctuate. Sensory avoidance can also become stronger as you age.

Understanding and learning to navigate your sensory preferences with more ease will make life a lot more pleasant and free up energy to continue on your healing journey. By knowing the things that may be overstimulating to you and making adjustments where needed, you can prevent sensory overload and create tiny changes that will have a big impact over time. Likewise, strategically engaging in stimulating activities can help your nervous system organize itself and offset the impact of aversive stimuli. In chapter 6, I'll guide you in implementing these changes and introduce the specific activities that can help support your unique sensitivity.

HOW HIGHER SENSITIVITY CAN SUPPORT YOUR HEALING JOURNEY

If you are highly sensitive, you may feel like you have more work to do, or have a longer healing journey ahead of you. But higher sensitivity can actually be a great advantage when working to regulate your nervous system.

Highly sensitive individuals are remarkably responsive to healing interventions, often bouncing back from dysregulation more quickly than their less sensitive counterparts. Like an orchid requiring the right conditions to bloom, sensitive individuals tend to respond readily to the right environment. This high responsiveness is precisely why embarking on a healing journey can make such a difference.

One of the leading sensitivity researchers, Michael Pluess, with his colleague Jay Belsky, coined the term "vantage sensitivity" to describe the heightened response some individuals show to positive interventions and supportive environments. In a 2018 review, Pluess and his colleagues found that, in line with the vantage sensitivity hypothesis, having higher sensitivity to the environment significantly predicted how well people responded to interventions. If you have high sensitivity and suffer from the physical and emotional symptoms of a dysregulated nervous system, you are likely to heal more easily than someone who is less sensitive, provided you take the right steps to support yourself.

You're naturally wired to thrive in positive and supportive environments and bounce back from dysregulation. If you capitalize on your vantage sensitivity, you can enjoy the benefits of being more sensitive, such as more creativity, empathy, awareness, and openness, without becoming dysregulated.

The more sensitive you are, the more essential it is for you to recognize how to manage stress levels and regulate your emotions. Mastering these skills can halt the negative effects on your physical and mental health and even reverse previous damage. By learning how to regulate their nervous systems, highly sensitive people can not only experience comparable or even better physical and mental health than other less sensitive people but also make use of their unique gifts for a happier and fulfilling life.

Sensitivity is a multifaceted trait that affects people differently. How it manifests in your life depends on an intricate mix of factors, including genetics, environment, and your life experiences. Your journey up to this point, marked by these factors, may have led to a dysregulated nervous system and the symptoms you're currently experiencing. To move forward and lay a foundation for your path to regulation, you need to understand how you got here. In the next chapter, I will guide you through understanding how your unique mix of sensitivity, difficult life experiences, and stressors all came together and led to your particular set of symptoms.

4

The Tipping Point: How Stress and Fear Lead to a Dysregulated Nervous System

IN THE LAST TEN YEARS, there has been an explosion in stress and fear research, with the COVID-19 pandemic serving as a massive catalyst. This influx of studies has allowed scientific researchers to gain a greater understanding of how our bodies respond to and cope with stressful moments, giving us invaluable insight into how the stress response and fear response all play into nervous system dysregulation.

One of the essential breakthroughs that the scientific community has made from the recent surge in research on stress and fear is the realization that our physiological stress response is much more complex than previously thought. Older theories of stress and trauma focused on simpler isolated processes. For example, some theories focused mostly on the autonomic nervous system, a branch of the nervous system responsible for regulating involuntary processes like heartbeat and digestion, and the hypothalamic-pituitary-adrenal (HPA) axis, the bodily system responsible for releasing the stress hormone cortisol. Other theories focused mostly on large areas or layers of the brain. But recent research has shown that the stress response involves not only the autonomic nervous system and HPA axis, but also various groups of neurons throughout the brain. These groups of neurons aren't just in one part of the brain but are scattered across many different areas. They work together to coordinate your stress response when you face a threat or challenge.

Along with illuminating the complexity of our stress response, recent stress research has demonstrated that we each have a unique and individual response to stress. The diversity of our reactions to stressors, both minor and major, is remarkable.

Some of us may spring into high alert at the slightest hint of a problem, whereas others remain seemingly unaffected in even the most challenging situations.

One important component of the differences between your stress response and other people's is your biology—the genes you were born with and your innate level of sensitivity. But your response to stress isn't purely biological—it's also shaped profoundly by your environment. That means that all your past experiences have contributed to how you respond to stressors now.

The key to healing dysregulation is understanding and addressing the individual differences in your stress response. Understanding how your genetic makeup and personal experiences influence your stress response will help you recognize what makes your response unique. Then you can apply targeted, practical solutions for healing that support your unique stress response. Ultimately, supporting your unique stress response is the path to a thriving body and mind and a regulated nervous system.

In this chapter, I will give you a tour of the stress response and fear response systems. Then I'll delve into how these systems can become overwhelmed and dysregulated, and how environment and genetic predispositions contribute to these changes in your nervous system. This journey of understanding is a vital step toward healing, paving the way to reclaim your health.

DECODING STRESS: AN INSIDE LOOK AT YOUR BODY'S AROUSAL LEVELS

Stress is how your nervous system responds to challenge or demand. Your body is always in some state of stress arousal. Even right now, as you read this book, your body is experiencing a certain level of stress. Maybe you're relaxed, breathing deeply and feeling at ease in your body. Maybe you're feeling tense, and frantically trying to get through this chapter and on to the next. If you had an accurate map of different levels of stress arousal, it would be much easier to recognize your current level of stress and see how it's shaping your present-moment experience.

Stress researchers have documented various brain states associated with different levels of stress arousal. Research from Elissa Epel and her team at the University of California, San Francisco summarized much of this research on brain states, describing four distinct levels of arousal. Other research has verified a different type of physiological response to extreme stress, the freeze response, which is associated with a part of the brain called the periaqueductal gray. The research team at Heal Your Nervous System and I have incorporated this data into a new model of stress alertness, specifically designed to support your work with dysregulation: The Alertness Elevator.

The Alertness Elevator

Imagine your stress response as an elevator, moving through varying arousal levels as you respond to life's circumstances. Each "floor" represents a different state of arousal of the body and mind, from deep rest on the ground floor to high alert on the top floor.

The Blue State: Deep Rest and Cellular Regeneration

At ground level is the blue state, a state of deep rest. Here your body and mind are in deep relaxation mode. This happens during activities such as meditation or deep sleep, where your body can regenerate cells and restore itself. This state is marked by minimal stress levels, increased parasympathetic activity—the "rest-and-digest" mode of your nervous system—and enhanced cellular health, promoting relaxation and restoration.

The Green State: Relaxed and Focused

Moving up with the elevator, you enter the green state. It's your "flow" state—where you are focused and relaxed and your body is at ease. This state allows you to be engaged in an activity while maintaining a sense of relaxation. Stress levels are high enough for you to stay focused and low enough that you can stay simultaneously relaxed. Your heart rate and respiration support active engagement in the task at hand, and attention is heightened. It's a state with a balance of activity in the sympathetic branch of your nervous system, which helps rev you up, and the parasympathetic branch, which helps cool you down.

The Yellow State: The Treadmill of Cognitive Overload

Riding up you reach the yellow state, a state of alertness and mental exertion, where your mind and body experience a moderate level of stress. This state is characterized by a heightened mental load that feels like your mind is on a nonstop treadmill. It's a state of cognitive overload, where your thoughts may race, often consumed by worry, self-criticism, or feelings of shame. This state is a result of the extra mental effort needed to complete a task, which often leads to decreased performance and increased frustration. You might notice your heart beating faster and your muscles tensing up, signs that your body's stress response is in an activated, persistent mode.

The Red State: Acute Stress Response and Full Alertness

Reaching the top, you find the red state, a state of acute stress. Here, you are on full alert, ready to either fight or run away. It's your body's response mechanism to a full-blown threat. In the red state, your heart beats faster, pumping more blood to your muscles and organs, and your breathing speeds up to get more oxygen into your

The Alertness Elevator: Understanding Your Body and Mind States

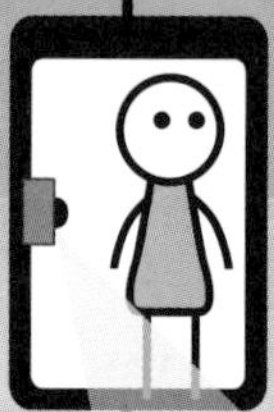

	Your Body May Feel	Your Mind May Feel	You See the World As
Red	Pounding heart, shallow breathing, muscle tension, sweating	High-alert, fear-driven, threat-focused, hypervigilant, anxious, tense, catastrophizing	An unpredictable battlefield filled with threats and chaos
Yellow	Quickened pulse and chest breathing, muscle tension, heightened senses	Increased anxiousness or nervousness, racing or ruminating thoughts, unconsciously feeling unsafe.	A challenge of demanding tasks, incessant change, and pressure to constantly adapt
Green	Steady pulse, breath reaches your belly, muscles are relaxed	Focused, relaxed, efficient, engaged, positive, calm, harmonious, open	A place of opportunity where challenges are manageable and engagement with tasks is fluid
Blue	Calm, relaxed, gentle heartbeat, slow deep breath	Peaceful, serene, replenished, safe, content, at ease, restful	A peaceful sanctuary where safety prevails and harmony exists

Purple

Body
Immobilized, slow heartbeat and breathing, loose muscles

Mind
Disengaged and inert or overwhelmed, helpless, frozen

World
An overwhelming chaos, unbearable, paralyzing

system. Your body increases your blood glucose levels, giving you an energy boost. At the same time, more blood is drawn away from your gut and toward your muscles, readying you for action. In this state, your senses are heightened and you're more alert than ever, making it easier for you to react quickly and effectively to the threat at hand. It's your body's way of giving you the best chance possible of handling the situation.

The Purple State: Emergency Freeze and Immobility

Imagine the purple state as an emergency stop button in the elevator. It's like hitting pause when you sense extreme danger, making your body freeze, essentially becoming immobile. When the level of threat or danger increases significantly, your body switches to a defensive mode, like freezing or tonic immobility (passing out). In this state, your heart is slowed and you feel like you can't move. Both freezing and tonic immobility are reactions to threats. Freezing is an active response that allows you to "stop, look, and listen" and prepares you to fight or flee, whereas tonic immobility is a passive response, resembling a state of physical and mental paralysis.

The Two Sides of Stress

Stress gets a bad rap, but it's not always a problem. Scientific research indicates that low to moderate stress can enhance resilience. If your nervous system is regulated and you encounter a stressful situation, you will transition through the red and yellow states and return flexibly to the green and blue states when the stressor disappears. Stress like this, even though it may feel very intense when you're in the red or yellow state, is not a problem and can even be beneficial for your health and growth.

Spending an appropriate amount of time in the red and yellow states, where your body's defenses are mobilized, can teach your body and brain to handle stress better in the future. And when the stressor is removed and you transition back to the green and blue states, your body gets a chance to recover and rejuvenate. This cycle of adaptation is a key part of building resilience.

However, if you're stuck in a constant loop of red and yellow states, the story changes. Chronic, repeated stressors can damage your body and mind and increase your risk of disease. In chronically stressed individuals, research has shown that simply anticipating a stressful event can cause significant stress. So, it's not just the stressful event itself that causes the problem, but even the *anticipation* of it triggers stress responses and can lead to health issues. Over time, chronic stress may change your nervous system's wiring, contributing to a spiral that is increasingly difficult to break free from.

To end this painful cycle, you must learn to manage your "alertness elevator." You need to be able to return to the green and blue states as your baseline for recovery. There's nothing wrong with shifting through the red and yellow states in demanding situations, but it's crucial to give your body and mind enough time back in the green and blue states to recover. The ability to navigate your states can be the difference between a resilient response to stress and a debilitating one.

What Chronic Stress Does to Your Body

Prolonged stress, spending too much time in the red and yellow states without enough time to recover in the green and blue states, can have a severely negative impact on your health. When you have a prolonged or chronic stress response, three parts of your body's normal stress response can get derailed and cause serious problems for your health: cortisol, oxidative stress, and inflammation. Here's how it happens.

1. **Cortisol:** When you are in the yellow and red states, your HPA axis (hypothalamus, pituitary gland, and adrenal glands) produces a stress hormone called cortisol and sends it around your body. Cortisol signals to other body systems, such as your immune system and liver, to prepare for stress. Cortisol is beneficial in moderate doses, but when your body continually produces high levels of it, a range of health problems emerge—from weight gain to a weakened immune system.
2. **Oxidative stress:** Chronic stress can also lead to oxidative stress, which causes cell and tissue damage. This happens when there's an imbalance in your cells between the production of harmful waste molecules, called reactive oxygen species (ROS), and your body's ability to detoxify these molecules or repair the resulting damage. High levels of ROS can damage cells, proteins, and DNA in your body.
3. **Inflammation:** Chronic stress can result in persistent inflammation. Inflammation is a normal immune response designed to protect your body in times of illness or injury. However, if inflammation becomes constant, as it can in response to chronic stress, it can lead to health problems, including heart disease and arthritis.

Excessive cortisol, oxidative stress, and inflammation can also disturb the mitochondria in your cells, inhibiting their ability to make energy. Mitochondria are the powerhouses of your cells and are responsible for producing the vast amount of energy your brain and body need to function. Over time, chronic stress can damage mitochondria and cause them to stop working properly. All your cells, particularly your brain cells, need the energy they produce to function; without it, your cells begin to fail to do their jobs properly.

Returning to the pinball effect from chapter 1, you can start to see in more detail how the series of causes and consequences unfolds, which makes your game of pinball go awry. Chronic stress disrupting the function of mitochondria, blocking energy production in your cells, is a key factor in the complex set of causes and consequences that lead to nervous system dysregulation and the development of a wide range of painful body and mind symptoms.

UNPACKING THE FEAR RESPONSE: A BIOLOGICAL SURVIVAL MECHANISM

The stress response and the fear response are like cousins—closely connected and able to influence one another. In fact, the way you experience and express fear can change depending on your stress levels.

Both the fear response and the stress response use similar pathways in the brain, engaging key areas such as the amygdala, hippocampus, prefrontal cortex, and thalamus. In the context of fear, these brain areas work together to create, store, and bring up fear memories, and in the context of stress, these same areas help manage the body's stress response.

Your body's fear response can be thought of as a protective reflex, a generic "go-to" that kicks in lightning fast as soon as you perceive danger or potential harm. However, this natural reflex does not come with an instruction manual that explains which stimuli you should respond to and which you should disregard. Rather, it is designed to rapidly and efficiently learn what's dangerous from your environment. Your life experiences train your fear response for what you should find scary.

From an evolutionary perspective, this can be a tremendous advantage because it enables our species to survive and adapt to changing environments. Humans are equipped to learn quickly from their experiences to be afraid of anything that can cause harm. But for the individual, this ability to learn so quickly and easily to be scared of things can cause you to become activated not just by actual threats, but also by less threatening situations, such as unfamiliar social situations or thoughts and memories from the past. One of the most common ways that your nervous system learns to be scared is by experiencing something that makes you feel helpless or overwhelmed. These experiences are called "traumatic stressors."

The concept of psychological trauma has gained widespread attention over the past few years. However, I have found the term "trauma" often leads to considerable confusion and misconceptions of what's actually going on in your nervous system.

Recent research even suggests that the way you understand the concept of trauma can have a direct impact on your nervous system.

For example, in a 2022 study at Harvard University, researchers experimented with giving people tasks that led them to believe the concept of trauma encompassed either only very extreme events or almost anything emotionally distressing. The group that was led to believe that the concept of trauma included almost anything distressing felt more intense negative emotions after going through an emotionally distressing experience themselves. Research like this indicates that using a vague word like "trauma" to talk about a wide variety of distressing experiences can make already-disturbing experiences even worse. Gaining a more detailed and specific understanding of the impact that distressing experiences have on your nervous system can increase your resilience and nervous system regulation.

To understand the impact of distressing experiences on your nervous system, it's important to carefully differentiate between traumatic stressors, post-traumatic stress disorder (PTSD), and the embedded alarms that are, sometimes, left behind in your nervous system after experiencing traumatic stressors.

Traumatic Stressors

A traumatic stressor, an extremely painful or disturbing event that made you feel an intense sense of danger or helplessness, is one of the worst experiences people can go through. A traumatic stressor could be as horrific as being the victim of assault or abuse, and as common as a breakup, feeling embarrassed in front of a crowd, or feeling neglected by your caregivers as a child. What makes a situation into a traumatic stressor is not an objective measurement of how horrible it is compared to other people's experiences, but how much it overwhelms *your* capacity to cope.

After a distressing experience like this is over, your nervous system usually requires a period of recovery. Sometimes this can last just a few minutes whereas other times it might last weeks or even a few months. During this recovery period, you may have intrusive memories of the event come into your mind and feelings of fear and helplessness come into your body seemingly from out of nowhere. These intrusive memories or feelings can suddenly throw you back into a red or yellow state. Your nervous system is reliving or reexperiencing aspects of the traumatic stressor events in order to integrate them and heal. Overall, during the recovery period, you may spend a significant amount of time in red and yellow states. This is a normal part of the recovery process. Nothing is going wrong here. In fact, human nervous systems have an incredible capacity to integrate and recover from even the most horrific experiences.

According to George Bonanno, a trauma researcher at Columbia University, for the vast majority of traumatic experiences, these intrusive memories fade over time as your body and mind integrate the experience and go through the recovery process. In a small minority of cases, though, intrusive memories stay the same or get worse over time. If intrusive memories don't fade over time, it can be diagnosed as PTSD.

PTSD: When the Fear Response Misfires

Traumatic stressors and PTSD are hot topics of scientific research right now. As more research comes out, new ways of understanding traumatic stressors and PTSD in the brain and body will likely further clarify our understanding and help us respond most effectively to each person's unique needs. However, based on Bonanno's trauma and resilience research, making a clear distinction between a normal recovery process (which can be extremely difficult) and PTSD can clarify your experience and aid in your recovery.

Going through a high-stress period of recovery and integration after an overwhelming experience is totally normal and demonstrates your body's incredible capacity to keep going even after very difficult experiences. Even extreme traumatic stressors don't necessarily lead to nervous system dysregulation. They may lead to a prolonged period of red and yellow states and feeling deep pain, but as the intrusive memories fade, your nervous system will spend more and more time in green and blue states and recover from any cellular damage accumulated during and after the event.

In the case of PTSD, though, the intrusive memories don't fade, and the nervous system stays on high alert indefinitely. This is one way the nervous system can get dysregulated.

One reason this distinction is important is that when you know that it's normal to experience a period of intrusive memories along with increased yellow and red states after a traumatic stressor, and that in the vast majority of cases it will fade as your mind and body integrate the experience, that knowledge can actually help the healing process and increase your resilience.

If you're still dealing with intrusive memories after a few months, it might be time to get professional help. The practices in this book will support your journey to resolving PTSD, but if these memories are seriously affecting your everyday life and ability to function, reaching out to a medical professional is a crucial next step.

Embedded Alarms: Unlearning the Fear Response

Not all traumatic stressors leave a lasting impact on your nervous system. Sometimes after a traumatic stressor, all you need to feel resolved and let it go is to have a good cry, let yourself feel angry or upset while you think through what happened, or spend some quality time with a loved one. But other times, because your fear response is so well adapted to learn quickly, an experience in which you felt overwhelmed or powerless is enough to embed this memory in your nervous system. The memory gets stored in a part of your brain called the hippocampus, which is closely connected to a part of your brain that plays a major role in the fear response, the amygdala. Memories of less intense traumatic stressors can also get embedded in your hippocampus if the stressor was repeated over an extended period of time.

When a memory gets embedded in your nervous system, your brain creates a "snapshot" of the experience your body went through and this too gets stored in your hippocampus. Along with storing all this detailed information, your brain learns to raise the alarm more quickly in situations similar to the traumatic stressor experience. Research has shown that your neurons actually physically adjust themselves—known as synaptic potentiation—to make it easier to raise the alarm in associated situations. I call this an *embedded alarm*.

An embedded alarm isn't necessarily problematic and can even save your life. That's why evolution has oriented your nervous system so strongly toward learning to be scared, even after just one overwhelming experience. Imagine that, as a child, you came very close to being hit by a car. The experience was a traumatic stressor, and your nervous system embedded an alarm for situations it perceives as similar. Let's say that, as an adult, you're walking down the street looking at your phone and you accidentally start to veer toward oncoming traffic. Your embedded alarm picks up the danger, activates the red state, and, suddenly fearful, you look up in time to step back from an oncoming car. Your embedded alarm saved your life.

But consider a situation where there's no actual danger. Something in the environment—a sound, a smell, or a particular situation—resembles some aspect of a past traumatic stressor. As you experience this new situation, your embedded alarm goes off and your nervous system is thrown into the red state, even though there's nothing threatening. You may have conscious memories and physical reactions associated with the original traumatic stressor come rushing back, or you may have no conscious memories at all. Sometimes you might relive bodily memories of the event, whether or not you consciously remember the experience that led to this embedded alarm. For example, you might feel a sudden pain or tightening in an area of your body that was injured during the original traumatic stressor when you learned this fear response.

If your nervous system embedded this alarm after an overwhelming event in early childhood, you may not have any narrative memory of the traumatic stressor—but the alarm is still present in your neurons. Narrative memories typically start forming around age three, but bodily memories of fearful situations can form before that, and alarms can be embedded in your nervous system linking only to the bodily memory. In a present-moment situation, when there's no real danger, perhaps you don't even realize that the reason you're suddenly in the red state is because something in the environment caused your nervous system to set off an embedded alarm.

Experiencing your embedded alarms going off in a safe situation isn't necessarily a problem. In fact, realizing that you're in a safe situation while an embedded alarm is triggered can help flush that embedded alarm out of your nervous system. However, a large number of embedded alarms going off in a wide variety of situations can contribute to nervous system dysregulation.

Just like the pinball effect from chapter 1, these embedded alarms can be both a cause and a consequence of dysregulation. They can contribute to dysregulation by consistently putting you into the red or yellow state, increasing a background sense of danger. They can also be a consequence of dysregulation because, if your nervous system is already dysregulated, it may be more likely to feel overwhelmed in more situations and embed even more alarms. Additionally, the normal process of unlearning fear and removing alarms that are no longer useful can be hampered if your nervous system is stuck in the yellow state and can't come back to the feelings of safety in the green and blue states.

Fortunately, you are not powerless in the fear response. In fact, just as your nervous system *learns* the fear response, it can also *unlearn* it. Any time an alarm goes off and you consciously recognize that, despite feeling fear, you are actually safe, it will help your nervous system unlearn that particular embedded alarm. Knowing this can remove the danger and mystery from your fear response and puts you back in charge.

In the following chapters, you'll learn how to slowly and gently allow your nervous system to feel safer. As your nervous system feels safer, you can become more aware of your embedded alarms and meet them with a physical experience of regulation, thereby "deprogramming" and replacing the embedded alarm with a new experience of safety and agency.

WHY DO STRESS AND FEAR AFFECT PEOPLE DIFFERENTLY?

Why is there such a wide variation in the ways people respond to stress and fear? Why do some of us seem to cope well in the face of adversity, whereas others become overwhelmed more easily and even develop PTSD as a result? The answer lies in understanding the juncture at which your nervous system loses its capacity to respond flexibly to stressors and starts becoming dysregulated, remaining stuck in the yellow and red states of alertness and fear.

Nature and nurture work together to determine the tipping point—the point when your nervous system stops flexibly responding to stress and fear and becomes dysregulated. Your nature, or genetic makeup, provides the blueprint for your individual characteristics and inherent stress responses. Meanwhile, nurture, or your

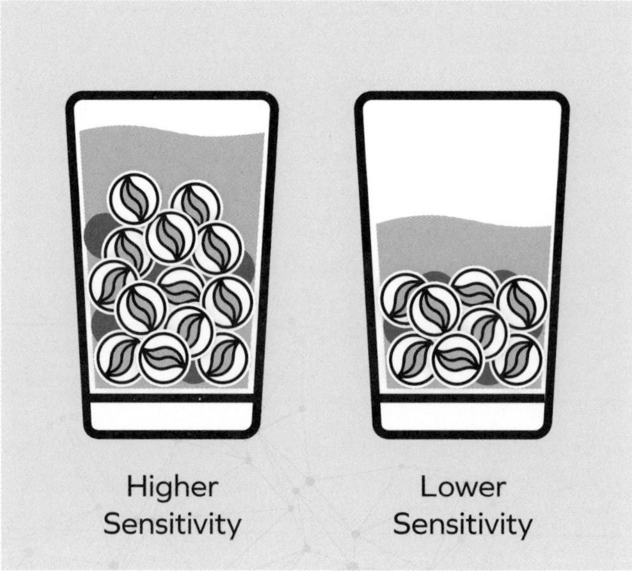

environmental influences, encompasses your upbringing, life experiences, and current circumstances, all of which shape how your genetic blueprint is expressed.

Imagine for a moment that you're holding a cup filled with marbles and water. The marbles symbolize your inherent sensitivity to fear and stress. The water represents your stress response. When you experience a stressor, it's like adding more water to your cup. Spending time in the green and blue states, where your body can rest and repair, is like draining water from your cup. As long as your cup doesn't overflow, your nervous system remains regulated. But if you pour too much water into your cup without also draining it—too much time in the red and yellow states, without enough green and blue—your cup will overflow and your nervous system will tip into dysregulation.

If you have more marbles in your cup, you may react more intensely to stressors. As discussed in the previous chapter, higher nervous system sensitivity is not necessarily a problem and, in the right conditions, can be a great strength. It can allow you to process your thoughts, feelings, and experiences deeply, sometimes leading to profound insights, appreciation, and understanding of things other people miss. But having higher sensitivity also means you're more likely to activate your stress response.

Now think about the size of the cup itself, which represents your capacity to deal with stressors. The good news is, the size of your cup is not fixed and can change over time. Although your innate sensitivity—your number of marbles—is at least partially coded in your genes and unlikely to change, many things can influence the size of your cup and give you more capacity to handle stressors.

Imagine your upbringing and childhood experiences as the base material of your cup. If you grew up in an environment that was relatively safe and learned healthy emotional regulation skills during these formative years, you likely have a sturdy and spacious cup. In other words, you're well equipped to handle larger amounts of stress. But even if your cup is smaller as a result of a more challenging childhood, as an adult, you still have a great deal of control over how big your cup gets.

For example, as an adult, getting proper sleep and regular exercise can make your cup larger, improving your capacity. Learning emotional regulation strategies that you may have missed learning from your caregivers as a child can also have a profound impact on the size of your cup as an adult. Conversely, a stressful lifestyle may make your cup smaller, lowering your tolerance. Hormonal changes and aging can also reduce your cup size.

When it comes to handling stress and determining your tipping point, you are not simply at the mercy of your genetics or circumstances. You might have an inherent sensitivity to stress based on your genetic blueprint, but your choices, your self-understanding, and the techniques you learn and practice as an adult have a major impact on the size of your cup. In the following chapters, I'll show you how to use all of these to expand the size of your cup and reverse your dysregulation.

Improving nervous system regulation involves understanding and implementing techniques to navigate the interplay between your thoughts, emotions, and physical sensations so you can move flexibly between the different levels of arousal, instead of spending the majority of time stuck in yellow and red states. By doing so, you're not just managing your stress but also actively improving your capacity to handle it. This is where your real power lies: not in avoiding stress, but in enhancing your ability to deal with it when it does arrive. And that's exactly what I aim to equip you with through this book.

HOW CHILDHOOD EXPERIENCES AFFECT YOUR STRESS RESPONSE

Your childhood played an important role in shaping your present-day response to stress: It influenced the current size of your cup, representing how much stress you can handle before it tips over into dysregulation.

Your childhood also played an important role in how your elevator functions, which brings you up and down between different levels of stress, moment by moment, throughout your day. If, during your childhood, your nervous system was not trained to respond flexibly to stress, moving you back to a relaxed green state after a stressor has passed, it might still struggle to do that now in adulthood.

These factors are not fixed or unchangeable, however. Plenty of research indicates that your stress response and your capacity to handle stress with a regulated nervous system can change during adulthood. Understanding which factors from your childhood may have contributed to your current level of regulation can help you make sense of how you got here. Simply understanding what happened can increase the organization of your nervous system, what psychologists call "coherence of mind," which can dramatically improve your nervous system regulation.

Your Environment in Early Childhood

In 2014, Dr. Marco Del Giudice and colleagues proposed a model to explain how different levels of stress responsivity develop over a person's life-span. They called it the "adaptive calibration model" of stress responsivity. According to their model, your nervous system periodically adjusts how sensitive you are to stress based on how dangerous your environment feels.

The process starts while you're in the womb. Even before being born, your nervous system used the information it had available, such as how many calories you were getting and how much stress hormone your mother was sending you, to predict how risky your environment would be. It set an initial level of stress responsivity based on this level of risk.

Your stress responsivity continued to get major calibration updates throughout childhood. During childhood, when the brain develops most rapidly, your environment had a strong impact on your nervous system's responsivity. Even as an adult, each life transition serves to calibrate your responsivity to stress, bringing it closer to being optimal for your current environmental conditions.

During each major phase of development, such as birth, the transition from childhood to adolescence, and the transition to midlife or menopause, your nervous system has another opportunity to adjust its stress responsivity. Additionally, your responsivity to stress doesn't recalibrate only during major developmental milestones. Any significant life event that marks a change from an old version of yourself to a new version can be enough to cause your stress responsivity to recalibrate. For example, starting a new job, leaving school, and getting married could all potentially trigger an adjustment in your stress responsivity.

Let's say you were raised in a dangerous, unpredictable, or neglectful environment as a child. Your stress response may have been significantly more sensitive than if you were raised in an environment where you generally felt safe and cared for. The adaptive calibration model says that your higher sensitivity to stress is not the result of anything going wrong in your development. In fact, it was highly adaptive for your nervous system to internalize the sense that your environment felt unpredictable and dangerous. This background sense of danger makes you more alert and wary, which can increase your chances of survival in an unsafe environment.

The adaptive calibration model describes four different patterns of stress responsivity:

1. Sensitive
2. Buffered
3. Vigilant
4. Unemotional

Sensitive pattern: As a child, if your nervous system assessed your environment to be safe and low stress, you were most likely to develop a sensitive nervous system that is open and highly responsive to the environment.

Buffered pattern: In a moderate-stress environment, your nervous system will have a moderate level of stress responsivity. You may actually be less sensitive to stress than the child raised in an extremely low-stress environment. Many researchers believe this pattern—having a background sense of safety but still experiencing moderate stress—leads to the highest levels of resilience in children and sets them up well to thrive later in life.

Vigilant pattern: In an unsafe or unpredictable environment, you are likely to develop high responsivity to stressors so you can react quickly to threats and protect yourself. This pattern causes your nervous system to stay vigilant. Although it is well adapted to unsafe environments, like a dangerous neighborhood, staying in this pattern consistently can wear out your body and mind quickly and lead to dysregulation more easily.

Unemotional pattern: In a severely stressful environment that regularly overwhelms your ability to cope, your nervous system adapted by reducing your sensitivity to stress to very low levels. This pattern is the least sensitive to stress, likely because, tragically, in the traumatic environment you grew up in, reacting to stress wasn't helpful. It was best to just tune it out as best you could and conserve calories.

You may resonate with one of these patterns, but it's not necessarily important to figure out exactly which pattern you had. In fact, because circumstances can change throughout childhood, it can be difficult to fit your childhood into just one of these descriptions. But the adaptive calibration model shows two important things: It explains biologically how different people can experience different levels of stress during their childhood and how that, along with their innate genetic blueprint, can contribute to surprisingly different levels of stress responsivity later in life; it also shows that, although your childhood environment played an important role in shaping your current stress responsivity, your responsivity can continue to be updated throughout life. You are not destined to live within the patterns you developed during childhood. This is very clear from the scientific literature and it's a critical message I want you to hear before moving to the next sections.

Your Upbringing

One of the most important parts of your nervous system's environment during childhood was your relationship with your parents or other primary caregivers. Scientific research in the field of attachment theory shows that a child's relationship with their primary caregivers during childhood plays a critical role in training their nervous system to handle stress.

Attachment researchers consider a bond between a child and their caregivers to be "secure" if the child seeks closeness and comfort from their caregivers during stressful situations, and the caregivers are consistently able to comfort their children enough that the child is ready to play again once the stressor has passed. An infant-caregiver bond is considered "insecure" if the child either does not seek closeness and comfort in a distressing situation, or the child seeks comfort but can't be soothed even when the stressor has passed.

If you developed secure attachment as a child, you're likely to have an easier time regulating your emotions and handling stressors. You can flexibly move into red or yellow and then come back down to the green state once you're no longer in a stressful situation. On the other hand, if you have an insecure attachment status, you may find it harder to manage your emotions and cope with stress. For example, you may get stuck in the yellow state for long periods of time after a stressor and have trouble coming back to the green state.

The good news is that, even if you missed parts of this nervous system training in childhood, you can still give your nervous system this training as an adult. All of the practices in this book will help retrain your nervous system to handle stress flexibly. In chapter 9, I will revisit attachment theory and show you specific techniques to fill the gaps in nervous system regulation training that you may have missed from your primary caregivers as a child.

PUTTING IT ALL TOGETHER

In this chapter, I have shown you that both fear and stress are normal and important functions of the human body. However, when fear and stress become chronic, they can lead to dysregulation. How easily this happens for you is influenced by your genetic blueprint and your life experiences. While you can't change your genetic blueprint, you *can* change how your nervous system handles stress, which is enough to reverse nervous system dysregulation. You can unlearn fear responses, add the missing pieces to nervous system regulation training that you missed during childhood, and expand your capacity—the size of your cup—to handle more stress in the future without tipping over into dysregulation.

In the next chapter, I will show you how to combine all of these pieces, and put them in the right order, so you can systematically implement all the necessary steps to get your nervous system working smoothly again.

5

The 5-Stage Plan to Reverse Nervous System Dysregulation

IN THE PREVIOUS CHAPTERS, I helped you see how your nervous system got dysregulated. I introduced nervous system dysregulation as the missing factor in a wide range of painful symptoms that show up in the body and mind. I reviewed the complex set of factors that may have contributed to your nervous system becoming dysregulated—from your current sensitivity levels, to your innate genetic blueprint, to all the life experiences that have left an imprint on your body and mind. Now it's time to put the theory into practice to reverse your nervous system dysregulation. In this chapter, I share a straightforward, practical approach to healing nervous system dysregulation. I call this the 5-Stage Plan.

INTRODUCING THE 5-STAGE PLAN

The "quick-fix cycle," introduced in chapter 2, is pervasive in our culture. As such, many people struggle to make progress on their healing journey, instead feeling as though they are running in circles exploring traditional, alternative, and integrative medicine—from yoga and meditation to acupuncture and hypnosis. These various healing approaches can be life-changing for the right person, but without a cohesive plan for their use, they aren't likely to result in full nervous system regulation. Often, these interventions either quickly burn you out, or they never get off the ground because you don't know where to begin and which to prioritize in your specific situation.

I believe that a simple, straightforward strategy for healing nervous system dysregulation is missing in this equation. Through extensive work with many people trying to

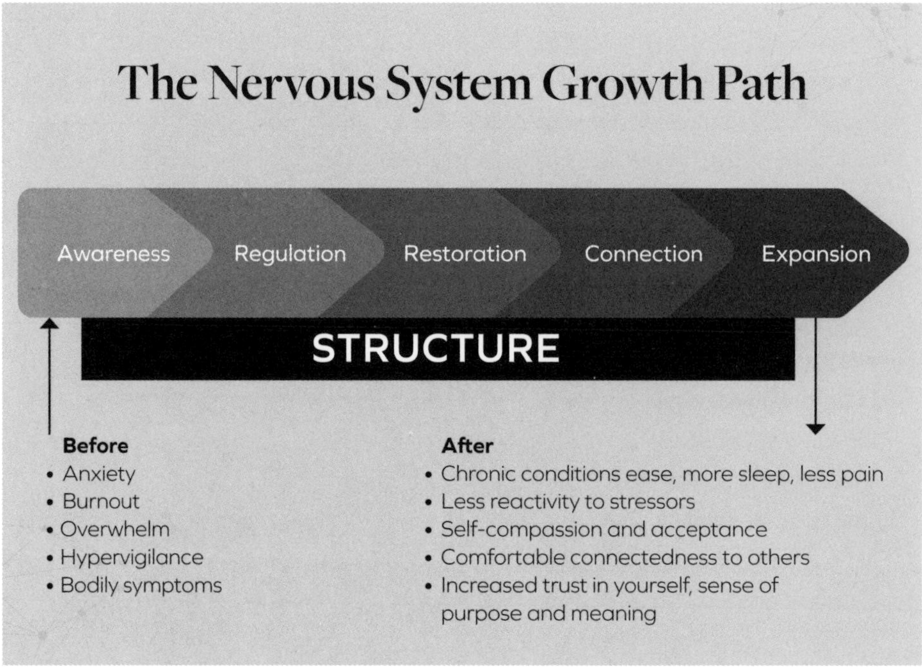

regulate their nervous systems, I've found that building a regulated nervous system follows a specific sequence, a series of stages that break down the process into manageable, actionable pieces. That's why I developed this 5-Stage Plan: to fill a void in the way we approach healing nervous system dysregulation.

The Nervous System Growth Path
Awareness
Regulation
Restoration
Connection
Expansion
STRUCTURE
Before
• Anxiety
• Burnout
• Overwhelm
• Hypervigilance
• Bodily symptoms
After
• Chronic conditions ease, more sleep, less pain
• Less reactivity to stressors
• Self-compassion and acceptance
• Comfortable connectedness to others
• Increased trust in yourself, sense of purpose and meaning

The 5-Stage Plan heals nervous system dysregulation by systematically rejuvenating the 4 Pillars of Nervous System Health—body, mind, connection, and spirituality—in a targeted, step-by-step process. Each stage of the plan intentionally addresses and builds on these pillars in a sequence that promotes sustainable healing and growth. This methodically nurtures and repairs each pillar, addressing any existing gaps, and ultimately leads to a well-regulated and healthier nervous system. The 5-Stage Plan is not just about overcoming dysregulation; it's about strengthening resilience and enhancing your capacity to handle life's challenges.

In this visual of the 5-Stage Plan, you start on the left with symptoms like anxiety, burnout, and chronic physical conditions. One or more of your 4 Pillars are relatively weak. On your healing journey, you'll start by laying a foundational structure that will support you throughout the five stages. Then you'll progress through the stages sequentially, each stage building on the previous one and ending with a regulated nervous system that can respond flexibly to stressors. You'll feel confidence and self-trust, and your chronic symptoms will likely have eased. Each of the 4 Pillars will be strong.

In the following chapters, I'll walk you through each stage in detail, showing you specific practices that will help accomplish the goals of that stage. But first, I'll share an overview of the 5-Stage Plan, and what you'll be able to accomplish in each stage. The five stages to reversing nervous system dysregulation are:

1. Awareness
2. Regulation
3. Restoration
4. Connection
5. Expansion

Stage 1: Awareness

This is the starting point of the plan. In the Awareness stage, you may be feeling overwhelmed and frustrated; you may feel confused about why your physical or mental symptoms do not seem to go away even though you have been receiving treatment or professional advice. You may even feel like an open wound, frustrated that your sensitivity has caused such extreme challenges in your life. It can be easy to blame yourself for these feelings, especially when you're told that the cause of your pain is something you should supposedly be able to "just let go" of, like your way of thinking or feeling, limiting beliefs, mental suffering, or even your ego.

This stage is all about *slowing down* your habitual response and becoming clearer about what's happening, moment by moment, in your nervous system. That means establishing a greater awareness of your thoughts, emotions, and physical sensations in real time, strengthening the mind pillar in the 4 Pillars of Nervous System Health. This stage is essential to complete first because you can't release the alarm in your nervous system without first becoming aware of what the alarm feels like in your mind and body. Just like in the story of Milarepa from A Field Guide to Nervous System Regulation (see page 6), the famous Buddhist yogi who learned to bow to his demons, saying, "Eat me, if you wish," you'll learn to open up to and become curious about your thoughts, feelings, and sensations, even when they feel uncomfortable or scary.

In the Awareness stage, you'll also learn to recognize where you are on the alertness elevator at any given moment. You'll start to recognize when you're in the red state, the yellow state, the green state, and the blue state. This is especially important because it allows you to reconnect with your internal sense of how your body feels. You aren't just becoming aware of your thoughts, but also becoming aware of your physical responses to stressors and recognizing them as normal, healthy, and even helpful.

Stage 2: Regulation

This stage is all about releasing the internal sense of alarm and reestablishing a sense of trust between you and your body. Here you'll learn about somatic, or body-based, practices that create feelings of safety and help build a felt sense of self-confidence. By implementing these somatic practices, you'll strengthen the body pillar of the 4 Pillars and you'll be able to face triggers with less fear and anxiety.

While working through this stage, you'll also work on your ability to regulate emotions such as the fear response. As you build the ability to regulate emotions, you'll feel more confident addressing challenging situations with curiosity and openness instead of automatically seeing them as a threat.

The Regulation stage in the 5-Stage Plan teaches you how to mitigate stress and anxiety as it arises *in the moment*, putting you back in the driver's seat of your own mind and body. Often, when people experience this new sense of control, they are shocked with their ability to actually guide their body instead of being at its mercy. This may be a profound shift for you, particularly if you have struggled with conditions like anxiety and panic attacks. With this new sense of safety, you can meet your thoughts, emotions, and physical sensations, and feel all your feelings, without being consumed or overwhelmed by them. Your nervous system can finally relax into a new sense of safety, allowing it to flush out the alarm it has been holding on to.

Stage 3: Restoration

This stage is all about coming home to yourself and meeting challenges with flexibility. In the previous stage, you learned to regulate stress as it arises in the moment, gaining a new sense of control over your nervous system. During this stage, you'll discover how to respond more flexibly to a wide range of stressors, so those stressors put you only temporarily into red or yellow states and no longer lead you back into nervous system dysregulation.

This is also the stage in which you can heal some of the deeper underlying wounds and patterns that may have contributed to your dysregulation. You will learn techniques to shift to a more secure attachment status and let go of dysfunctional coping strategies—you know, the "hard stuff." This is also a good time to work with a practitioner or community on releasing your embedded alarms from old traumatic stressors. This deep work becomes infinitely more achievable and effective when you nurture safety within your mind and body through the previous two stages—Awareness and Regulation.

It can be tempting to go straight for the deep wounds to get quick results, but this approach often backfires. If you go straight for the hard stuff, without setting up a foundation of awareness and in-the-moment regulation, you're likely to become overwhelmed, experience an increase in symptoms, and stop following the plan. To see lasting change, you must progress slowly and diligently through each stage, building your new healing journey as a set of healthy habits rather than quick fixes.

This Restoration stage is all about restoring and regenerating your nervous system flexibility. It seeks to undo the negative effects of past experiences that have created pain, stress, and fear as your responses to stress. It focuses primarily on combining both the mind pillar and the body pillar of the 4 Pillars of Nervous System Health, but in the background also starts to work on the connection pillar. At this point, surrounding yourself with supportive people is hugely important—whether a practitioner, mentor, friend, or family member. Support may also come from a community or group setting, such as an online forum like the Heal Your Nervous System community, meditation class, or group therapy.

Stage 4: Connection

By this stage in the plan, you are feeling much more confident to manage your inner energy safely and calmly. You feel a growing sense of self-trust as you're no longer thrown off balance at the whim of every stressful thought, feeling, or embedded alarm, and so it's time to bring your nervous system into deeper connection with the world around you, including connecting with a sense of purpose, other people, nature, and beauty. This stage also helps you strengthen the connection pillar of the 4 Pillars of Nervous System Health.

You'll learn to shift from feeling what others are feeling, and sensing their emotions without boundaries (empathy), to being genuinely compassionate toward them while maintaining control of your feelings. You'll become more assertive, set more explicit boundaries, and start attracting healthier relationships into your life. You'll also begin to feel more comfortable in social situations and find that you're no longer as drained after being around people.

Feeling alone, isolated, and disconnected from the world around us weighs heavily on our nervous system. Developing a special bond with the natural environment, uncovering our innate sense of beauty and creativity, and connecting with our purpose can drastically redefine our relationship, in the most positive way, with the world. Nature, especially, is intrinsically connected to the human nervous systems. Reestablishing the ancient bond between your nervous system and the natural world can restore the sense that you are interconnected with all beings, and not as isolated as you fear. The Connection stage of the 5-Stage Plan brings a deep sense of stability, insight, and plentiful joy to be shared with others.

Stage 5: Expansion

The final stage in the 5-Stage Plan offers the opportunity to increase your ability to understand, feel, and cope with stressors in more positive ways. You've come a long way since stress was a source of threat and danger. Now you'll learn to use stress as an ally to expand your nervous system's capacity, build even more daily energy, and keep growing. You'll also learn how to expand your capacity with experiences of awe, which can act as a gateway to the fourth pillar of nervous system health, spirituality, or connection with something larger than yourself.

As you move through this stage, you might notice that your day-to-day thoughts, feelings, and approach to life start changing. You see the world in a different light and are facing life with an attitude of curiosity and courage. You might notice a natural sense of abundance and generosity start to arise, feeling like you have a lot to offer others.

In the Expansion stage, you develop a deep sense of trust—not only in yourself and your ability to navigate whatever comes your way but also in the unfolding of life itself, appreciating the beauty and opportunity even in challenging experiences. You develop a sense of purpose and meaning, and you're driven by a desire to share your gifts with the world.

THE 4 PLEDGES FOR HEALING NERVOUS SYSTEM DYSREGULATION

The team of practitioners who lead the Heal Your Nervous System community and I have had the honor of supporting thousands of people on their journey to nervous system regulation. Among the people we support, certain issues come up again and again that can get in the way of healing. To set yourself up for success, consider each of the four pledges following. If it seems reasonable and supportive for your journey, choose to commit to it and take the pledge before moving forward with the practices and strategies in the following chapters. These pledges can help keep you on track, even when things get challenging. Write them down on a notepad to keep near your computer, post them on your fridge, or leave them next to your bed so you can be reminded of them when you first wake up.

Pledge 1: I Will Take Small Actions, Many Times

Nervous system regulation happens in the context of everyday life. You still go to school, have a job, take care of your loved ones, or whatever other important life activities fill your day. You don't need to commit long hours every day to doing the practices that will help regulate your nervous system. In fact, if you have a dysregulated nervous system, you probably don't have the time or energy to devote to a whole set of new practices. Your cup of marbles is likely already overflowing.

The key to regulating your nervous system is not in doing long, complicated practices but, rather, doing simple, short, straightforward practices *consistently*.

Eventually, you will gain mastery of the skill of keeping your nervous system regulated. But gaining mastery of any skill takes time, and that's especially true for mastering nervous system regulation. Sure, there will be sudden breakthroughs and moments when it seems you can increase your abilities and progress rapidly, but the truth is, consistent practice will take you further than anything else.

Consistent, short repetitions of the practices in each stage of the 5-Stage Plan will build new neural pathways that allow your nervous system to regulate reliably and flexibly. At times, progress may seem slow, but every repetition of the practices creates a compounding effect until, eventually, you're reaping the rewards for all your effort.

Staying on Track

A related obstacle we sometimes see people experience is getting stuck in planning and analyzing, rather than implementing the practices.

Nervous system regulation is not a cognitive process. Of course, you do need your mind involved to learn about and follow a quality plan, like you're doing now. However, cognitive processes alone, like planning, strategizing, and analyzing, won't regulate your nervous system. That's why we emphasize *small* actions. Even just one small action, taken every day, will help you see results and feel an increased capacity in your nervous system.

Pledge 2: I Will Take It Slowly

Another common misstep we see people make when just starting out is biting off too much at once and then getting burned out. The upcoming practices you'll learn in the 5-Stage Plan are not complex—most can be done in just five to fifteen minutes, and you might find yourself wanting to move quickly and take on many of these practices at once. Resist that temptation and, instead, proceed at a slow and steady pace.

Starting to heal a dysregulated nervous system is a journey, not a race. It can be challenging to maintain this perspective, as many of us are haunted by a sense of urgency and become frustrated when we don't move quickly. It can be disappointing to feel like you're not healing as quickly as you'd like. You might find yourself asking questions like, "Why am I still here? When will the pain end?"

Staying on Track

People often tend to give themselves timelines and create expectations that are simply unrealistic, which can lead to feelings of disappointment or even guilt. But success isn't better based on how quickly you progress from one stage of the 5-Stage Plan to the next. Pushing yourself to do too many practices at once or moving too quickly through the five stages can actually create even more unneeded stress and anxiety and block your progress.

In the first stage of the 5-Stage Plan, Awareness, you'll learn about the practices that will help you listen to your body. Often, the desire to go faster is driven by an internalized sense of urgency. You might notice a clenching or tightness in your body, maybe in your heart or your gut, that tells you you're in danger and you need to heal faster. Don't let that sense of urgency define your journey. Instead, be gently present with it, recognizing it as an old, embedded alarm, and meet it with a sense of safety and soothing, just like you might do with a child scared of monsters in the closet.

Pledge 3: I Will Do One Thing at a Time

Multitasking is associated with the yellow state on the alertness elevator. Your mind is using working memory heavily as it tries to keep track of multiple things at once and meet lots of different demands. Don't let the 5-Stage Plan be another thing that sends you into the yellow state.

Instead, complete one stage of the 5-Stage Plan at a time. And within each stage, choose just one practice to do at a time. In the Heal Your Nervous System online community, we give people just one practice each week to do, to help them keep this steady pace and not become overwhelmed. I recommend keeping a similar pace, doing just one practice each week. And if you find a practice that helps, slow down even more and keep doing that practice for as many weeks as you want. Give yourself permission to go as slow as the most sensitive parts of you want to go.

The most sensitive parts of your nervous system are also the most easily overwhelmed. Counterintuitively, by going slowly, you actually reduce your tendency to get overwhelmed, which leads to a more regulated nervous system.

Imagining yourself in the final stage, Expansion, feeling regulated, connected, and deeply trusting in your body to respond to stress appropriately might seem a long way off, but following my 5-Stage Plan, doing just one practice at a time, allowing each practice to build on the previous one, makes the work surprisingly simple and straightforward.

Staying on Track

One common obstacle that this pledge helps protect against is chasing shiny new techniques to avoid facing the challenges in your healing journey. Don't get me wrong: Trying new practices is fun and can be helpful at times. With an abundance of books, courses, and resources available on the topic, there is no shortage of solutions to explore.

But constantly seeking a new practice, hack, or habit eventually becomes a way to avoid actually doing the work to heal and regulate your nervous system. Don't be fooled: this is yet another manifestation of the "quick-fix cycle" we discussed in chapter 2. Be aware when the tendency to seek shiny, new techniques arises and remember that, although this tendency is a normal part of the healing journey, you'll make more progress by letting it go and coming back to the practices that have been shown to be able to take you through the hardest parts of the journey.

Pledge 4: I Will Face Obstacles as Challenges

Healing a dysregulated nervous system is a serious undertaking, and it's absolutely inevitable that you will face obstacles along the way. It might require more time than you anticipated to get a handle on the initial awareness practices and begin to experience their positive effects. As you begin to regulate your nervous system better, you might feel like life keeps throwing more stress your way. Or, just when you start feeling stable and grounded daily, a major stressful event happens, completely disrupting your balance.

Stress researchers have uncovered two different ways that people orient to the unexpected events and stressors that—inevitably—interrupt their plans:

1. Viewing new, unexpected events as a threat: People feel angry, resentful, or fearful because this new obstacle got in the way of their carefully laid plans.
2. Viewing new, unexpected events as a challenge and an opportunity for growth: Research shows that people who see new obstacles as challenges are much more resilient than those who see them as threats.

The first part of this pledge recognizes there will be obstacles. You can't anticipate what they will be, but whenever they show up, you can say to yourself, "Ah yes, I was expecting that," and whatever it is will be much less likely to lead to overwhelm.

The second part reframes your view of those inevitable obstacles—when they do come, you can approach them as another challenge, another opportunity to practice your awareness and regulation skills. Learning is a process of trying, failing, and trying again. We learn *because* of our mistakes and the obstacles we encounter, not despite them. And, with each obstacle you overcome, your nervous system's ability to handle stressors will grow.

Staying on Track

Related to this pledge is the common tendency to chase unattainable ideals or hold unrealistic expectations. Be aware of any parts of yourself telling you you're not doing it "right." Pay special attention to any perfectionistic tendencies—don't fall into the trap of thinking that unless something is perfect, it isn't worth doing.

Rather than comparing yourself to others, compare yourself to yourself. Right now, your nervous system is dysregulated. That's your baseline. Any improvement from that baseline, even a couple moments of green state, or a few more minutes of restorative deep sleep in the blue state than you usually get, is a huge win. Any improvements from your baseline are causes for celebration and appreciating your progress.

COMMON QUESTIONS

Here are some common and important questions I hear from people as they go through the 5-Stage Plan to Reverse Nervous System Dysregulation. Asking questions is a valuable part of the process. When questions like these come up, it can be a sign you're growing in your understanding and ability to grapple with the complex issues of your health. Come back to this section at any point during your healing journey to review.

Q: How long will regulating my nervous system take?

A: It's taken your nervous system years to develop dysregulation, and it will take time to reverse it. How long? Everyone is different, so it's difficult to say how long it will take *you*, but by following the 5-Stage Plan, you can significantly accelerate the process compared to approaching your regulation process haphazardly. With that in mind, here are some guidelines about how long it often takes people using the 5-Stage Plan:

- On average, people start experiencing relief, feeling calmer, and responding differently to triggers after four to six weeks of implementing practices in the Awareness and Regulation stages.
- In four to six months, the results you're experiencing become anchored and longer lasting.
- Deeper issues, such as embedded alarms, extreme burnout, and attachment wounds, usually require more time to heal. Some estimates based on scientific studies suggest that one to two years of short, daily practices can lead to fundamental shifts in these deeper issues, but much will depend on your particular situation. Don't get discouraged if it takes you longer; that's not uncommon.

Just like mastering a martial art, achieving mastery of nervous system regulation requires dedication and lifelong commitment to meeting your own needs. But you don't have to master everything at once! Start small, commit to learning and healing, and enjoy the journey as it unfolds. On the other side of your commitment is a newfound sense of freedom and peace that will last a lifetime.

Q: Will the 5-Stage Plan work for my diagnosis or symptoms?

A: When managing physical or emotional problems, people often feel anxious and unsure of whether anything will help. As you will see in the following chapters, the practices and techniques for regulating your nervous system have been shown in scientific studies to have positive effects on a variety of health conditions. Regulating your nervous system is critical so that you fix the underlying cause of the issue, but it's also important to work with your doctor on any medical diagnoses you have.

Q: Can I heal from a dysregulated nervous system?

A: Yes! Your nervous system does not have to remain stuck in a pattern of chronic stress. It holds the potential to reverse its own dysregulation. The practices I've included here are based on scientific research. There is a growing body of scientific evidence supporting the efficacy and benefit of practices we use to reverse nervous system dysregulation.

Q: Can I follow the 5-Stage Plan if I already use other practices, like somatic treatment, talk therapy, CBT, EMDR, etc.?

A: Integrating different practices can be highly beneficial when tackling complex issues like nervous system dysregulation. These forms of therapy can bolster and support your progress on the 5-Stage Plan and vice versa, resulting in a more powerful combined effect.

However, be mindful of the pledges discussed in the previous section. Don't overcommit to too many different practices and methods all at once, and don't get stuck in planning and strategizing about which practices you are going to do without actually getting started.

If you're already working with a practitioner on a modality such as CBT, EMDR, or talk therapy, I recommend consulting with them before starting the 5-Stage Plan. They could be a useful ally, one of those supportive people you surround yourself with, as you start to implement these new practices.

Sometimes it's best to complete your current cycle of work before adding any fresh elements into the mix. This is especially true if the work you're doing is already putting a heavy burden on your nervous system, such as reprocessing traumatic stressors. But once you have the capacity, starting to implement the 5-Stage Plan alongside your current practices can accelerate both.

Q: Is nervous system dysregulation a mental or physical diagnosis?

A: Nervous system dysregulation is *neither* a mental nor a physical diagnosis. It is a framework to help you better understand your symptoms and take consequential actions to improve them. As such, following the 5-Stage Plan and regulating your nervous system is not a replacement for working with your medical provider to diagnose and treat diseases such as viruses, infections, diabetes, and cancer. Working with a medical professional can be an important part of the body pillar in the 4 Pillars of Nervous System Health. Any underlying health conditions could be part of what's causing your nervous system dysregulation and must be evaluated by a certified medical professional as part of healing your nervous system.

I use the framework of nervous system dysregulation to help you understand the interconnectedness and inseparability of the mind, body, relationships, and spiritual connection to something larger than yourself. By shifting from simply seeking separate treatment for each symptom to seeing how everything in your body—biology, psychology, and lifestyle—interacts with the other, you're empowered to work on all the aspects of your life that affect your health.

Q: Why do I see improvements in some areas but other symptoms get worse?

A: It is entirely normal to have a fluctuating array of symptoms during the initial stages of working to heal your nervous system. This may happen because restoring energy levels can cause cells to become hyperexcitable, leading to disruptions in the body as it strives to recalibrate to the restored levels of energy.

Experiencing fluctuating symptoms is often a sign that things are improving. Throughout the healing process, it is essential to be patient, consistent, and kind to yourself as you witness these fluctuations and transitions on your journey toward improved health.

Q: Can I follow the 5-Stage Plan and heal my nervous system alone?

A: Taking the lead in your healing journey is a critical step toward recovery, but it is not something to tackle completely alone. Recovery inevitably involves ups and downs, which can be challenging to manage without support from others—whether through working with a practitioner or engaging with an online or in-person community. If you can find and afford a good practitioner, I highly recommend hiring them. Working with someone trained in the process of healing provides support, accountability, and insight to keep you moving along the path and can help you get out of your own way.

However, not everyone has access to regular one-on-one support from a professional who can guide them along the healing journey. Working with a community of other journeyers can provide enough support to keep you going. Talking to peers about their healing journeys, in a safe space, is a valid option to help maintain momentum and perspective on your journey. Online communities, like the Heal Your Nervous

System community, provide a way to connect with others even if you don't have access to a local support group.

With a solid support system, you can weather the ups and downs of the journey while still remaining in the driver's seat of your healing process.

Q: Can I regulate my nervous system while I'm on medication?

A: Absolutely. Medications save lives and are a vital part of many people's healing journeys. Some people require lifelong medication to support their healing journey, whereas others can taper off medication once their nervous system is consistently in a regulated state, with the proper guidance and support from a medical professional. Remember, *making any modifications to medications must always be done under medical supervision.*

NO FINISH LINE: THE ONGOING JOURNEY OF NERVOUS SYSTEM HEALING

Healing a dysregulated nervous system can often feel like an overwhelming and daunting task, but the 5-Stage Plan provides clear direction on how to move forward. Unraveling, and mastering, each stage—Awareness, Regulation, Restoration, Connection, and Expansion—is like piecing together an intricate puzzle that gradually reveals a big, beautiful picture. Although the sequence of the stages may initially appear rigid, it is flexible enough to be adapted to fit your individual circumstances. Healing is never linear, so it's essential to find what works for you. But keep in mind that the order of the stages has an important purpose, with each stage building upon the previous stage.

You'll notice that, although you move through the stages sequentially, there isn't an end point. What started as a journey of healing eventually becomes an ongoing adventure, one in which the stages become deeper and richer as you move through them. When practiced over time, the process can be an incredibly rewarding and life-changing experience. With patience and commitment, you can learn to master this process and create a thriving and healthy nervous system.

Before you dive into the five stages, it's crucial to first establish a structure of foundational elements that will bolster your nervous system health. I call this an underlying structure to support your nervous system, and it is the topic of the next chapter. Without this, the techniques presented in the five stages might not be as effective. However, when accompanied by this structure of daily habits, your nervous system will be better equipped to handle even the most challenging parts of your healing journey.

6

A Structure to Support Your Nervous System

MY 5-STAGE PLAN TO REVERSE NERVOUS SYSTEM DYSREGULATION starts with implementing an underlying structure that supports your nervous system throughout your healing journey. Structure and predictability can help your dysregulated nervous system feel a little safer and more relaxed. It can also help organize the different forms of stimulation coming in. And it sets up your current environment to support your regulation rather than work against it. Providing structure doesn't have to be complicated or difficult, but it does have huge rewards.

In this chapter, I share how you can start building a simple structure that will support regulation throughout the 5-Stage Plan and beyond. The structure, primarily in the realm of the body pillar in the 4 Pillars of Nervous System Health, consists of building routines in four areas of your life that are most central to your nervous system: physical sensations, sleep, fuel, and home. You'll learn how to set up routines to support sensory stimulation and movement, sleep and circadian rhythm, blood sugar regulation and gut microbiome, and feelings of ease and simplicity in your home.

CREATING A SENSORY STIMULATION ROUTINE

If you are highly sensitive, you may have learned to avoid certain sensory stimuli or try as much as possible to immerse yourself in sensory stimulation that's notably soothing, like taking long warm baths or listening to your favorite music. Even if you're not innately highly sensitive, nervous system dysregulation can temporarily increase your sensitivity to certain stimuli and similarly cause you to seek certain stimuli and avoid others.

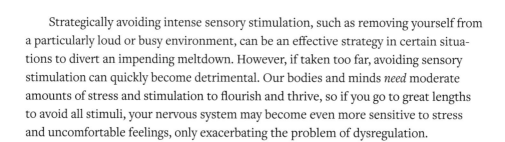

BUILDING MOMENTUM

IMPLEMENTING STRUCTURE PRACTICES INTO YOUR DAILY LIFE

The following practices, our first set, could easily become overwhelming if you don't stick to the four pledges (see page 76). Remember to *take it slowly* and *do one thing at a time*. You do not have to do all of this at once to make progress.

I recommend starting with sensory stimulation because this will have the biggest effect on the nervous system for most people. Once you've built a routine around sensory stimulation, move on to sleep and fuel.

You don't have to perfect these structure practices before moving on to the 5-Stage Plan. You can follow the sequential stages of the 5-Stage Plan even while you continue to work on your daily structure. But, if at any time it starts to feel like too much, just dial it back. It's okay to come back to doing only sensory stimulation practices if you start to get too tired, anxious, or overwhelmed after adding sleep, or fuel, or home. Remember, taking small actions many times is the path to nervous system regulation. Every few weeks or months, consider revisiting this chapter and adding a little more structure to your routine.

Strategically avoiding intense sensory stimulation, such as removing yourself from a particularly loud or busy environment, can be an effective strategy in certain situations to divert an impending meltdown. However, if taken too far, avoiding sensory stimulation can quickly become detrimental. Our bodies and minds *need* moderate amounts of stress and stimulation to flourish and thrive, so if you go to great lengths to avoid all stimuli, your nervous system may become even more sensitive to stress and uncomfortable feelings, only exacerbating the problem of dysregulation.

Similarly, you may have seen advice suggesting that you engage in "soothing practices," such as pampering yourself at a spa, going for a peaceful walk in a botanical garden, or taking a long hot shower, every time you start to feel uncomfortable. "Soothing practices" are a noninvasive way to get a momentary breather from sensory overload, and they can be lovely if you enjoy them, but they are not appropriate for regulating your nervous system or working with sensitivity.

Rather than react to your nervous system's sensitivity, your goal should be to gently teach your nervous system to manage a greater variety of stressful stimuli, stretching and expanding your capacity instead of contracting and retreating from stimulation.

A **sensory stimulation routine** is a selection of activities and experiences that offer the right amount of sensory input to help keep your nervous system stimulated—without becoming overwhelmed. It includes gently stimulating the senses of touch, taste, smell, seeing, and hearing as well as the sense of balance and body awareness in space. It's like filling your cup with the right blend of sensory experiences and activities that stimulate your nervous system and help it recalibrate to different types of stimulation. It's easy to implement, can be done while engaging in other activities, and will work like magic on your nervous system. It's important for anyone experiencing dysregulation, regardless of their sensitivity level.

In a dysregulated state, your nervous system feels unsafe, which can show up as difficulty concentrating, feeling anxious, or struggling with sleep patterns. A sensory stimulation routine provides a clear message of safety to the nervous system. By incorporating sensory experiences that are calming and grounding, a sensory stimulation routine signals to your nervous system that your body is secure and well connected to its environment. This security can encourage your nervous system to switch from a high-alert yellow or red state to a green state, where you feel ease and relaxation.

If you have lower sensitivity, you may often find yourself understimulated and seeking additional sensory input. A tailored sensory stimulation routine can provide you with much-needed stimuli in a controlled way, helping your nervous system stay alert and responsive.

In contrast, if you have higher sensitivity, you might be prone to sensory overload. Your nervous system can become overwhelmed easily by the multitude of sensory data in your environment. The purpose of a sensory stimulation routine is to introduce sensory experiences gradually, and in a manageable quantity, thereby expanding your nervous system's capacity while avoiding overwhelm.

By staying consistent with your routine, you'll find that you don't need to rely as often or as heavily on coping strategies such as withdrawing, or immersing yourself in soothing stimuli to avoid other, uncomfortable, feelings.

People living with chronic conditions, such as chronic fatigue or chronic pain, often tell me they don't think they have enough energy to do anything, let alone engage in a stimulation routine. If this sounds like you, start small, with one thing at a time, and add more activity as your energy gradually increases. I have seen this approach work wonders, even for those whose lives are particularly hard hit by their chronic issues.

Creating and Implementing Your Sensory Stimulation Routine

Creating a sensory stimulation routine is an individualized process—what works for one person may not work for another—and what works today may not be what works tomorrow. The process is dynamic and needs room to change as your life circumstances and needs change. Although the initial establishment of a routine may provide noticeable improvements, it is not a static or one-time solution. Instead, consider it an ongoing commitment to your health.

Just as your body changes, grows, and adapts, so should your sensory stimulation routine. With time, you might find that some activities aren't as beneficial for delivering the optimal level of nervous system stimulation—the level that feels most comfortable in your body—as they used to be. Or new challenges might necessitate different types of sensory stimulation. This isn't a sign of failure, but rather an indication of your growth and the dynamic nature of your sensory needs.

Regular assessment and adjustment are key to keeping your routine effective and relevant. This might mean replacing an old activity with a new one, adjusting the duration or intensity of certain exercises, or experimenting with new forms of sensory input that might better cater to your evolving needs. It's not about creating a perfect routine, but about understanding your body, recognizing its needs, and being flexible enough to adjust your sensory stimulation routine accordingly. This process is about nurturing an ongoing conversation with your body and its sensory experiences, using that understanding to inform and adjust your routine.

With patience, observation, and a willingness to adapt as needed, you'll find that a sensory stimulation routine is not a short-term fix but a lifelong commitment to fostering flexibility and harmony within your nervous system.

To start building your sensory stimulation routine, pick two or three options from the following lists of sensory input and spend ten to twenty minutes each day engaging in these activities. You can choose to do different things each day or each week, as variety will help keep the practice fresh and interesting, or stick to the same ones if that feels better to you. You can fit most of them into your regular daily routine without having to carve out extra time.

>> DO THIS

VESTIBULAR AND PROPRIOCEPTIVE INPUTS

Vestibular input, related to the sense of balance, and *proprioceptive input*, related to internal body sensations, are the most important inputs for organizing the nervous system. Each day:

- Start with vestibular input, active proprioceptive input, and passive proprioceptive input. Aim for at least three minutes of stimulation for each of these sensory systems, and aim to eventually work your way up to ten minutes each.
- After a few days or weeks, when you're ready for something more, add some tactile input to stimulate the sense of touch
- For many people, daily proprioceptive, vestibular, and tactile input will be enough. But if you are very sensitive to sounds, smells, lights, and textures, begin adding those inputs to gently stimulate your nervous system in a safe way.
- End with some additional passive proprioceptive stimulation to ground the nervous system.

Remember, try different things until you find a combination that works for you. The following lists are great places to start, but don't be limited by them. They are not meant to be comprehensive.

Continue to experiment with different activities until you find certain ones that feel good in your body. They'll all be helpful for you, but certain ones might be exceptionally good for your nervous system, and your body will tell you that because something about it will feel good. Once you find those that feel good, stick with them for a while, if you like, or keep experimenting.

Vestibular Input

Vestibular input stimulates the vestibular system, located in the inner ear, which is primarily responsible for maintaining *balance, coordination, and spatial orientation.* Activities that stimulate the vestibular system, such as swinging, spinning, or rocking, can be extremely helpful for organizing the nervous system, enhancing concentration, improving balance, and developing more spatial awareness.

- Perform head rolls, side-to-side movements, and up-and-down motions while seated or standing.
- Spin in a chair or make circles with your arms extended outward.
- Swing on a swing set or in an adult-size hammock.
- Do yoga poses that involve balancing, such as the tree pose.
- Move quickly between postures, such as jumping jacks or star jumps, while standing.
- Play games, like tag, that involve moving rapidly in different directions.
- Rock back and forth while seated on a yoga ball, fitness ball, exercise cushion, etc.
- Jump rope, alternating between two-foot and one-foot jumps.
- Do trapeze exercises using a pull-up bar, rings dangling from the ceiling, etc.
- Dance to fast-paced music.
- Roll down a hill or inclined plane.
- Engage in repeated back-and-forth motions, such as rocking in a rocking chair.
- Ride a bike, scooter, or skateboard, or rollerblade, etc.
- Position yourself upside down with your feet against the wall or weight-bearing on your hands.

Active Proprioceptive Input

The proprioceptive system, composed of sensory receptors in our muscles, tendons, and joints, provides feedback about your body's *position, movement, and force.* Active proprioceptive input involves doing activities that stimulate feelings of changing body position, muscle movement, and resistance. Actions such as jumping, climbing, or pushing and pulling heavy objects stimulate the proprioceptive system, and can help ground your nervous system, promoting motor control, enhancing body awareness, and fostering a sense of physical strength and capability.

- Do wall push-ups or arm push-ups against a wall or other stable surface.
- Play tug-of-war with a large exercise band while sitting, standing, or doing body-weight exercises.
- Push against a wall, heavy furniture, or weighted blankets.
- Vacuum.
- Wash windows.
- Take out the trash.

- Carry heavy items, such as laundry baskets, up and down stairs.
- Perform weight-lifting exercises using jugs filled with water as weights.
- Use elastic exercise bands to engage in strength and resistance training while seated or standing.

Passive Proprioceptive Input

Passive proprioceptive input involves *receiving sensory feedback about body position and movement without exertion or force.* It can include activities like wearing a weighted vest, using compression clothing, or receiving deep pressure massages. These experiences stimulate the proprioceptive system in a different way from active proprioception, emphasizing sensations related to grounding, calming, security, and stability.

- Use massage tools, like a pressure point stimulator, vibrating roller ball, or massaging brush.
- Do deep pressure squeezes with pillows, stuffed animals, rope toys, etc.
- Wear weighted vests and belts while doing daily activities.
- Use a weighted blanket at night or for a nap.
- Squeeze your arms and legs, self-hugging, or engage in play fighting with your kids or pets.
- Use compression clothing or compression sheets.
- Get a deep-tissue massage.
- Lie underneath big pillows or cushions, feeling their weight.
- Wrap yourself in a blanket like a burrito.

Tactile Input

Tactile input stimulates sensations related to *skin contact with the external world.* It is useful for organizing your nervous system's detection and interpretation of texture, temperature, pressure, vibration, and pain.

- Brush your skin with a soft-bristled brush.
- Take a warm shower or bath.
- Manipulate textured objects, such as sandpaper, bubble wrap, velvet fabric, or foam blocks.
- Apply body lotions with various textures and scents.
- Apply ice packs on skin areas that need relief from pain or stress.

- Spin different types of fabric, such as silk, cotton, or wool, between your fingers.
- Garden, or do any tactile outdoor activity that involves touching plants and soil.
- Play with modeling clay or play-dough with different shapes and textures.
- Work with a pet, such as brushing their fur or feathers.

Olfactory Input

Olfactory input stimulates your *sense of smell*. Your olfactory system plays a vital role in detecting and interpreting odors in our environment, which can influence your behavior, emotions, and memory. Include olfactory input in your sensory stimulation if you are particularly sensitive to smells or if you enjoy these activities.

- Take walks in nature and use nasal breathing to take in various smells from plants, trees, and flowers.
- Bake different recipes and take in the aromas of spices, herbs, and other ingredients.
- Sniff coffee beans or tea leaves.
- Play games with scented items, such as socks or washrags with different odors, such as lemon, lavender, or peppermint, during blindfolded smell tests.
- Find interesting smells while outdoors, such as from mud puddles, wet grass, or rotting wood.
- Experiment with creative uses for familiar scents, such as mixing baking soda and vinegar to make a fizzy science experiment.
- Visit farmers' markets or stores that specialize in herbs and spices to sample different aromas.
- Create arts and crafts projects with materials that have distinct smells, like paint, papier-mâché, clay, etc.
- Use culinary items, like citrus fruits or fresh herbs, to create homemade potpourri.
- Cook meals with strong-smelling herbs, such as basil, oregano, and thyme, and spices like paprika and cinnamon.

Oral and Gustatory Inputs

Oral and gustatory inputs engage your *sense of taste* and the *physical functions of the mouth and jaw*. Your gustatory system is crucial for identifying and processing flavors and textures in food, which plays a role in appetite, nutrition, and the overall process of fueling your body. Although tasting and eating are part of everyone's daily routine, a focus on oral and gustatory inputs is particularly important if you are highly sensitive to tastes, textures, or temperatures in food.

- Eat crunchy snacks, like carrots, tortilla chips, or pretzels.
- Suck on hard candies, such as peppermints, lemon drops, or jawbreakers.
- Eat foods that require mouthing and licking, such as ice pops, applesauce pouches, or baby foods.
- Drink from differently shaped containers, like sports bottles or sippy cups, or use straws.
- Use a variety of utensils, like spoons, forks, chopsticks, or your hands, to eat.
- Experiment with foods at different temperatures, like warm soup or cold sherbet.
- Blow bubbles with carbonated drinks or flavored syrups.
- Eat crunchy salads with ingredients like nuts and seeds.
- Drink warm beverages, like herbal tea or hot cocoa.
- Create savory dishes that combine multiple flavors, like stir-fries.

Auditory Input

Auditory input activates your *sense of hearing*, which can influence your emotional state, attention, memory, and communication with others. This type of input is important to add to your routine if you are often distressed by different types of noises.

- Listen to your favorite music or audiobooks using headphones.
- Explore soundscapes in the area by taking a sound walk.
- Participate in auditory activities, like riddles, tongue twisters, and storytelling.
- Play rhythmic instruments, such as drums, the xylophone, or cymbals.
- Sing nursery rhymes, folk songs, hymns, or karaoke.

Visual Input

If you are highly sensitive to certain types of light, colors, or visually busy environments, incorporating calming visual stimuli into your routine can help make different types of visual input less disrupting to your nervous system.

- Look at fractal art, such as the Mandelbrot set or other mathematical patterns.
- Observe picturesque panoramas, and take in the sights of wide-open spaces.

- Examine intricate details in close-up photographs of everyday objects.
- Watch videos of calming natural scenes, such as sunrises or sunsets.
- View artworks, noticing the small details and shapes in each.
- Go on a photography walk and capture interesting images from your environment.
- Search for interesting patterns to explore in unexpected places, like the pavement, clouds, or plant leaves.
- Explore abstract paintings and interpret the symbolism of their shapes and colors.

Assessing Your Sensory Stimulation Routine

With your sensory stimulation routine, your primary goal is to signal to your nervous system that your body is secure, well connected to its environment, and able to transition easily from a state of high alert to a state of calm. Measuring the effectiveness of your routine is not about ticking off completed activities on a checklist, but rather gauging your internal responses to these sensory experiences. Look for signs of relaxation, grounding, and a heightened sense of well-being. Do you feel calmer after certain activities? Do you notice improved sleep or a greater ability to focus? Are feelings of anxiety or stress diminished?

The process of monitoring the effectiveness of your routine involves paying close attention to these changes and noticing the impact of the practices on your nervous system. You might find it helpful to keep a journal documenting your activities and responses, noting any shifts in your mood, focus, and overall state of being.

Moreover, consider your level of comfort and connection with your environment. After implementing your routine, do you feel more comfortable? Are you finding it easier to engage with those tasks that previously caused discomfort or sensory overload? These improvements are indicators that your sensory stimulation routine is helping ground you and foster a sense of safety.

Remember, the ultimate effectiveness of your sensory stimulation routine lies in its ability to bring about a sense of calm, grounding, and enhanced well-being. By carefully observing your responses and adjusting your practices accordingly, you can cultivate a routine that continues to nurture a harmonious relationship between your body and its environment.

SLEEP: SETTING UP AN EFFECTIVE DAILY CYCLE

Our bodies are governed by an internal clock that follows a twenty-four-hour cycle known as the circadian rhythm, which regulates sleep and various other physiological processes. This master clock, located in the brain's suprachiasmatic nucleus, is set and adjusted by signals from our nervous system, such as the release of neurotransmitters.

This circadian rhythm is essential to the human body's functioning and is especially important for nervous system regulation. Because it plays such an important role in nervous system regulation, maintaining a consistent circadian rhythm is extremely helpful as you go through the 5-Stage Plan. If you have sensory processing sensitivity, your nervous system may be even more sensitive to changes in the circadian rhythm, and you may find it even more beneficial to stick to a predictable, stable schedule.

Your circadian rhythm is influenced by many factors, including external light or darkness, temperature, food intake, and movement. All these cues that adjust your circadian rhythm have been honed by evolution over millions of years to help us stay alert, focused, and productive during the day, and rest, heal, and sleep properly at night. Our ancestors' bodies had to learn how to read these cues correctly to survive, so we have evolved ways of being incredibly attuned to them. Understanding how the environment can affect this cycle will help you maintain a consistent circadian rhythm and make it much easier to regulate your nervous system.

Maintaining a consistent circadian rhythm doesn't mean becoming overly dependent on your routine and fearing any slight disruption to it. Some unexpected changes to your routine or a few nights of bad sleep are not enough to create chronic dysregulation. However, allowing your body to settle into a routine that you maintain most of the time will significantly boost your success in all stages of the 5-Stage Plan and help your nervous system regulate.

Anxiety and Sleeplessness

Sleep problems are often one of the first signs of a dysregulated nervous system. Sleep problems have become increasingly common. One reason for this increase is that modern lifestyles and habits, such as staring at your phone or computer late at night, interfere with your circadian rhythm and interrupt your natural sleep-wake cycles.

The importance of sleep for health has been recognized for centuries, yet it remains one of the most mysterious aspects of human biology. Scientists have long debated why we need sleep and what happens during it that makes it so important for our health and well-being—a necessity for survival so great it has withstood millions of years of evolution! What mysterious process does sleep bring about to be worth doing it for a third of our lives?

It's now widely accepted that sleep plays a critical role in consolidating memories, regulating hormones, restoring energy levels, repairing damaged cells, remodeling neurons, boosting immunity, and reducing stress levels.

Our ancient ancestors must have been able to get a good night's sleep despite the dangers and threats they faced. They had a much closer connection with nature and its rhythms, which would have helped them regulate their sleep-wake cycle better than we do today, and they lived in tribes that helped keep them protected from dangerous predators at night.

A dysregulated nervous system can be one of the underlying causes of sleep struggles and, eventually, lead to chronic insomnia. Burnout, embedded alarms, high-functioning anxiety, chronic conditions, having young children, and many other circumstances can make it difficult to get a good night's sleep. Although you can't necessarily know which came first, working on regulating your nervous system and addressing the underlying causes of dysregulation will lead to improved sleep. And even small improvements in sleep quality will help regulate your nervous system.

Regardless of the initial source of sleeplessness, for many people, sleep challenges take on a life of their own and become an additional problem. This is called sleep anxiety, and it can even make going to bed a trigger that causes further nervous system dysregulation. Even if you feel perfectly relaxed and ready to fall asleep, if you have sleep anxiety, it will start to kick in the minute you get into bed. Your mind starts spinning with thoughts like, "What if I don't fall asleep?" "What if I don't get enough rest to function tomorrow?" "How will the lack of sleep affect my health, my relationships?"

Lack of sleep and sleep anxiety create a vicious cycle. Like the pinball effect, where causes lead to consequences, which then become new causes, lack of sleep can further dysregulate the nervous system, which, in turn, contributes to sleep anxiety. Ultimately, the solution to this cycle is to fix the underlying causes of nervous system dysregulation, which we'll do in the following 5-Stage Plan. But creating a structure for regulation to assist and reinforce your circadian rhythm is a critical step to reversing nervous system dysregulation and improving sleep quality along with it. In the next sections, I share some simple interventions that help reestablish a healthy circadian rhythm and can lead to better regulation.

Sensitivity to Light and Dark

Electric lighting has enabled major advances in human productivity, but along with it comes a darker side. We now have the ability to stay up later, but this exposure to light after dusk can have massive implications for our circadian clock and throws off our body's natural cycle of day and night. Production of melatonin, a hormone that triggers sleep and suppresses neuron activity, is significantly affected by light. If your melatonin production is too low, that can cause you to have trouble falling asleep or staying asleep. Studies have found that even light as low as 30 lux (comparable to electronic devices or typical indoor lighting) could reduce melatonin production by up to 50 percent.

Although most people's circadian rhythms are affected by nighttime lighting, some individuals may be more sensitive than others. There seems to be considerable variation in the degree to which nighttime lighting can cause circadian disruption, with some people being up to fifty times more sensitive than others.

For example, one study found that different levels of light intensity elicited the same reduction in melatonin production in two groups: people with low sensitivity required 400 lux (equivalent to the light typically found in a well-lit office or classroom during the day) to cause a 50 percent reduction of melatonin, whereas individuals with high sensitivity needed only 10 lux (equivalent to the light emitted by a candle from a distance of about one yard [one m]) to cause the same drop in melatonin. Recent studies also found that even very dim blue light, such as from electronic devices, can suppress melatonin production.

It can be difficult to determine whether you are vulnerable to sleep disruptions caused by artificial light. Because light sensitivity is so variable, it's best to err on the side of caution and, as much as possible, dim artificial light after sunset and cut it entirely by 10 p.m. In the next section, you'll learn how to manage your light intake throughout the day to help reset and maintain a healthy circadian rhythm that will support your nervous system regulation.

Reset Your Circadian Rhythm

Although you have little direct control over your circadian rhythm, recent research has revealed there are ways to manipulate its functions. By exposing yourself to the correct external cues, such as light/dark cycles, you can effectively tell your body when it should be ready to sleep, eat, and perform other vital functions.

There are three steps to using light and darkness to establish a healthy circadian cycle to support nervous system regulation: morning sunlight, afternoon sunlight, and dim lights after sunset.

1. Morning Sunlight

This foundational step is to get bright light in your eyes, ideally from sunlight, within the first thirty to sixty minutes after waking—even better if you can do this within five to fifteen minutes of waking. This action sets off a chain of events that readies your body for the rest of the day. The chain reaction starts with the release of cortisol, which helps adjust your internal clock to the correct morning schedule, wakes up your brain and body, and prepares you for falling asleep later. Solid scientific evidence shows that viewing light early in the day is the most powerful cue for wakefulness and helps you fall and stay asleep at night.

2. Afternoon Sunlight

Do the same thing outside later in the afternoon. Being outside for ten to thirty minutes, depending on how cloudy it is, when the sun is at a low solar angle, signals to your internal clock that it's evening and almost time to go to sleep, helping anchor your brain and body to the current time. The wavelengths of light you see that look yellow, blue, and orange before and during sunset tell your brain and body that night is coming, easing the transition into nighttime. Afternoon sunlight is particularly helpful if you plan to watch television, use the phone, or socialize with friends in bright artificial-light settings at night. Soaking up some late-afternoon sunlight can partially offset the negative effects of exposure to nighttime lights.

3. Dim Lights after Sunset

The third step to establish a great structure to support sleep is to dim artificial lights of any color after sunset and, particularly, avoid artificial light during the nighttime hours between 10 p.m. and 4 a.m. Depending on your lifestyle, achieving this might be the most difficult thing to do. Even a small amount of light late at night can be enough to disrupt your circadian rhythm and your sleep, especially if you are highly sensitive to light.

Overhead artificial lights are the worst, so if you need lights on in the evening try to position them as low to the ground as possible. Dim screens and TVs, and try to keep phone usage to the absolute minimum. For a tranquil atmosphere, some people prefer candlelight or moonlight.

USING NUTRITION TO SUPPORT SENSITIVITY

Understanding how food and nutrition affect your level of stress is an extremely powerful step to supporting sensitivity and regulating your nervous system. Although nutrition is important for everyone, sensitive people, especially, can benefit from fueling their bodies with the appropriate nutrients. Recent studies have continued to highlight the connections between diet and mental health. Proper nutrition helps regulate your nervous system by providing reliable building blocks for your cells to do their jobs.

Nutritional choices are highly personal decisions guided by a variety of factors such as health needs, income, preferences, cultures, tastes, and beliefs, and even more important, what works for your body and nervous system and what is sustainable *for you*. Although it would take an entire book to cover the wide range of available strategies, I will suggest a few you can consider incorporating into your structure. We'll discuss food cravings, managing blood sugar, and establishing and maintaining a healthy gut microbiome as part of the structure of nutrition to support your nervous system.

It is always wise to consult your doctor before making any changes to ensure they are safe and appropriate for you. Don't be afraid to ask questions and then take action: Taking ownership of your nutrition will pay significant dividends in terms of physical and emotional well-being.

>> DO THIS

SUPPORT YOUR NATURAL CIRCADIAN RHYTHM

Aim to do this five or six days per week:

- Go outside. Staring through a window won't cut it. Eyeglasses or contact lenses are okay, but skip the sunglasses. For the fullest benefits, go outside within thirty minutes of waking up—even sooner if you can.
- Expose your eyes to enough light: on sunny days, five minutes is enough. Scale up to ten minutes if it's partially cloudy, or thirty minutes if heavily clouded.
- Go outdoors and do the same before sunset, if possible.
- If you wake before sunrise, turn on artificial lights, but get outside when the sun rises.
- If sunlight is unavailable, selfie ring lights or another bright artificial light can help.
- Make up for a lost day the following day. Getting natural outdoor light in your eyes has a cumulative effect.
- Limit the use of electronic devices after sunset, specifically those with screens.
- Dim the lights after sunset and position them as low to the ground as possible.
- Try red light bulbs, which have been shown to have a lesser impact on melatonin production.
- Create a consistent sleep routine: go to bed and wake up at the same time, or within about thirty minutes of that time, each day to help regulate the body's circadian rhythm and promote healthy sleep patterns.

Food Cravings with Dysregulation and Sensory Sensitivity

You may tend to seek out highly palatable foods with lots of sugar and salt—particularly chocolate, sweets, and energy-raising drinks like sodas. Although anyone can fall into a pattern of eating foods that are engineered to give us pleasure, if you have a dysregulated nervous system or heightened sensitivity, you may be especially susceptible to cravings.

Studies suggest that high sensitivity to sweetness can be linked to an increased preference for carbohydrate-dominated or sweet foods in sensitive people. This heightened response can also lead to a greater sense of reward when consuming these types of foods, which is seen by increased brain activation in areas related to food-reward processing when exposed to sweet or high-fat food odors.

You may find yourself craving these types of foods when under emotional distress or experiencing anxiety. This is due to the activation of the brain's dopamine reward center, which happens in all brains but seems to be particularly challenging for the highly sensitive brain.

Managing cravings and avoiding overconsumption of sweets and sodas can be a daily challenge, especially if you have heightened sensitivity. The interaction between stress, sensitivity, and food craving can look like this: You feel overwhelmed. The stress of the day takes its toll on you, and you feel angry, sad, and exhausted all at once. To soothe these feelings, you reach for the sugary treats or the drink you know will give you an instant energy boost. The resulting dopamine surge sends a wave of pleasure through your body, and for the first few moments after indulging in that sweet treat, everything feels good again.

Although these sugary snacks provide a boost of energy and a better mood, this quickly fades, leaving you feeling sluggish and tired, and struggling to focus on anything other than the craving for *more sugar*. By now, you likely need to consume an increased number of sugary treats and beverages just to relieve the intense discomfort. This creates an endless cycle of cravings that can be hard to break.

Staying away from processed foods, which are practically everywhere, can be daunting, and the cravings they spark often prove too intense to dismiss. Processed, highly palatable foods are popular for a reason: their convenience, taste, and appeal in a busy world. They are often created with flavors and textures designed to please sensitive people. Unfortunately, the big food industry is keenly aware of our susceptibility and knows how to exploit these vulnerabilities for its own profit. By flooding the market with cheap, highly processed foods and drinks loaded with sugar, salt, and unhealthy fats, they reinforce an addictive cycle that keeps us coming back for more.

To combat cravings and the need to lean on sugary foods and drinks as coping strategies, it is essential to slowly tackle the various aspects of regulation—with food being one of the most crucial yet difficult elements.

It's hard or impossible to beat cravings solely with willpower, yet with a tailored strategy and a comprehensive plan, you can break out of this vicious cycle of craving sugary foods, which leads to further dysregulation. To break this cycle, you need to approach your cravings indirectly, without trying to use willpower to overcome them.

One intervention you can start using right now is to pay more attention to how your body feels when you eat. Stress researcher Elissa Epel studies food cravings and binge eating. She emphasizes the importance of fostering awareness while eating and introducing healthy stimulation of the nervous system.

Epel's research has shown that increasing your awareness of the sensory experience of eating makes you more attuned to your body's signals of hunger and fullness. This, in turn, can lead you to make better food choices and reduce the likelihood of binge eating. Whether you're eating something highly nutritious or getting a boost of sugar from your favorite snack, get curious about the full sensory experience of eating. Let yourself enjoy the pleasant aspects of it, and also pay attention to any unpleasant or neutral aspects. You might be surprised by how much this relatively effortless intervention leads to changes in your dietary habits without the use of willpower.

More broadly, though, you are relying on these sugary snacks and treats to make you feel better because you regularly feel overwhelmed. Your body is too often in yellow and red states and doesn't spend enough time in green states. Your cravings will ease significantly when your nervous system can relax into a green state easily and you can feel good without needing to reach for sugar. This is exactly what we will focus on in the 5-Stage Plan to Reverse Nervous System Dysregulation. In other words, instead of trying to fix the cravings, the solution to eliminate cravings is to create conditions that support your inherent sensitivity and lead to a regulated nervous system.

Take Control of Your Blood Sugar Levels

Ever felt *hangry*? When your blood sugar dips too low, you might get grumpy and irritable, a mix of being hungry and angry, or what some people call "hangry." Evidence has been mounting over the past few years of a strong connection between blood sugar, or glycemic levels, and mood. It's not surprising. After all, the brain runs mostly on glucose, the primary type of fuel in our blood.

As more research is conducted into the correlation between food and mood, it is becoming increasingly clear that those with hypersensitivity and chronic nervous system dysregulation can also be highly prone to glucose fluctuations. These shifts in blood sugar levels can trigger a wide range of symptoms—from irritability and anxiety to headaches and fatigue.

When you eat a meal high in carbohydrates and low in fiber, glucose rushes into your bloodstream and triggers the release of insulin from your pancreas to shuttle that glucose into cells for energy. This can lead to quick changes in mood and can even trigger anxiety symptoms or depression. The carbohydrates you ate were digested too quickly, leaving you with a sudden crash in blood sugar levels once digestion is complete.

In contrast, when you eat a meal rich in fiber and protein, the absorption rate of glucose from your meal is slowed, making it easier for your nervous system to regulate mood and energy. Consuming meals rich in fiber and protein can help you feel more satisfied with your meals and reduce dramatic blood sugar spikes. This will help you cut down on processed foods, which, as you just learned, only intensify your dysregulation and create further cravings.

Regulating blood sugar levels is an important part of creating a structure for regulation in your daily life. It also helps keep your mitochondria healthy. Mitochondria, as I shared in chapter 1, are the parts of your cells that turn glucose into the energy your cells need to function properly. Mitochondrial dysfunction plays an important role in the pinball effect leading to dysregulation, and is linked to problems with hormones, metabolism, moods, emotions, and overall health. Keeping your blood sugar relatively stable, most of the time, nurtures your mitochondria so they can provide the necessary energy for smooth cellular functioning.

The way each individual's metabolism responds to different foods and activities can vary significantly, something scientists call "carbohydrate tolerance." Monitoring your glucose levels throughout the day can be an eye-opening and empowering experience because it helps you understand how *your body* is uniquely sensitive to different foods and activities. Having this knowledge makes it easier to maintain optimal glucose levels, preventing big dips and spikes that could lead to cravings and dysregulated metabolic processes.

Using a continuous glucose monitor (CGM)—even for just two weeks—can be an enlightening experience, providing valuable information about how your body responds to changes in blood sugar levels and changing the way you think about your metabolism.

A CGM measures glucose levels through a tiny sensor inserted under your skin, usually on your arm. Typically, the sensor has a life-span of fifteen days before needing to be replaced. This sensor measures your interstitial glucose level, which is the amount of glucose in the fluid between cells. This information provides real-time readings of your glucose levels throughout the day and night.

With this information, you can understand, for example, how a certain food affects your glucose, or identify a certain habit that causes glucose levels to drop or

>> DO THIS

KEEP BLOOD SUGAR LEVELS STABLE

Even if you don't have a CGM, you can still effectively keep your glucose levels in check by using some simple strategies.

- Consume fiber-rich foods, such as green veggies, at every meal. This will create a matrix of fiber in your digestive tract that will help slow the body's digestion of starch and sugar. A simple solution is to add a mixed green salad or steamed veggies to each meal.
- Include some protein and healthy fats in each meal and snack. When eating foods such as rice, bread, or pasta, eat them last. The order in which you consume food impacts how your body absorbs these nutrients, so eating carbohydrates alongside or after fats and proteins, rather than before, can help slow the absorption of the carbohydrates and prevent large spikes in blood sugar.
- If you want a sweet treat, eat it as dessert at the end of a meal rather than as a snack. Sweet drinks and treats should never be consumed on an empty stomach, as this can lead to big glucose spikes in the blood.
- After a big meal that includes an abundance of carbs, activate your muscles to absorb some of the glucose that's rising in your blood. Go for a brisk ten-minute walk or do some of your sensory diet heavy-lifting activities, like house chores.

rise too quickly. Armed with this knowledge, you can make the necessary changes and adjustments in your lifestyle that will help regulate your glucose levels—and, ultimately, help regulate your entire nervous system.

Unfortunately, CGMs aren't yet easily accessible for all: They may require a doctor's prescription or exceed your budget. Knowing that, here are several ways to identify a spike in blood sugar levels without relying on a CGM:

- Experiencing difficulty concentrating or mental fog
- Experiencing sudden fatigue or energy slumps
- Feeling hungry shortly after eating
- Feeling jittery or anxious
- Feeling thirsty more often than usual

- Having frequent headaches
- Having strong cravings for sweet foods or drinks
- Having trouble falling or staying asleep

Foster a Healthy Gut Microbiome

Thousands of years ago, the human gut was home to a vibrant bacterial ecosystem teeming with thousands of different microbial species, or microorganisms. A study published in the journal *Nature* analyzed ancient DNA from coprolites—or preserved feces—from between one thousand and two thousand years ago found in rock shelters in Utah and Mexico. The analysis revealed an astonishing extinction event: the human gut has become significantly less diverse over the past millennium.

Gut health is essential for keeping our bodies healthy, especially when it comes to regulating our nervous system. That's because the brain and gut are connected in a two-way relationship called the gut-brain axis. This is a complex interplay between the gut lining, the immune system, the gut microorganisms, and the part of the nervous system located inside the digestive system, called the enteric nervous system. This relationship demonstrates a *direct link between what you eat and the regulation of your nervous system.*

The gut microorganisms play an essential role in this relationship: The microorganisms are intricately connected with the entire human body, and when they become disrupted from things like antibiotics, chronic stress, diet, or lack of sleep, your nervous system, immune system, and other bodily systems can feel the effects. If your gut microbiome is thrown out of balance entirely—known as dysbiosis—the whole gut-brain axis can start to fall apart. This imbalance can be likened to taking away one card from a house of cards—it throws off the entire structure and causes it to collapse. In a similar way, disrupting the gut microbiome can cause dysregulation throughout the entire brain-body system.

Disruptions in the intestinal microbiota have been linked to various brain conditions, including Parkinson's disease, Alzheimer's disease, autism, anxiety, and depression.

The pinball effect plays a role here as well, where a trigger like taking an antibiotic to heal an infection gives rise to a consequence, like gut dysbiosis, that produces more triggers and causes, like chronic stress and nervous system dysregulation. Nervous system dysregulation can further shift the composition of the gut microbiota, leading to even more dysregulation of the nervous system and an increase in overall symptoms.

Scientists who study the connection between the gut microbiome and mental health have introduced the concept of a "psychobiotic diet": a diet tailored to the needs of your gut microbiome. Implementing a diet that supports your gut microbiome can have enormously positive benefits for your nervous system. Fostering a strong and

>> DO THIS

HEAL YOUR GUT MICROBIOME

- Introduce low-sugar or sugar-free fermented foods into your diet, such as yogurt, kefir, fermented cottage cheese, kombucha, and vegetable brine drinks; fermented vegetables such as sauerkraut and kimchi; and fermented vinegars like apple cider vinegar. Begin with two 1-cup servings each day, increasing that to four and, eventually, six portions.

- Introduce foods high in prebiotic fibers, like onions, leeks, cabbage, apples, bananas, and oats. Aim for six to eight servings per day of fruits/vegetables; five to eight serving per day of grains; and three to four serving per week of legumes.

- Try a psychobiotic diet for four weeks to see the difference in how you feel. Check with your doctor or health-care provider first to ensure it won't interact with any medications or existing conditions.

diverse ecosystem of friendly beneficial bacteria living in your gut promotes a cascade of positive events in the brain and body, like calming inflammation and reducing stress.

How you choose to fuel your body is extremely personal and providing detailed guidance about your individual dietary needs is beyond the scope of this book. The vast majority of people will benefit from slowly introducing sugar-free fermented foods, such as yogurt or sauerkraut, and higher-fiber prebiotic foods, like onions and oats. But your dietary restrictions, sensitivities, or preferences may not allow you to introduce a psychobiotic diet as I suggest here. If you have dietary restrictions or sensitivities that inhibit you from eating the foods on this list, or if trying them causes digestive symptoms to worsen, check in with your health-care provider to work on a more specialized and individualized plan.

CREATING A SIMPLER HOME ENVIRONMENT

The more cluttered and disorganized your environment is, the more your attention must multitask to take in your surroundings. Your nervous system must filter out this excess data, which increases the likelihood that you'll stay in the yellow state while you're at home, rather than moving back to the green state.

By simplifying your home environment, you can significantly reduce the amount of sensory input your brain has to process, which can help reduce feelings of overwhelm and fatigue and give you more capacity to take care of your responsibilities and lead a meaningful life. Having fewer items in your home that are more meaningful to you, rather than a wide array of items that you don't care about, can help your nervous system find more relaxation in the safety of your home.

Simplifying your home doesn't mean adhering to a particular design trend, giving up your love for colors, or sacrificing creativity. Simplicity is about reducing the amount of "stuff" you have around you, so you can focus on what brings peace to your nervous system. With a more organized space, it's easy to add decorative elements without overwhelming your nervous system.

Having children can add significantly to the number of things in your home. As a mom of four, I know all too well how much stuff comes with raising children—and the resulting chaos it can bring to my life. Keeping my sanity despite the mess and clutter often feels like an uphill battle. But I've learned that I don't need to fill my space with a lot of different things for children to be happy and living a simpler lifestyle doesn't mean denying them the things they need and love.

Adopting a simpler lifestyle revolves around concentrating on what truly adds value to your life. This approach emphasizes the importance of giving priority to essential items. Instead of accumulating many low-quality possessions, consider investing in fewer, but better-quality, items when your budget allows. This is about mindful consumption, where quality takes precedence over quantity. Just like adults, children's nervous systems also benefit from being surrounded by fewer objects, which can create a sense of safety and relaxation in the home.

Additionally, the stress caused by clutter and disorganization in the home has been shown to profoundly affect caregivers, with some studies suggesting that these stressors can have detrimental effects on a caregiver's quality of life. This, in turn, leads to increased levels of stress for their children, which can negatively affect the children's health and life satisfaction. It can also make it more difficult for parents to regulate their child's nervous system, because their own capacity is quickly saturated. These findings highlight the importance of having a sense of order and routine in the home, creating an environment free from too much clutter.

Being intentional about new purchases or bringing new items into the home can help lighten the load on your nervous system, allowing you to manage your stress levels better and feel more in control of your environment.

>> DO THIS

DECLUTTER YOUR HOME

- Intentionally commit to buying less and keeping unnecessary items out of your house.
- Before buying something, ask yourself whether you need it or whether it will add to your home's sense of dysfunction.
- Create a budget and stick with it to avoid impulse buying.
- Whenever possible, invest in higher-quality items that will last longer.

IMPLEMENTING YOUR NEW DAILY RHYTHMS

Our modern culture has become disconnected from the natural world in many ways. The rhythms that are common in our culture, such as eating processed food on the go and staying up late staring at screens, go against the evolutionary rhythms of the human body built over millions of years. We spend most of our days inside, often moving very little, and relying on artificial light to guide our schedule. I'm not suggesting that you go live in a cabin in the woods. You can still enjoy the benefits of modern technology and stay in most of the same rhythms of the people around you. But the practices in this chapter, backed by extensive scientific research, will help you align enough with your body's evolutionary rhythms so that your nervous system can stay sustainably regulated for the long term.

Begin your journey by selecting and executing a single option from what I provide here. As described in the sensory diet section, I recommend starting with proprioceptive and vestibular input from movement, followed by ensuring that your circadian rhythm is in place. As you progress to the next stages of your journey toward regulation, include more aspects of this structure in your life. It's essential that you take things slowly and start with baby steps. This will ensure you have laid a strong foundation to support the deep dive into repairing your dysregulation in the forthcoming chapters.

Once you've established enough structure that you feel ready to add something else without getting overwhelmed, it's time to start the 5-Stage Plan. The first stage, Awareness, is all about seeing what's really going on in your nervous system without getting caught up in it. It's only when you see what's happening that you can start to intervene at the right moments to regulate your nervous system.

7

Stage 1: Awareness—Recognizing Your Nervous System Patterns

YOU'RE AT WORK and have a meeting scheduled with your boss. As you enter the room, you notice that your boss has a scowl on their face. Your nervous system immediately activates the red state. Your heart races, and your palms get sweaty. Your boss speaks in a condescending tone and criticizes your recent work. You try to defend yourself, but your boss interrupts you and continues to berate you. Feeling trapped and helpless, you snap and lash out at your boss. You yell and accuse them of being unfair and unreasonable. Your boss, taken aback by your reaction, ends the meeting abruptly and asks you to leave.

As you walk out of the room, your heart still racing, your mind replays the events—you keep thinking about what you could have said or done differently and how you could have handled the situation better. You feel angry at your boss and frustrated with yourself for losing control, perhaps even embarrassed about how you behaved.

Hours go by, and you're still unable to let go of the situation. You try to distract yourself with work, but your mind keeps wandering back to the meeting. You feel stuck in the yellow state and unable to move on from what happened.

Your body's stress response is still blaring its sirens and stopping you from returning to a calm state, or what you learned previously is the green state. So, you might find yourself constantly replaying the fight over and over in your head. Your mind might even start making up worst-case scenarios, like losing your job or being ostracized at work. This could keep you up all night, tossing and turning, and struggling to find some peace.

But here's how things would be different with a regulated nervous system. Instead of getting stuck in a loop of worry and physical distress, you are easily able to navigate back to your green state. It's not that the argument didn't affect you—it did. But your nervous system is able to stop those alarming "what if" thoughts from spiraling out of control.

You might still replay parts of the argument in your head, but you do so constructively. You think through what went wrong and how you might address it the next day. You might call a friend or use another coping strategy that helps you reach an understanding of the situation and feel better about it. Physically, you might feel a bit restless, but it doesn't rob you of a good night's sleep. You know you've been wronged, but you're also confident that you can handle this bump in the road. You may even remain upset about how your boss treated you, but you're not overwhelmed.

This is where stage 1 of the 5-Stage Plan comes in. In this chapter, I will delve into the first and most essential step on the journey to healing nervous system dysregulation—Awareness. By learning to track the patterns and signals that your body sends you moment by moment, you can train your stress response to become unstuck from the yellow state and spend more time resting and recovering in the green and blue states. By understanding the different states of activation your nervous system typically goes through and what they feel like in the body, you can learn to recognize when you're in a state of heightened arousal and take steps to regulate yourself—before you reach the point of lashing out or getting stuck in rumination.

Monitoring your physical sensations, emotions, and the state of your nervous system introduces a valuable pause, what I refer to as the *gap*. This gap serves as a buffer between the moment you feel the sting of a stressful situation and your reaction to it—sort of like slowing a knee-jerk reaction. You intentionally create space to fully absorb and process the myriad of feelings, thoughts, and sensations happening in the present moment.

It takes a fair bit of patience and perseverance, as it's all too easy to revert to your default habits, like tuning out, bypassing, or rushing to fix things. However, with practice, you'll be able to resist these urges and stay present. You'll be able to approach whatever arises with curiosity and self-compassion, like a kind friend sitting with you through a tough time.

Practicing the gap can be uncomfortable, even downright scary at times. But by opening yourself up to your experiences, you're effectively rewiring your brain, creating new connections that put you in control of your nervous system's alarms. In doing so, you're teaching your nervous system how to return to its calm state after it's been stirred up, helping and retraining it to self-regulate.

For many years, scientists believed that adult brains were more or less fixed and no longer underwent significant changes. Recent advances in neuroscience, however, have challenged this notion, revealing that our brains continue to evolve throughout our lives. This means you are not destined to be stuck in whatever stress patterns and embedded alarms currently contribute to your dysregulation. By staying aware of and tracking your body and mind's responses and feelings, your brain can change in a way that will allow your nervous system to regain its natural flexibility.

But recognizing what's happening in your body and mind from moment to moment can be challenging, especially when your attention is frequently scattered across various tasks and distractions. It's easy to become disconnected from your emotions and your body's subtle signals. You might find yourself on autopilot, navigating life's challenges with ingrained habits and coping mechanisms that may not serve you in the long run. When these habits lead to nervous system dysregulation, a cascade of unwanted consequences that wreak havoc on your mind and body can be the result.

Tracking and becoming more aware of your sensations, feelings, and behavioral patterns will allow you to replace old coping strategies that no longer serve with healthier, more effective ones, leading to improved nervous system regulation as well as a greater sense of control and agency of your body and mind. Embarking on this journey is a courageous act, and it all begins with a single, powerful choice: to be present and attentive—and aware—of the ever-changing landscape of your inner world.

EXPANDING THE GAP BETWEEN TRIGGERS AND RESPONSES

When you experience difficult feelings, it seems natural to attempt to get rid of them. Whether it's an angry reaction or the craving to light a cigarette, your instinct may be to push away or suppress these negative feelings. However, what happens when you pause and pay close attention to them instead? Scientific research into mindfulness suggests that simply noticing these feelings in the body can create enough space for you to respond more appropriately.

Many behaviors that contribute to nervous system dysregulation are the result of habit, and you have more control over them than you might realize. For example, imagine someone cuts you off in traffic. Your nervous system interprets this as a threat, pushing you instantly into the alert red state. You're filled with anger and your body prepares for a fight. Being in the red state is uncomfortable, and because there's no actual fight to engage in, naturally, you yearn to revert back to the peaceful, green state.

Your nervous system knows that sugar can provide temporary comfort, leading you to automatically reach for a candy bar in your glove compartment. After taking a

BUILDING MOMENTUM

IMPLEMENTING AWARENESS PRACTICES INTO YOUR DAILY LIFE

Integrating the awareness practices into your life is not time-consuming and does not require much of your precious energy, which may already be limited. All it requires is for you to become a curious observer, noticing the way your bodily sensations, thoughts, and emotions occur and change throughout the day and then journaling about them briefly at the end of the day. I recommend a dedicated notebook for keeping track of this.

This combination of practicing awareness, moment to moment, throughout the day and reflecting on your observations at the end of the day is enough to accomplish the goals of this stage: revealing your patterns of bodily sensations, thoughts, and emotions.

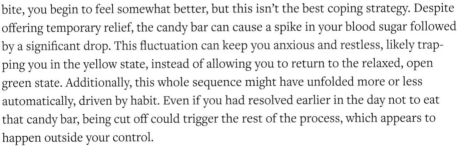

bite, you begin to feel somewhat better, but this isn't the best coping strategy. Despite offering temporary relief, the candy bar can cause a spike in your blood sugar followed by a significant drop. This fluctuation can keep you anxious and restless, likely trapping you in the yellow state, instead of allowing you to return to the relaxed, open green state. Additionally, this whole sequence might have unfolded more or less automatically, driven by habit. Even if you had resolved earlier in the day not to eat that candy bar, being cut off could trigger the rest of the process, which appears to happen outside your control.

So how can you break this cycle, ensuring that random incidents, like reckless driving by others, don't trigger a chain of responses that keep you in the red and yellow states for the rest of the day?

Eventually, in stage 3 of the 5-Stage Plan, Restoration, you'll work on cultivating a profound sense of safety in your body so that, when another driver cuts you off, you don't necessarily get angry or upset at all. And in stage 2, Regulation, you'll learn how to use simple body-based techniques to come back to the green state when you do get upset, so instead of reaching for the candy bar, you can reach for a more adaptive tool like your breath—a better strategy that can provide long-term improvement, consistently bringing you back to the calm green state, instead of keeping you stuck in the yellow one.

But right now, in the Awareness stage, your task is to deepen your understanding of what's really going on in your nervous system, informed by your direct experience. Building awareness is about allowing yourself to become fully present in the moment, *nonjudgmentally* observing your thoughts, feelings, and sensations without attempting to change or fix them. This simple act of witnessing can help you recognize your habitual patterns, feelings, and urges and create enough distance to insert a more useful response, rather than respond in a habitual way that's contributing to your dysregulation. Without awareness, your nervous system's responses are set on automatic mode and you'll end up doing whatever old habits have worked in the past to help you feel a bit better, even temporarily. But adding awareness is like switching to manual mode, giving you the opportunity to try responding differently.

Moreover, simply by observing your feelings in a nonjudgmental way, you become more receptive to them rather than avoiding them or pushing them away. This receptiveness can help you become more compassionate and kinder to yourself, which helps shift the nervous system down to the green state.

Observing nonjudgmentally can be difficult. Self-judgment, an attitude that's harsh, shaming, or punitive, is endemic in our culture, so it may seem normal or natural to judge yourself. However, self-judgment is stressful for your nervous system and can throw you into the yellow or red state. On the other hand, letting go of judgment and becoming more curious, open, and accepting of your sensations and emotions are keys to recognizing and becoming aware of what's happening in your body and creating a safe space for regulating your nervous system.

This is why reversing nervous system dysregulation starts with developing awareness of the *sequence* of events that can lead to dysfunctional coping strategies and ongoing nervous system dysregulation. Awareness, combined with a nonjudgmental attitude, is necessary to create the gap between your feelings or sensations and your habitual reactions to them. Only when you create the gap can you choose to insert a more functional coping strategy, such as the ones I'll show you in the following stages of the 5-Stage Plan.

For example, imagine you've made plans to catch up with a friend over coffee, and they cancel at the last minute, which makes you feel a rush of disappointment. Their cancelation hits an existing sore spot—it feeds into your self-doubt and stirs up inner wounds, making you feel like you aren't important enough to them.

Normally, this emotional cocktail of disappointment, feeling unimportant, and self-doubt would send you up your alertness elevator and into a higher state of stress.

You might lash out with a passive-aggressive text, or you might withdraw and ice them out for a while. This reaction is a threat response. You're in the yellow or even red state on the alertness elevator, with your body and mind responding to this perceived threat.

But now that you're incorporating awareness into your life, you don't have to respond in this habitual way to stressors. When you receive the cancellation text, you pause. You acknowledge the physical sensations of disappointment, the pang of feeling unimportant, and the self-doubt that's been stirred up. You notice your usual urge to fight back or retreat, but instead of reacting, you take a deep breath and observe these reactions with compassion and understanding. *This is the gap.*

Within this gap, you created space to make a conscious choice to react to your stressors differently. When you feel ready, you calmly communicate your feelings to your friend: the disappointment about the canceled plans, the sense of feeling unimportant, and the insecurities it all dredged up. By using the gap to respond from a place of honesty and calm, you prevent the situation from escalating, protect your friendship, and teach your nervous system a more helpful way to respond.

In stage 2, Regulation (chapter 8), you'll learn some widely applicable practices to take advantage of these gaps to come back to the green state. But you start by creating the gap, which means practicing awareness.

A fascinating example of the power of awareness to alter habitual responses and build new neural pathways comes from a 2013 study by Hani Elwafi and colleagues with people looking to quit smoking. In their study, participants who felt an urge or craving to smoke were asked to practice being aware in the present moment. They practiced paying close attention to their breathing and observing their thoughts, feelings, and sensations without judgment. Although they still experienced the craving to smoke, those who practiced awareness were able to stop responding to the craving by smoking. Instead, they created a "gap" to observe the craving and respond to it in a different way. Over time, the intensity of their craving began to reduce naturally.

At the beginning of treatment, there was a strong positive correlation between daily cigarette use and self-reported craving for cigarettes. However, by the end of the four-week treatment period, the relationship between cigarette cravings and smoking had significantly weakened. This "decoupling" process happened because the participants practiced awareness. In other words, when you build awareness, you are no longer at the whim of your habits and cravings. Instead, you have more agency to make a different choice, even when you feel a craving or habitual response. Although the craving or habitual response may remain for a while, if you don't act on it, it eventually fades.

After just four weeks of working on widening the gap, participants were able to decouple the relationship between the trigger and the response. These findings, along with more than one hundred other studies showing a wide array of benefits for building awareness, suggest that, in a relatively short period of time, you can build a functional gap between the trigger and the response. Ultimately, this new gap will allow new feelings and behaviors to emerge in your nervous system, and lead to more regulation.

From Dog Mind to Lion Mind

From dog mind to lion mind is a simple yet powerful open monitoring technique that helps you shift your perspective and approach to difficult emotions and thoughts. It is based on a compelling Tibetan metaphor used to describe two different ways of encountering situations—the dog's way and the lion's way.

Imagine you have a bone in your hand. If you stand in front of a dog and wave the bone in front of him, then toss the bone away, the dog will immediately start chasing the bone.

Now imagine standing in front of a lion, waving that same bone from side to side. The lion is poised, watching you with a steady gaze that sees beyond the bone. He understands that the bone is just a small piece of a much larger reality. The lion may decide to pursue its prize—that bone—or may keep his gaze on you. Worse still, it might even make a meal of you!

But the dog cannot see beyond the bone, so by controlling the bone, you control the dog's reality.

Now, imagine the bone represents a story or an emotion you are experiencing, like the thought "I'm not good enough," or the feeling of anger. As the bone is held in front of you, consider how you will choose to respond. Will you, like the dog, chase after the bone? Or can you take a moment to create space between yourself and the bone, displaying the attitude of the lion?

This simple shift can create a massive change at a neurobiological level. Consistently choosing to respond to emotional challenges by switching to "lion mind" begins to remodel the synapses that trigger unhelpful coping strategies.

Imagine your current response as a 5G-level connection—strong, fast, and almost instantaneous. This high-speed connection represents how quickly your nervous system gets triggered by challenges, leading to those reactions you want to change. By consistently switching to lion mind, you can start to reshape those synapses.

The process of reshaping the synapses is similar to transforming your 5G-level connection into a slower signal like sending Morse code. This slower communication reduces the intensity of your habitual responses and gives you time to pause, reflect, and replace unhelpful responses that increase dysregulation—like reaching for the

>> DO THIS

CULTIVATE LION MIND

To switch from dog mind to lion mind, follow these simple steps:

1. When a difficult emotion or thought arises, take a moment to notice it.
2. Imagine the emotion or thought as a bone being waved in front of you.
3. Ask yourself, "Am I in dog mind or lion mind right now?"
4. Take a deep breath and create a little space between you and the bone.
5. Observe the emotion or thought with curiosity and without judgment.
6. Try to shift your perspective and see the bigger picture.
7. Stay present and continue to observe without getting carried away.

candy bar—with new, more helpful ones. It is a journey from dog mind to lion mind—from being controlled by our emotions to mastering them.

So next time a trigger arises, ask yourself, "Am I showing up as the dog, focusing on and chasing after the bone, or am I choosing to be the lion, seeing beyond the bone and staying grounded in the larger reality?"

APPROACHING YOURSELF WITH GENTLE CURIOSITY

The importance of being open, curious, and nonjudgmental to nervous system dysregulation as you explore your thoughts and emotions cannot be overstated.

Imagine yourself as a kind and nurturing caretaker, observing a small child in your care. You want to approach the child with a warm and compassionate eye, understand their needs, and provide comfort when necessary.

Similarly, in building a safe and nurturing environment for your nervous system to become regulated, you need to approach yourself with the same gentle curiosity and compassion. It's essential to let go of the need to fix or explain away your experiences and, instead, simply acknowledge, be aware of, and track them.

In the early stages of your journey, you may find it tough to approach yourself with compassion and empathy, especially if you tend to be severe in your self-judgment.

This critical inner voice can create additional resistance and stress, making it more challenging to work on reversing nervous system dysregulation.

However, as you gently nurture self-compassion and understanding, you can start to relieve this inner critic of its duty. Your inner critic has been trying to protect you, to keep you safe by making sure you don't make mistakes. But as you cultivate awareness, you can start to unburden your critic. You can show it that you've got this, that you're capable of keeping yourself safe. It's like taking a heavy backpack off your inner critic's shoulders, leaving it more free and less stressed.

This creates a nurturing, supportive environment for the next steps on your healing journey. Having an inner critic is normal: Retraining your nervous system to shift from self-judgment to self-compassion takes time and effort, but with patience and persistence, it can lead to substantial healing.

>> DO THIS

NURTURE SELF-COMPASSION

1. Treat your coping mechanisms with understanding and compassion. Although they may not always be the most effective or healthy, you can acknowledge that they have served a purpose in helping you navigate life's challenges and difficult moments. Even self-judgment is a coping mechanism, so the same process applies if you notice yourself being judgmental.

2. Pay attention to your emotional and physiological states as you would with a child, without attempting to judge, explain, or distract yourself from them. Instead, allow your awareness to rest on them gently, observing how they arise and how they affect your emotional and physiological states.

3. Recognize your natural inclination to cling to certain emotions, experiences, or coping mechanisms, just as a child might hold on to a favorite toy or resist bedtime, and patiently work on easing this grip. It's normal to judge yourself when you cling to old patterns, but that can contribute to a rigid, inflexible nervous system and perpetuate feelings of stress and anxiety. By fully accepting these tendencies, without judgment, you gradually learn to soften your grip on them.

THE JOURNEY UP AND DOWN THE ALERTNESS ELEVATOR: CREATING YOUR PERSONAL MAP

The alertness elevator provides a great visual representation of your different states of arousal. With that in mind, I'll show you how to map your typical experiences in different arousal states. This map will become an important tool for monitoring your nervous system's shifts throughout the day, which will increase your awareness and help you expand the "gap" between getting triggered and reacting habitually and allow for more helpful responses instead.

When you're on a journey, a map helps you know where you are, understand the path you've taken, and navigate where you want to go. Similarly, mapping your typical behaviors against the alertness elevator allows you to gain a clearer understanding of your reactions, helping you identify patterns, triggers, and your habitual reactions to various situations.

The goal here isn't to judge yourself for being in a yellow or red state, nor is it to try to constantly stay in the green or blue state. The goal is to increase your awareness and understanding of yourself. This practice is about noting, "Oh, this situation has pushed my 'elevator' up to the yellow state," or "I seem to be spending a lot of time in the red state recently; what's causing that?"

It's important to remember that there's no right or wrong state to be in. Each state has its role and purpose—from the deep restorative rest of the blue state through the relaxed focus of green, the slight activation of yellow, the acute stress response of red, to the protective immobility of the purple state.

As you become more adept at mapping your states, you'll be aware of and able to recognize patterns more quickly. You'll see the situations, thoughts, or emotions that tend to push your elevator to higher, more stressed states. Likewise, you'll start to understand what helps you return to calmer, more regulated states. With this understanding, you can explore strategies that support your nervous system's regulation, making your journey through life more flexible and resilient.

This practice is a significant step toward self-awareness and building agency over your nervous system, the foundation for the healing journey ahead. This is *your* map. It will be unique to you and will evolve and change over time as you continue to learn, grow, and navigate your life's path.

The Blue State

In the blue state, you are in a state of deep rest and relaxation. Your body is in the restorative blue state during deep sleep, but it's also possible to reach the blue state while you're awake during periods of immense tranquility. For example, entering a deeply meditative state, going on retreat, or an hour in a float tank can all potentially

>> DO THIS

CREATE YOUR ALERTNESS ELEVATOR MAP

Here's a step-by-step guide to creating your alertness elevator map. A blank elevator map can be found on page 120.

1. **Find a quiet moment:** Start by setting aside some uninterrupted time for yourself. Choose a moment when you're alone and can afford to relax and focus on yourself. Make sure the environment is calm and quiet.
2. **Activate your states:** Except for the purple state, try to recall a past experience or situation that typically brings you to each of the alertness elevator states: blue, green, yellow, red. To evoke the blue state, you might recall the feeling of drifting off to sleep or sinking into deep meditation. A time that you've felt calm, open, and attentive could help you remember the green state. And a mildly stressful situation could help you tap into the yellow or red state. Concentrate on the emotions and sensations that come up as you recall each scenario.
3. **Note your observations:** Pay close attention to how your body feels and reacts in each state. What physical sensations do you notice? What emotions are tied to each state? Write down your observations in your journal. Your notes should be personal and meaningful to you and serve as clear reminders of what each state feels like in your body.
4. **Return to calm:** Exploring these states might stir up intense feelings, especially when you're tapping into the higher-stress states. If you find it hard to come back to a more relaxed state after the exercise, take a few moments to engage in a calming activity, such as a guided relaxation exercise, going for a gentle walk, having a comforting chat with a friend, or losing yourself in a piece of soothing music.
5. **Handle the purple state carefully:** If you have previously experienced the purple state, one eliciting an emergency response such as freezing or immobility, it may be beneficial to note any sensations associated with it, but only if this doesn't cause you too much discomfort. If during the exercise the purple state arises spontaneously, causing extreme discomfort, stop the exercise and practice calming and grounding exercises. Do not try to activate the purple state intentionally during this exercise.
6. **Use your map regularly:** Once your map is ready, use it as a daily check-in tool. Regularly ask yourself, "Where am I on the map right now?" Refer to your notes to identify your current state. Doing this can help heighten your awareness of your nervous system's responses and equip you with the information you need to more effectively regulate your state.

Remember, your map is not a static document. It's a living tool that will evolve as you continue to grow and understand yourself better. Keep updating it as you gain new insights about your responses and states.

Riding the Alertness Elevator: Recognize Your Body and Mind States

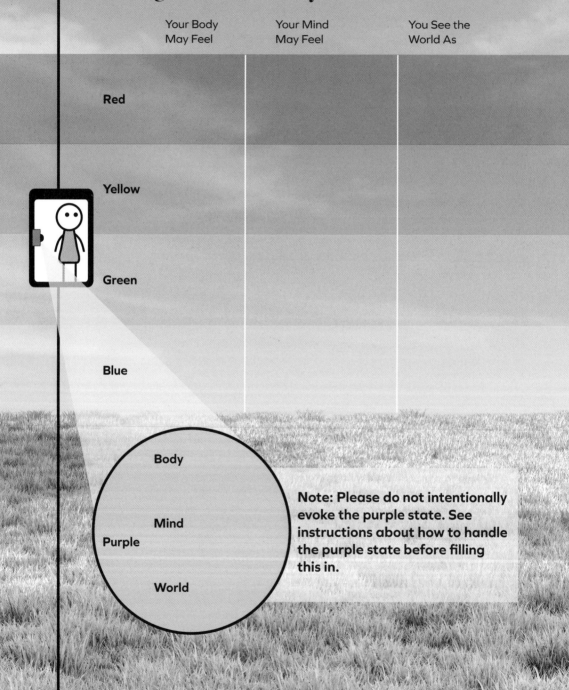

	Your Body May Feel	Your Mind May Feel	You See the World As
Red			
Yellow			
Green			
Blue			

Purple

Body

Mind

World

Note: Please do not intentionally evoke the purple state. See instructions about how to handle the purple state before filling this in.

put you in the blue state. Here are some common feelings and experiences associated with the blue state:

- You feel at peace, calm, and tranquil.
- Your breathing is steady and slow, and your heart rate is lower than usual.
- Your body feels heavy and completely relaxed.
- Your mind is quiet, with minimal thought activity.
- You may experience a sense of disconnection from your surroundings as you're deeply relaxed or even asleep.
- You may experience a sense of restoration and rejuvenation upon waking from sleep.
- Physical sensations are typically muted as your body is in a state of rest.

The Green State

In the green state, you feel safe and connected with yourself and others. Here are some common feelings and experiences associated with the green state:

- You feel calm, content, and relaxed.
- Emotions like joy, wonder, curiosity, affection, compassion, and confidence are common.
- Your breathing is slow and deep, and your heart rate is steady.
- You feel connected to your body and emotions.
- You have a clear mind and can think and plan effectively.
- You feel social, and it's easy to interact with others.
- You may feel creative, inspired, and motivated.
- You sleep well and wake feeling rested.

The Yellow State

In the yellow state, you feel alert and a bit on edge. Here are some common feelings and experiences associated with the yellow state:

- You feel tense, restless, or anxious.
- Emotions like annoyance, impatience, contempt, and a sense of being uninterested are common.

- Your heart rate and breathing may be slightly increased.
- Your muscles might be tense, and you may feel apprehensive or uneasy.
- Your thoughts may be racing, or you may be excessively focused on problem solving.
- You may feel social, but interactions can be strained or stressful.
- You may have trouble relaxing or winding down to go to sleep.
- After a while in this state you may feel "tired and wired," like you're fatigued but have trouble resting.
- You may have a sense of urgency and feel as though you need to constantly do something.

The Red State

In the red state, you are in a state of high alert or stress. Here are some common feelings and experiences associated with the red state:

- You feel stressed, anxious, or panicked.
- Emotions like fear, dread, aggression, rage, or hatred are common.
- Your heart rate is significantly increased, and your breathing is fast and shallow.
- You may experience muscle tension, a "knot" in your stomach, or other intense physical sensations.
- Your mind is likely racing with thoughts of what could go wrong or what needs to be done.
- Social interactions may be difficult or avoided altogether as your focus is primarily on the perceived threat.
- You may have trouble sleeping due to heightened arousal.
- You may feel a strong urge to fight, flee, or freeze.

The Purple State

In the purple state, your body and mind are in a state of extreme alert, often frozen due to perceived threat. Remember, the purple state is an intense stress response that typically occurs when you face extreme threat or trauma. It's not something to intentionally invoke, but recognizing the signs can be beneficial in understanding your nervous system's reactions. Here are some common feelings and experiences associated with the purple state:

- You may feel a heightened sense of fear or dread.
- Your body may feel frozen or paralyzed, unable to react or move.
- Your heart rate may slow significantly.
- You may experience a sense of disconnection from your body and emotions.
- You might feel as if you're watching yourself from the outside, almost as if you're in a dream or movie.
- Your mind may feel foggy, confused, or blank, unable to think clearly or plan.
- Social interactions may seem impossible or overwhelming, and you might feel isolated.
- Your sleep may be disturbed, marked by nightmares or insomnia.
- You might feel stuck or trapped, as if unable to escape the perceived threat.

EMBRACE FLEXIBILITY, FORGET BALANCE

There is a widespread misunderstanding that being regulated means you remain calm at all times, instead of flexibly moving among and between different states. But actually, it is entirely normal and healthy for your nervous system to spend time in various states, including even very high-stress red states that can feel extremely uncomfortable.

You may have been told that to live a good life you must seek "balance." We're told to pursue work-life balance, emotional balance, and even stress balance to achieve physical well-being. Many people make the mistake of trying to "balance" their nervous system, believing the ultimate goal of a regulated nervous system is to avoid activating their survival responses and going into their associated yellow or red states.

But trying to avoid the yellow and red states can inadvertently have the opposite effect, causing your nervous system to become rigid and tense and, ultimately, keeping you stuck in a cycle of dysregulation.

Instead, picture a regulated nervous system as a fern that bends and sways gracefully in response to external stressors. Regulation isn't about maintaining constant calm or relaxation but, rather, about learning to flow with life's inevitable ups and downs.

The key to a healthy nervous system lies in its flexibility, not balance. Embracing the natural ebb and flow of life and allowing yourself to experience different emotional states is essential for fostering regulation. A regulated nervous system can adapt to varying circumstances with ease, whereas a dysregulated one remains stuck, constricted, and unyielding.

Accepting this can be both daunting and liberating. It challenges you to accept that fluctuations are a natural part of life while at the same time freeing you from the pressure of striving for an ideal and unattainable state of neutral balance where you never get scared or stressed.

If you have a highly sensitive nervous system, this adaptability is especially important for navigating the challenges that your sensitivity presents without becoming overwhelmed or dysregulated. By focusing on flexibility and adaptability, you can build a resilient nervous system that quickly rebounds from stress.

For example, imagine you are facing a particularly demanding period at work, such as an upcoming event or deadline. During this time, it's natural for your nervous system to become highly activated. You might feel more anxious, have difficulty sleeping, and experience other stress-related symptoms. In fact, this heightened state can be beneficial, as the extra adrenaline your body produces in response to the stress can help you focus, potentially boosting your productivity and performance.

Problems arise when you are unable to bounce back to a regulated state once the stressful situation has passed, or when the stress becomes chronic and surpasses your ability to cope.

Aim for a flexible nervous system. It is not only healthy but also practically useful to regularly experience the whole range of levels on the alertness elevator as you navigate life's challenges. The goal is to cultivate the ability to *adapt* to the challenge and then *return* to a regulated state once the circumstances change and ease.

Most people spend a few weeks to a few months in the Awareness stage just practicing shifting from dog mind to lion mind, learning to recognize and track movements up and down their alertness elevator, and bringing a more kind, compassionate, and nonjudgmental attitude to their observations. Although these practices are not complex, don't underestimate their power. These simple shifts can create profound change in your nervous system. But you also don't need to perfect them to continue on to the next stage. Each stage builds upon the next, so once you start practicing regulation in the next stage, you'll still continue building awareness. Over time, these awareness practices will become second nature, much like driving a car was once a complicated task that required all of your attention but is likely now something you can do without much thought or effort.

In the next stage, Regulation, you'll switch your primary focus to the body pillar and I'll show you how to use body-based practices to shift down to the green state. This is also when you start gaining a sense of agency over your emotions, reactions, and states of alertness. You'll learn the tools to not just be at the whim of your feelings but also to shift and change them using your body to feel better.

>> DO THIS

FOSTER FLEXIBILITY

As you embark on your path of self-discovery and healing, remember that regulation *is* flexibility. By fostering a flexible nervous system, you open the door to a more vibrant, resilient, and fulfilling life experience.

- Embrace the idea that it is normal and beneficial for your nervous system to experience a range of emotions and reactions.
- Let go of the notion that a regulated nervous system must always be balanced and calm.
- Strive for flexibility and adaptability, allowing yourself to navigate life's challenges with grace and agility.

8

Stage 2: Regulation—Building Agency through Embodied Safety

Picture yourself waking up each morning with a profound sense of safety, inner peace, and tranquility, ready to embrace the day with confidence. It may sound like an elusive dream, but it is achievable when you consistently practice nervous system regulation.

As you worked on creating a structure, you set the groundwork for keeping your nervous system settled into its natural rhythms with the right amount of stimulation. In the Awareness stage, stage 1 of reversing your nervous system dysregulation, you learned to shift from dog mind to lion mind and see the bigger picture of what's happening in each moment. Part of that bigger picture was your nervous system's state and noticing when you experience a green or yellow state, or go from green to red, and back. Now that you've had some practice with awareness of your various states, it's time to learn stage 2, Regulation, and how to intentionally take the elevator back from red, yellow, or even the purple state to the safe and relaxed feeling of the green and blue states.

In this chapter, I show you how to return to a sense of calm and safety within your body and mind. The capacity to return to a state of calm and safety, consistently and effectively, cultivates a powerful sense of agency, which, in turn, allows you to trust in your ability to regulate your emotional states. You'll learn to cultivate embodied safety—a state that transcends a purely mental concept of security—developing into a tangible feeling of being secure, open, and comfortable within your own body. This represents the next level of strengthening the body pillar in the 4 Pillars of Nervous System Health.

Learning to cultivate an embodied sense of safety is a fundamental skill for anyone with a dysregulated nervous system, but it is especially important if you have heightened sensitivity. Your intense emotional experiences make it even more essential that you are able to rely on your body's natural regulation mechanisms to come back to the green state, rather than trying to use your mind alone to think your way out of states of high alertness.

I'll also dispel a common myth about emotions so you can have more moments of joy, wonder, and relaxation and fewer moments of fear, anger, or jealousy. The belief that emotions are purely mental processes is outdated. Current research emphasizes that emotions are an intricate dance between the mind and the body.

Emotions aren't just "in your head"; they are deeply connected to the body's reactions. They emerge from the dialogue between your brain and body, optimizing how you use your energy resources in response to the world around you. They're not housed in particular parts of the brain. Instead, emotions are dynamically constructed across the entire brain and deeply tied to bodily sensations.

So to truly improve your emotional well-being, it's essential not to just address the mind but also to ensure the body feels safe and open. This goal is at the heart of the body-based practices we'll explore in this chapter. Importantly, these insights underscore that you're not simply at the mercy of your emotions. *You have the capacity to learn, change, and influence your emotional life*, and gain a greater sense of control over your experiences.

Throughout the chapter, we will delve into various techniques, which I call "portals," that can help regulate both your body and your mind. These techniques lay a firm foundation of acceptance and safety, which forms the bedrock for the rest of your healing journey. By understanding and applying these strategies, you will learn to harness the power of your own body to create a secure and reassuring internal environment, bringing a profound and enduring sense of calm and well-being.

PORTALS TO RESET THE NERVOUS SYSTEM

Portals represent gateways into your nervous system. Throughout this chapter, I'll show you how to use the portals of breath, muscles, touch, internal body sensations, and movement as doorways into the nervous system that allow you to directly organize your nervous system's responses and shift your alertness elevator to a lower, calmer, floor. Think of these portals as access points through which you can engage in targeted practices that help retrain your nervous system. The goal is to shift from a persistent state of alarm or stress toward a more open and relaxed baseline, offering you the flexibility to effectively handle challenges and demands.

By leveraging cues that signal safety to your nervous system, you can encourage your body to let down its guard and relax. This, in turn, allows for the release of

BUILDING MOMENTUM

IMPLEMENTING BODY-BASED EXERCISES INTO YOUR DAILY LIFE

Practicing awareness isn't something you tick off a list and complete, but, rather, an ongoing process that continues in the background even as you transition into the subsequent stages of this healing journey. If journaling proved beneficial for you, it's a good idea to carry on with the practice. Consider setting aside some time each evening to briefly jot down your observations about your nervous system's behavior throughout the day. This practice of conscious observation and reflection can remain a consistent part of your routine throughout all five stages of your journey.

In stage 2, Regulation, I will introduce you to brief, body-focused exercises designed to create tangible sensations of safety, calmness, and ease within your body. Each exercise requires five to ten minutes to complete, with the ideal practice routine being twice a day—once in the morning and once in the evening. You have the flexibility to either repeat the same exercise for each session or try a different one. However, it's crucial to remember that this isn't about perfection, it's about progress. Don't turn this into another task you feel you must do perfectly, leading to guilt when you skip a session. Keep in mind the four pledges you made in chapter 5 and take your journey as slowly as you need to. This isn't a race.

Initially, you may experience some resistance toward these exercises—that's perfectly normal. With continued practice, these portals will soon become more comfortable and enjoyable. They may even quickly evolve into a highlight of your day.

accumulated tension and redirects your cellular energy toward crucial repair and maintenance activities. In essence, you are teaching your body to recognize and respond to signals of safety, thereby encouraging a state of relaxation and enabling your inherent healing processes.

Each time you travel downward on the alertness elevator, you create and reinforce new neural pathways in your brain. These experiences become part of your implicit memory, which your nervous system uses to control automatic unconscious processes, such as automatically moving up and down the alertness elevator. As you practice intentionally moving to green, you reinforce the neural pathways that lead to regulation and create new implicit memories of how to get there. Over time, your nervous system will start to rely on these new implicit memories to automatically respond more flexibly to stress. The shift to the green state will start to feel increasingly natural and effortless. Eventually, you'll find your nervous system autonomously shifting into this calmer state without any conscious effort on your part.

Each portal supports a plethora of different practices that can directly influence your nervous system. Many of these practices are backed by scientific research, validating their effectiveness in facilitating regulation of the nervous system. I share some of the most widely recognized ones here, but each nervous system is unique, so you'll need to experiment to identify which ones resonate with you most and yield the best results. Finding the perfect combination may take some time, so it's crucial to approach this process with patience and curiosity.

FROM ENERGY DRAIN TO REPLENISHMENT

A dysregulated nervous system can deplete your body's energy reserves, impacting overall bodily function and making it harder to deal with everyday stressors.

In a healthy, regulated state, your nervous system naturally cycles through different levels of alertness throughout the day. It uses up energy during the high-alert red and yellow states, but it replenishes this energy during the restful green state and, especially, the deeply restful blue state. However, when your nervous system is dysregulated, you tend to get stuck in the energy-consuming yellow and red states, which become your default states, with little time spent in the energy-replenishing green or blue states. This pattern has a substantial effect on your mitochondria, your cells' energy-producing factories.

Staying stuck in the yellow and red states doesn't allow your mitochondria adequate restful periods to generate the energy needed for optimal functioning. Consequently, they can't work at full capacity, leading to a significant reduction in overall energy production when compared to a well-regulated nervous system. This decrease in overall energy production plays a major role in many of the symptoms associated with nervous system dysregulation, such as fatigue, anxiety, muscle tension, skin issues, digestive problems, and more.

So imagine learning how to transition from the energy-depleting red and yellow states to the restorative green and blue states, which allow your energy reserves to replenish and your mitochondria to function at their best. Regulating your nervous system is the practice of mastering this transition, so you're not constantly in high-alert states—unless necessary. Applying techniques to regulate your nervous system allows you to flexibly transition from states of heightened alertness to states of rest and rejuvenation. This shift permits your body and mind to recharge and operate at their best. With this practice, you can ensure that your body has the energy it needs to handle all its tasks efficiently.

Developing the ability to regulate your nervous system is crucial for fostering a sense of agency and self-trust. The essence of life is to be exposed to unpredictable events and circumstances beyond your control, which can be challenging to navigate, especially when your energy is depleted. As you commit to the practice of understanding and managing your body's response to these stimuli, you take an active role in your physical and emotional well-being and begin to gain influence over your nervous system's states.

One of the quickest ways to influence your nervous system state is through the breath portal. This is not only an age-old concept but also an extensively researched one.

The Breath Portal

Your breath is special because it works in two ways. Most of the time, it happens naturally without you even thinking about it, just like your heart beating. But unlike your heartbeat, you can also control your breath if you want to. You can choose to breathe slower, faster, deeper, or even hold your breath. This means you can use your breath to help you relax and calm down whenever you need to.

Dr. David Spiegel, professor of psychiatry at Stanford University, describes breath as a "bridge between conscious and unconscious states." Breathing is a direct portal to influencing various aspects of your nervous system, including your heart rate and sense of safety.

There are various breathing techniques and exercises that can help you use your breath to condition your nervous system. Research from Andrew Huberman and David Spiegel's labs at Stanford University has shown that the physiological "sigh" can have a significant impact on the regulation of the nervous system during moments of high stress and anxiety.

The physiological sigh, also known as cyclic sighing, is a type of controlled breathing that involves taking two sharp inhales of breath, typically through the nose, followed

>> DO THIS

PRACTICE THE PHYSIOLOGICAL SIGH

Switch from dog mind to lion mind. Pay attention to your body and mind, recognizing when your nervous system becomes activated or when you're experiencing anxiety. Some common signs of anxiety include increased heart rate, shallow breathing, muscle tension, and racing thoughts. Once you become aware of these sensations, take a moment to acknowledge that you are experiencing anxiety or stress, and make a conscious decision to help calm your nervous system by practicing the physiological sigh exercise. You can close your eyes for this exercise if it helps you feel less distracted and more relaxed.

1. **Inhale.** Take a sharp, deep inhale through your nose, filling your lungs with air. Immediately follow this with a second, shorter inhale through your nose, further expanding your lungs.

2. **Slowly exhale.** After completing the two inhales, slowly exhale through your mouth. Allow the air to escape at a controlled pace and try to make the exhale longer than the combined duration of the two inhales.

3. **Repeat the process.** Repeat the physiological sigh pattern about five times, or as needed. You should begin to notice a calming effect on your nervous system as you continue to practice this breathing technique.

Just five breaths can start making a difference, but practicing for five minutes can allow a more fundamental shift in your nervous system state from red, yellow, or purple to green. Try this: set a timer for five minutes and keep up your calm breathing until the timer stops.

4. **Observe your body and mind.** After completing the physiological sighs, take a moment to notice any changes in your body and mind. You may feel more relaxed, focused, or present in the moment.

5. **Slowly return to your normal breathing.** Gradually transition back to your natural breathing pattern. Continue to focus on your breath for a few more moments before opening your eyes, if you closed them, and resuming your daily activities.

Practice the physiological sigh whenever you feel the need to calm your nervous system or reduce stress. With time and consistency, this simple breathing technique can become an effective tool for managing stress and promoting relaxation.

by a long, slow exhale through the mouth. This breathing exercise can lower anxiety and stress right away, moving you down the alertness elevator. A study published in 2023 on the physiological sigh showed that doing this practice for five minutes daily led to significantly more positive feelings throughout the day after just ten days. It also decreased rates of breathing at rest, which is a sign of overall body calmness.

THE BUILDING BLOCKS OF EMOTIONS: HOW TO GAIN AGENCY OVER YOUR EMOTIONAL EXPERIENCE

Emotions are integrally linked to the various arousal levels on your alertness elevator. This means that your emotional experience is often associated with your current state of alertness. For instance, when you're in a heightened state of alertness (red), you might typically feel anger, whereas a slightly lower state of alertness (yellow) could bring about anxiety, and a relaxed state of alertness (green) might be associated with feelings of joy or peace.

The intensity of these emotions in the various states of activation on your alertness elevator can vary widely among individuals. Some may not have very intense emotional responses, whereas others experience emotions very powerfully.

Just like a well-regulated nervous system fluidly moves through all states of alertness—red, yellow, green, blue—it also allows for a broad spectrum of emotional experiences. This means a healthy nervous system doesn't stick to just one emotion or range of emotions but allows for the entire spectrum, from happiness to sadness, from peace to anger.

Even in a well-regulated system, uncomfortable or distressing emotions, such as fear, anger, or jealousy, will still arise. They are a natural part of the human emotional experience. But these feelings wouldn't usually dominate your emotional landscape for long periods of time. Feeling frequently trapped in these distressing emotions for long periods of time is likely due to nervous system dysregulation.

Emotions are powerful motivators, and if you're feeling a lot of negative emotions, you probably want to do everything in your power to feel better. Traditional advice often proposes that to manage unpleasant emotions, you should change your negative thought patterns—for example, by thinking more positive thoughts. Although these techniques can be beneficial in specific contexts, they are based on an oversimplified understanding of how emotions function.

Traditionally, emotions were understood to be a direct result of our thoughts. They were also assumed to be universally experienced in the same way across different individuals and cultures. However, contemporary research provides a more nuanced perspective. One recent and widely respected theory of emotions is the "constructed emotion" theory proposed by neuroscientist and researcher Lisa Feldman Barrett.

Contrary to the traditional view, Barrett suggests that emotions are not universally experienced in the same way. Rather, emotions are individual and subjective experiences, constructed based on a combination of your present moment situation, your interpretation of the situation based on past experiences and cultural background, and your physical sensations in your body.

This means that your emotional responses aren't merely the product of your thoughts or the world around you. Modifying your thought patterns or trying to control the world around you may not be the most effective way to change how you feel. Instead, your emotions are deeply intertwined with your personal history, cultural context, and physical state. Modifying your physical sensations by using portals or working with your interpretations of your circumstances can sometimes be a much more effective way to shift your emotional state.

Just as your emotional experiences are individual and constructed from different aspects of your internal experience and external context, they also can't be tied to specific isolated regions in the brain. Instead, they involve a dynamic, interconnected network of brain regions, such as the prefrontal cortex, anterior cingulate cortex, insula, and amygdala, among others. These areas don't work in isolation but, instead, rapidly communicate and interact with each other in real time to create what you perceive as your emotional state.

Your brain can modify your experience of emotions in real time based on your memories of previous experiences and the context of everything happening in the current moment. For example, imagine you and a friend are both making toasts at a wedding. Your friend has a history of positive experiences with public speaking and comes from a culture that views speaking in front of strangers as a growth opportunity. She feels her pulse quicken and her nervous system feels the emotion of excitement. For you it's the opposite: Let's say you were laughed at when you got up in front of the class as a kid, and perhaps you come from a family or culture that views standing out from the crowd negatively. As you feel your pulse quicken before you give your toast, your nervous system feels the emotion of anxiety.

This simple example demonstrates how two individuals can interpret the same physical sensation (a quickened pulse) within the same external situation (giving a toast) as different emotions based on their unique histories and cultural backgrounds. One person interprets the sensation as excitement, whereas the other perceives it as anxiety.

In sum, contemporary research on the neuroscience of emotions shows that emotions are much more fluid and dynamic than traditionally thought. Emotions are a sophisticated process that continually adapts and responds to our experiences, context, and physical state. Most importantly, this research indicates that you have greater control over your emotions than you might realize.

WHY NERVOUS SYSTEM REGULATION STARTS WITH BODY-BASED PROCESSES

Barrett's theory of constructed emotions demonstrates that you can influence or modify your emotional experiences to have more positive emotional states and fewer negative ones. To modify your emotional experiences, you need to influence at least one of the three components that construct emotions:

1. Your current situation
2. Your brain's interpretation of the situation
3. The physical sensations you're experiencing in your body

Altering Your Current Situation: Changing Your Circumstances

The current situation is usually the first aspect people attempt to alter when they're unhappy. It means changing the circumstances in which you find yourself, and can include everything from moment-to-moment modification of your situation, like having a few drinks to calm your nerves or leaving a party when you feel anxious, to long-term life changes, like devoting your life to accumulating wealth to feel more secure or leaving a spouse because you feel unhappy. Let me be absolutely clear: If you're in a dangerous situation like an abusive relationship, you need to get out of it to feel better. Regardless of how much you work on understanding the past, or how much you try to regulate your current bodily sensations, if you're in real danger, emotions like fear and anger are natural reactions until you're safely removed from the situation.

But many people rely too much on trying to "fix" their present situation in the belief that this alone will alleviate uncomfortable feelings and pave the way to comfortable, pleasant ones. What they may not realize is that their immediate situation is only one piece of the puzzle in creating emotional experiences. Changing your surroundings may be a crucial step, but other components also contribute significantly to your emotional state.

Altering Your Brain's Interpretation of Your Situation: The "Top-Down" Approach

Another way to influence your emotions involves changing the way your brain interprets your current situation. This strategy is known as the "top-down" approach, as it starts with your thoughts and uses them to guide your emotional state. Meditation, visualization, and cognitive behavioral strategies are all examples of this approach.

However, trying to control your nervous system merely through thought is like attempting to ride a bike using just your mind. You might be able to visualize performing all sorts of maneuvers and stunts, but this won't actually get you moving. In other words, although cognitive strategies can be part of the solution, they can't do all the work on their own. Just as you need to physically pedal and balance to ride a bike, you also need to engage with your bodily sensations to effectively regulate your emotions.

Highly sensitive and perceptive individuals, in particular, often develop a strong analytical mind to help them manage their overwhelming emotions and stress responses. Over time, this heavy reliance on analytical thinking becomes a deeply ingrained habit as you continually sharpen your skills in dissecting and processing every detail of your experiences. Focusing on cognitive skills creates a sense of perceived control and temporarily reduces the body's intense reactions, but on its own does not lead to flexible regulation of your nervous system.

A typical pattern of using strong analytical thinking as a coping mechanism looks like this: Something activates your stress response and you find yourself in a high-stress red state. You use your cognitive skills, such as analyzing the situation or rationalizing everyone's behavior, to shift down to a somewhat less stressful yellow state. This transition might feel like an improvement because the immediate stressors are less intense, but it's not an ideal or sustainable state of being.

Using cognitive skills as a coping mechanism often involves ignoring or suppressing physical sensations and emotions, which are integral to a sustainable emotional experience. Without fostering a genuine sense of safety within your body, you'll remain stuck in the yellow state. Even though you've left the high-stress red state, you're still not entirely relaxed or at peace. The green and blue states, which represent tranquility and restoration, remain mostly out of reach.

In the short term, you can function reasonably well in the yellow state. You're managing your immediate stress and navigating life, but you're doing so with a constant undercurrent of tension and unease. This chronic strain can be incredibly draining, as it requires a high degree of energy to continually suppress the body's stress responses.

Over time, remaining stuck in this chronic yellow state can lead to physical and emotional exhaustion, or burnout. This sustained stress can eventually manifest as physical symptoms, like digestive issues or inflammation, or emotional distress, like chronic anxiety or depression.

Another form of the top-down approach to influence emotions involves revisiting and reinterpreting past experiences that have shaped your emotional responses. For example, consider the scenario where giving a speech induced anxiety because it stirred up a memory of being laughed at as a child. You might transform your emotional response to standing up in front of people by consciously revisiting that painful childhood memory while in a safe and secure state, such as in the presence of a loved one or therapist.

As an adult, you're not helpless or vulnerable like you were as a child. Recognizing this can allow you to bring compassion and warmth to your younger self and the feelings of shame and isolation that were experienced. As you offer this understanding to your past self, you can start to let go of those old, painful feelings, making room for new, more positive experiences. This process can help form new perspectives about public speaking that aren't rooted in fear and anxiety.

However, this practice of reflecting and reshaping past experiences is most beneficial for long-term regulation of your nervous system. It might not be as helpful if you are in the midst of nervous system dysregulation or an acute stress response. Before using a top-down approach to modifying your emotional landscape, the first and most accessible step is to establish a sense of safety and regulation at the physical level. Once this embodied sense of security is in place, you can effectively engage in deeper emotional work that involves reshaping past memories. I will delve into this process in the next chapter, when I discuss stage 3, Restoration.

Altering Physical Sensations: Managing Emotions Through the Body

To manage your emotions effectively, it's critical to address the third element that shapes them: physical sensations. The most effective and immediate way to influence your emotional state and create a stable foundation for emotional regulation is to engage in practices that cultivate a sense of safety within your body. Starting with a body-based approach is even more crucial when you're navigating the symptoms of dysregulation like anxiety, burnout, or other physical symptoms.

In 2023, Karl Deisseroth and his team at Stanford University conducted a study on mice, further underlining the direct connection between body sensations and emotional experience. They built a noninvasive mouse-size pacemaker to increase the heart rate of mice. When the experimenters made the mice's hearts beat faster, the mice displayed more anxious behavior, demonstrating this two-way connection between the brain and the heart and highlighting the intricate relationship between our emotions and our physiological state.

So as the Stanford team demonstrated in this experiment, the most effective and immediate way to influence your emotions at this stage of the 5-Stage Plan is by changing your body sensations, like your heart rate, breathing patterns as with the physiological sigh, and the tension you hold in your muscles via the portals I introduced earlier. They provide a direct approach to influence these bodily sensations, facilitating a transition to the green state on the alertness elevator and subsequently changing your emotional state. With consistent practice of these exercises, you will gain greater control over your emotions, fostering healthier and more adaptive responses to each moment.

One simple way to start getting out of an analyzing mind and back into your body is to harness the portal of muscles and touch.

The Muscles Portal

Anxiety, chronic stress, and nervous system dysregulation are interconnected factors that contribute to a chronic state of tension in the muscles. The most common muscles that carry tension in the body include the neck, shoulders, jaw, lower back, and hips. Chronic tension in these areas can lead to a range of issues, from pain and headaches to reduced mobility and stress-related illnesses.

Muscles are a powerful portal that allow you to enter your nervous system and move it back to the green state. Consciously releasing tension from these muscle groups improves blood flow, flexibility, and overall well-being. Moreover, using the muscles portal can help build awareness of how your emotions get constructed from contractions and sensations in different muscles.

The Touch Portal

Touch has always been an essential aspect of human life, playing a vital role in emotional bonding, communication, and overall well-being. In recent years, many treatment modalities have emerged that utilize the impact of touch on the nervous system to help the body move down to the more relaxed green state. Some studies have highlighted the functional connections between body tissues, internal organs, and touch-based therapies. These studies focused mainly on acupuncture, a technique targeting certain points on the skin, known as acupoints, which correspond to related organs in the body, according to traditional Chinese medicine. In the study, stimulating these points produced nerve signals that affected the organ's function. Not only did these studies experimentally validate some of the claims of traditional Chinese medicine, but they also demonstrated that physically touching your skin can directly impact the physical systems throughout your entire body.

Gentle and caring touches, like hugs and caresses, can help you feel physically safe and secure, which can be a very effective way to bring you back down to the green state. And not having enough physical touch in your life can lead to feelings of isolation, loneliness, and emotional distress.

Emotions such as joy and the feeling of safety often result from touch. Feeling good, even for a short period of time, can significantly and positively affect your nervous system, promoting stress relief and the move to the green state. However, for many people, touch can create a sense of discomfort or trigger embedded alarms from past traumatic experiences.

>> DO THIS

PRACTICE MUSCLE TENSION RELEASE

Neck and Shoulders Salamander Exercise

This series of movements, from author and body worker Stanley Rosenberg, progressively improves the flexibility in the thoracic spine, increasing your breathing capacity and reducing a forward head posture. Moving muscles in the head, neck, shoulders, and eyes in this particular way helps release chronic tension, signaling to your nervous system that you're safe and it's okay to shift down to the green state.

1. Start by sitting or standing comfortably.
2. Shift your eyes to look to the right, as if you're trying to look at your right ear but moving only your eyeballs, keeping your head facing forward.
3. Continue shifting your eyes to the right as you bend your neck so that your right ear moves down toward your right shoulder. Keep your shoulders down, moving only your ear toward your shoulder—not your shoulder toward your ear. Hold this position for thirty to sixty seconds. You should feel a stretch on the left side of your neck and shoulders, and, with your head at a 90-degree angle to the rest of your body, your eyes should now be looking toward the ground.
4. Come back to looking forward with your neck and spine in a neutral posture. Repeat the process on the left side, with your eyes looking to the left.
5. Repeat steps 2 through 4, with your eyes looking in the opposite direction. Hold for thirty to sixty seconds on each side.

Full Salamander Exercise

In the full salamander exercise, you flex the entire spine instead of just the neck. Flexing the entire spine can provide an even more powerful signal to your nervous system that it can relax, let go, and open into the green state.

1. Get down on all fours, making sure your weight is well distributed between the hands and the knees. You can also support your hands with a chair or a desk. Your head should be in one line with your spine, not above or below it. Lift and lower your head a bit to find the right alignment.
2. Look to the right like you did in the previous exercise, using just your eyeballs.
3. Hold your eyes in that position and tilt your head to the right. Continue bending beyond your neck just like a salamander all the way down to the bottom of your spine. Hold the position for thirty to sixty seconds and then return to a neutral position.
4. Do the same on the other side. Look left, tilt your head to the left, and then tilt the rest of the spine. Hold. Return.

>> DO THIS

PRACTICE SOOTHING SELF-TOUCH

Some ways to practice moving to a green state with self-touch include:

- **Self-massage:** Gently massaging tense muscles or applying pressure to specific points on the body can help relieve stress and promote relaxation.
- **Grounding techniques:** Placing your hands on your chest, abdomen, or another part of your body can help you feel more connected and present.
- **Mindful touch:** Focusing on the sensations of touch as you stroke your arm or hold your own hand can create a sense of comfort and security.

Although touch from another person can positively affect your nervous system, it's not always accessible, and if you have embedded alarms around touch, another person's touch could cause you to go up to the red state rather than down to green. Fortunately, you don't need someone else to harness the power of touch and move yourself down to green; you can also do it with self-touch.

INTEROCEPTION: THE FOUNDATION OF THE MIND-BODY CONNECTION

Growing up, you were probably taught that you have five senses: sight, sound, smell, taste, and touch. But it turns out that list is woefully incomplete. It's missing a whole array of different internal sensations that help your nervous system make sense of the world. For example, your vestibular system helps you balance and orient in space. Proprioception includes the sensations of muscle movements, such as contraction and stretching, and helps you know where each part of your body is at any given time. Interoception, which is sometimes referred to as the "eighth sense" after vestibular and proprioception, helps you understand your internal body state, such as temperature, pain, itching, hunger, thirst, and heartbeat. Emerging research is continuing to add more distinct interoceptive senses to this list.

Unlike the five senses of sight, sound, smell, taste, and touch, interoceptive sensations originate from within your body, providing a continuous flow of internal data about your physiological state, which is then sent to a part of your brain called the insula, which organizes the information and sends it on to other parts of the brain. For example, when you're hungry, sensations from your belly get sent to your insula, which organizes this information and passes it on to other parts of your brain that motivate you to go find some grub.

The Internal Body Sensations Portal

You may be surprised at how much information about your internal state is processed by your insula and is available to your conscious mind if you pay attention and look for it. Your cells and organs are constantly sending signals to your insula about their experiences, which makes interoceptive awareness a powerful "bridge" between your physical body's needs and your ability to take care of yourself. For example, if it's hot outside and you've been in the sun too long, your cells and organs will send signals to your insula conveying that they are feeling too hot. If you have weak interoceptive awareness, you might not realize what's happening and just know that you generally feel bad and uncomfortable. But if you develop strong interoceptive awareness, you will know that you feel uncomfortable because your body is too hot and you'll go find some shade. Developing strong interoceptive awareness enables you to adapt with flexibility to the changing world around you and your changing internal states.

Additionally, your insula and interoceptive sensations play a critical role in your nervous system's construction of emotions and feelings of pleasure, displeasure, arousal, and calmness. When your brain gathers data from your insula, it merges this with your past experiences and present environmental signals. Then it makes an educated prediction, or a "best guess," about how to make you feel to promote survival. Your brain's goal is to construct an emotional response, based on your history and your current situation, that is optimized to ensure efficient use of the body's energy resources, promoting survival and well-being.

Improving your interoceptive awareness can make it easier to be in the world without feeling overwhelmed or anxious. The better you're able to sense what's happening inside your body, the better you can handle your emotional and physical reactions, leading to improved emotional regulation, reduced stress, and higher levels of nervous system flexibility. In fact, when you become more tuned in to your body's internal signals, you are more likely to spend time in the green and blue states of calmness and joy, and less time in the stressful red and yellow states. This is because you're giving your brain more accurate data to make its "best guess" predictions about your emotional responses, leading to more appropriate, energy-efficient responses.

>> DO THIS

EXPLORE THE INTEROCEPTION PORTAL

This practice is designed to help you increase your interoceptive awareness by exploring various sensations in different parts of your body. By using the table as a reference, you can become more familiar with the sensations you might experience in each body part. This practice will also help you become more attuned to your body's signals and improve your ability to self-regulate.

1. **Find a comfortable position**. Find a quiet space where you can sit or lie down comfortably. Close your eyes and take a few deep breaths to center yourself and relax.
2. **Choose a body part.** Choose a body part from the following table as your starting point. You can begin with any body part and move through the list at your own pace.
3. **Focus on the sensations.** Bring your attention to the chosen body part and focus on the sensations you experience there. Use the table as a reference to help you identify different sensations you might be feeling. Try to stay with each sensation for a few moments, observing it without judgment.
4. **Move to a different body part.** Once you've spent some time exploring the sensations in the first body part, gently shift your focus to the next body part you choose. Repeat the process of focusing on the sensations you're experiencing in that area.
5. **Continue the exploration.** Continue working your way through the list of body parts, focusing on the sensations in each area. You can spend as much or as little time as you like on each part, depending on your comfort and interest.
6. **Reflect on your experience.** After you've explored all the body parts on the list, take a moment to reflect on your experience. What sensations stood out to you? Were there any surprises or new sensations you discovered? Consider how this practice might help you become more aware of your body's signals in daily life.

IDENTIFYING INTEROCEPTIVE SENSATIONS

Body Part: BRAIN • Alertness • Calmness • Clarity • Dizziness • Focus • Headache • Mental fatigue • Mental fog • Mental relaxation • Mental tension	**Body Part: FEET/TOES** • Coldness • Dryness • Foot cramps • Itching • Numbness • Pain • Sweating • Swelling • Tingling • Warmth	**Body Part: STOMACH** • Acid reflux • Bloating • Butterflies • Fullness • Gas • Gurgling sounds • Hunger • Indigestion • Nausea • Stomach cramps
Body Part: CHEST • Breathing rate • Chest pain • Deep breathing • Expansion and contraction • Fluttering sensation • Pressure • Rapid heartbeat • Shallow breathing • Shortness of breath • Tightness	**Body Part: HANDS/FINGERS** • Clamminess • Coldness • Dryness • Numbness • Pain • Stiffness • Sweating • Swelling • Tingling • Warmth	**Body Part: THROAT** • Choking sensation • Coughing • Difficulty swallowing • Dryness • Hoarseness • Itchiness • Sensation of a lump • Soreness • Swelling • Tightness
Body Part: EARS • Earache • Earwax buildup • Fullness • Hearing heartbeat • Itching • Muffled hearing • Popping sensations • Pressure • Ringing • Sensitivity to sounds	**Body Part: MUSCLES** • Cramping • Fatigue • Relaxation • Soreness • Spasms • Stiffness • Tension • Tightness • Trembling • Weakness	
Body Part: EYES • Dryness • Eyestrain • Heaviness • Itching • Pain • Pressure • Sensitivity to light • Tearing • Tiredness • Watering	**Body Part: SKIN** • Clamminess • Coldness • Dryness • Flushing • Goosebumps • Itching • Sensitivity to touch • Sweating • Tightness • Warmth	

Reclaiming *Body*fulness

Mindfulness has been the subject of extensive scientific research over the past few decades. There are now hundreds of studies showing its benefits. *Dog mind to lion mind*, from stage 1, Awareness, is an example of a mindfulness practice that you've already been doing. Unfortunately, the word "mindfulness" can sometimes be misleading. It is a translation of the word "*sati*" from the ancient Pali language and often understood in the West to mean "moment-by-moment awareness." However, this can sometimes lead people to think that mindfulness is mainly about focusing on your thoughts and your inner words. To regulate your nervous system, you not only need to practice being aware in the present moment of your mind but also of your entire bodily experience.

In our fast-paced culture, many factors contribute to widespread disconnectedness from our bodies. Your individual sensitivity can contribute to becoming more disconnected from your body as a defense mechanism, but there are also many cultural and environmental factors that push you toward disconnection.

Western religious and philosophical traditions have long valued the mind over the body, which has separated the two in Western thought. For example, Western medicine focuses almost entirely on physical manifestations of disease, often neglecting the role of emotions and thoughts in our overall well-being. The split between mind and body in our culture has led to a widespread neglect of emotions and bodily sensations.

There are also environmental influences of modern life that can make you feel disconnected from your body. For example, the intensity of life in bustling cities, without quiet time and direct access to nature, can overwhelm your body and nervous system, making it challenging to feel your emotions and sensations. As humans, we evolved in nature, and our bodies and minds still crave that connection.

In essence, your individual sensitivity, coupled with cultural and environmental factors, all work together to create a chronic disconnect between the mind and the body. But regulating your nervous system *requires* a strong connection between mind and body. We need to avoid the trap of having mindfulness become just another way we reinforce disconnection.

To avoid this trap and to emphasize the importance of experiencing the present moment in your body, I prefer the term "bodyfulness" over "mindfulness." Both terms describe the practice of staying aware of what's happening in the present moment, but bodyfulness emphasizes the importance of the rich and alive sensory nature of your moment-to-moment experience. Other terms, like "somatic awareness," "body sense," and "embodiment," are also emerging to help describe the experience of being in tune with our bodies and minds simultaneously.

>> DO THIS

BODYFULNESS CHECK-IN "ON THE GO"

You can adapt this bodyfulness check-in to any posture, including sitting, standing, walking, or even lying down. Make it a convenient practice to incorporate into your daily routine, even when you're on the go. Here's a simple step-by-step technique.

1. **Find a comfortable posture.** If you're standing, ensure your feet are hip-width apart and your knees are slightly bent. If you're walking, maintain a slow and relaxed pace, paying attention to the movement of your body. If you're sitting, sit comfortably upright, keeping your hips higher than your knees. And if you're lying down, lie flat on your back. You can also adjust any of these postures to accommodate your body's particular needs.

2. **Take a few deep breaths.** Inhale deeply through your nose, filling your lungs, and then exhale slowly through your mouth. Repeat this process a few times to help center your awareness and prepare your mind for the body scan.

3. **Focus on your legs and feet.** Bring your awareness to your thighs, knees, calves, ankles, and feet. Pay attention to any sensations or tension, and use your breath to release any tightness.

4. **Concentrate on your abdomen and hips.** Notice any sensations or tension in your stomach, sides, and hips. Use your breath to release any tightness you may feel in these areas.

5. **Move your attention to your chest and back.** Observe any sensations or tightness in your chest, upper back, and lower back. Take deep breaths and imagine any tension melting away with each exhalation.

6. **Shift your focus to your shoulders and arms.** Be aware of any tension in your shoulders, upper arms, elbows, forearms, and hands. Breathe deeply and visualize the tension dissipating with each exhale.

7. **Bring your attention to your head and face.** Notice any sensations or tension in your forehead, scalp, eyes, jaw, and neck. If you detect any tension, take a deep breath and imagine the tension releasing as you exhale.

8. **Take a moment to observe your entire body.** As you stand or walk, be aware of your whole body and any remaining tension. Breathe deeply and imagine tension leaving your body with each exhale.

9. **Finish with a few deep breaths.** Inhale deeply through your nose, filling your lungs, and then exhale slowly through your mouth. Repeat this a few times to help ground yourself and bring your focus back to the present moment.

As you practice being aware during body check-ins and portals, practice *bodyfully*. See what it's like to allow your whole body, not just your mind, to be present and aware moment by moment.

Remember, the key to a successful bodyful check-in and scan is to maintain awareness of your body and use your breath to help release tension. With practice, this technique can become a valuable tool for managing stress and promoting relaxation throughout your day.

The Movement Portal

Significant amounts of research have been done showing the profoundly positive effects that exercise and movement have on mood and the regulation of the nervous system. The benefits are not limited to those who are already physically fit or engaged in regular exercise—even people leading highly stressful lives or who have been physically inactive for years can benefit immensely from physical activity. Unless you already have a movement practice, while your nervous system is still dysregulated it is important to begin by introducing gentle activities. Before transitioning to more intense, vigorous movements, spend a few weeks just doing the active proprioceptive, passive proprioceptive, and vestibular inputs from the sensory stimulation routine I introduced in chapter 6 to help build a solid structure.

If you're experiencing severe dysregulation or have been inactive for a long time, diving straight into an intense exercise routine may do more harm than good. A gradual approach is essential to avoid injury, burnout, and further draining your body's energy before it can recharge. Gentle activities such as yoga and walking are excellent starting points, as they provide a low-impact way to engage muscles and elevate heart rate. These gentle exercises can be performed at various intensity levels, catering to your unique needs and abilities.

As you become more comfortable with gentle movements and your nervous system begins to regulate more effectively, it may be appropriate to introduce more vigorous exercise. These may include activities like running, swimming, or high-intensity interval training.

Like stage 1, Awareness, most people spend at least a few weeks focusing on the Regulation stage, and sometimes many months. You might be eager to move on, but remember your pledges from chapter 5: Take it slowly, and do one thing at a time. The next stage, Restoration, requires that you're able to use portals to help you come back to the green state when your nervous system gets activated. In the Restoration stage, you'll start working with some of the deepest triggers and root causes that contributed to your dysregulation. Working with these triggers and root causes can easily put you into the yellow or red states, and sometimes even in the purple state, so it's critical that you have the tools to come back to the green state before you start working on restoration. If you don't feel confident in your ability to shift back to the green state yet, keep practicing with the portals in this stage. Remember, this is not a race; the more you practice shifting down to the green state, the more you reinforce neural pathways of regulation, which will be helpful for the rest of your life.

When you feel ready to move on, stage 3, Restoration, contains some of the deepest and most profound work on your healing journey. You'll move to a combined focus on the mind and body pillars to address your coping strategies, attachment patterns, and embedded alarms that likely contributed most to your nervous system's initial dysregulation. This stage often feels like the hardest work for people on their healing journey, but it's also extremely rewarding as you start to let go of the deepest, most painful patterns in your nervous system and open up to a greater sense of fulfillment, meaning, and power throughout your life.

>> DO THIS

BEGIN AN EXERCISE ROUTINE

1. **Consult a medical professional.** Before starting any exercise program, consult with a health-care professional to ensure that the activities are suitable for your current health condition and to discuss any necessary modifications or precautions.

2. **Set realistic goals.** Establish clear, attainable goals for your exercise journey. Start with small objectives, such as walking for fifteen minutes a day, and gradually increase the time as you progress. This will help keep you motivated and focused on your overall wellness.

3. **Establish a routine.** Create a consistent routine that incorporates movement into your daily life. Choose a time of day that works best for you and dedicate that time to your physical well-being. Consistency is key to developing lasting habits.

4. **Begin with gentle movements.** Incorporate gentle movements into your routine, such as stretching, deep breathing exercises, or slow-paced walks. Focus on activities that are low impact and help improve balance, flexibility, and proprioceptive awareness. You can find some more ideas in the sensory stimulation routine inputs (see chapter 6).

5. **Gradually increase activity levels.** As you become more comfortable with gentle movements, slowly increase the intensity of your activities. For example, extend the duration of your walks, try a beginner's yoga class, or engage in light strength-training exercises using your body weight or resistance bands.

6. **Incorporate moderate exercise.** Introduce moderate exercises into your routine, such as brisk walking, swimming, or cycling for 150 minutes or more each week. Better to do it in three or more separate sessions than all at once, but experiment with different-length sessions and see what your body prefers.

7. **Add variety and challenge.** To continue challenging yourself and avoid getting bored, incorporate a variety of activities into your routine. Try different types of moderate exercises, such as dance or group fitness classes, or explore outdoor activities like hiking, biking, or kayaking.

8. **Monitor progress.** Keep track of your progress by recording your activities in your journal or using a fitness app. This will help you stay accountable, identify patterns, and adjust as needed.

9. **Introduce vigorous movement.** Once you have established a solid foundation of regular exercise and your nervous system is more regulated, gradually introduce more vigorous activities, like running, high-intensity interval training, or advanced fitness classes. Begin with shorter sessions and increase the duration and intensity over time.

10. **Stay in touch with your body's feedback.** Throughout your journey, stay attentive to your body's needs and limitations. Listen to your body and adjust your routine as necessary. Incorporate relaxation techniques, adequate sleep, and proper nutrition to support your overall well-being.

11. **Seek support and accountability.** Enlist the help of friends and family, or join a fitness group, to keep you motivated and accountable. Engaging in activities with others can make the process more enjoyable and increase your chances of making this a regular part of your life.

12. **Reevaluate and adjust.** As your fitness level improves, reevaluate your goals and adjust your routine as needed. Remember, your exercise journey is an ongoing process, and maintaining flexibility is essential for long-term success.

9

Stage 3: Restoration—Rebuilding Nervous System Flexibility

BARBARA, ONE OF THE MEMBERS of the Heal Your Nervous System online community, experienced severe abuse as a child and adolescent. The consequences of these repeated traumatic stressors manifested in adulthood as a wide range of symptoms, including chronic pain so severe that she ended up on disability. She also developed symptoms of dysregulation like substance abuse, binge eating, anxiety, rage outbursts, and harsh self-criticism. These challenges prevented her from living a full life, one in which she could set herself free from her past.

Barbara had been working one-on-one with a therapist for a couple of years and was making significant progress in reprocessing her embedded alarms from past traumatic experiences, but she continued to struggle with her recovery. Her physical symptoms persisted, and binge eating and emotional dysregulation remained a significant challenge for her.

Recognizing the importance of addressing her body's needs, Barbara sought a more comprehensive approach to her healing. She discovered the 5-Stage Plan to Reverse Nervous System Dysregulation, and went through the Awareness and Regulation stages to build a felt sense of safety in her body. By focusing on the somatic, or bodily, aspects first, and then coming back to her embedded alarms with the tools she had built in the previous stages, Barbara was able to regulate her emotions and address the physical symptoms that had been holding back her recovery.

Barbara's story illustrates one of the most important aspects of the 5-Stage Plan. It's very common for people to jump right into the hard stuff, like working on embedded alarms from past traumatic stressors or trying to fix harmful coping strategies like binge eating. However, that approach often increases your symptoms of nervous system dysregulation, causing you to spend even more time in the yellow and red states. By developing awareness and regulation first, you set yourself up to address the hardest parts without getting overwhelmed and needing to quit.

Stage 3, Restoration, is when you become more focused on the underlying beliefs, behaviors, and patterns of tension in the body that caused you to move toward dysregulation in the first place. This stage combines focus on the mind and body pillars in the 4 Pillars of Nervous System Health, strengthening both of them at once into one interconnected and stable support system for your ongoing nervous system health. During this stage, you can start to flush out some of the embedded alarms and underlying stress patterns that may have gotten stuck in your body from childhood or from distressing experiences you've been through as an adult. This is also the phase where you can look at your current coping strategies and learn to assess how well they're working and whether something else might be better.

During the Restoration stage, you might start to see some bigger shifts in your behaviors or beliefs about yourself that are no longer serving you. About six months into her journey, Barbara shared a remarkable update with our community: She had grown out of the identity of being a "trauma survivor" and now saw herself as someone who had met the challenge and overcome enormous suffering and hardship.

The transition that Barbara made was the result of all her work on the underlying patterns addressed in the Restoration phase. She confronted the old beliefs about herself and recognized that some of them were no longer true and were holding her back. This stage isn't easy, but if you're willing to do the work, the positive transformation that can result may astound you.

ADDRESSING THE UNDERLYING CAUSES OF DYSREGULATION

There are three primary underlying causes that may have contributed to your dysregulation that are appropriate to address during this stage:

1. Current coping strategies
2. Attachment patterns
3. Embedded alarms from traumatic stressors

These aren't entirely separate categories—they overlap to some extent—but they stem from different causes and are best addressed in different ways.

Your *current coping strategies* are the ways that your nervous system has learned to respond to challenging or demanding situations. For example, you may have learned to cope with stress by working out, praying, burying yourself in work, or drinking a big glass of wine. Although conventional wisdom might tell you that there are "good" and "bad" coping strategies, the scientific research on stress management says there are only more or less useful strategies. What makes one coping strategy better than another is simply how effective it is in meeting your short-term and long-term needs. In this chapter, I show you a tool called the Nervous System Navigator for helping you assess your current coping strategies and improve them, when necessary.

Your *attachment patterns* were shaped primarily in early childhood, up to two years of age, when your nervous system was first learning to regulate. In early childhood, through your attachment bond with your primary caregivers, your nervous system received training in how to navigate stressful situations and move between the different levels of the alertness elevator. The quality of the training that your nervous system received in those formative years varies considerably from person to person. If your parents' nervous systems could flexibly move up and down the alertness elevator, they probably showed your nervous system how to do that reasonably well too. However, if they didn't have very flexible nervous systems, they might not have known how to train your nervous system to be flexible either. But any training you missed in childhood is just as available in adulthood. In the section on attachment patterns, I show you a simple exercise so you can start retraining your nervous system's underlying patterns.

Your *embedded alarms* from traumatic stressors, introduced in chapter 4, are normal, learned fear responses to stimuli that remind your nervous system of dangerous or overwhelming events. When your nervous system is regulated and safe, embedded alarms that are no longer useful will often resolve on their own. Watching them come up and simultaneously recognizing or reminding yourself that you're totally safe and not actually in danger right now can result in the embedded alarm being unlearned. It may take several times of watching and noticing you're safe before it starts to release.

Sometimes, though, embedded alarms that are no longer helpful don't flush out of your nervous system on their own. They get stuck, and more processing is needed to make sense of the overwhelming or terrible experience you went through to unlearn the alarm. Working with embedded alarms that are no longer useful but still stuck in your nervous system, not resolving on their own, typically requires the help of a trained professional in a one-on-one or group setting. There are many therapeutic modalities for working with embedded alarms that have extensive anecdotal and scientific evidence supporting their efficacy, including internal family systems, somatic

BUILDING MOMENTUM

CONSIDER WORKING WITH A PROFESSIONAL FOR EMBEDDED ALARMS

If your nervous system only recently got dysregulated, you may be able to get back to sustainable regulation just by working with your current coping strategies or embedded alarms. For most people, however, working with attachment patterns is highly beneficial for maintaining long-term regulation.

The most important point for working at this stage is that you pace yourself. Working with attachment patterns and embedded alarms may bring up feelings that used to be too intense for you to handle, such as feelings of deep hurt, grief, or anger. The structure, awareness, and agency you built in the previous stages has given you the capacity to handle these intense feelings now, but the feelings may still be extremely upsetting. Using all your tools from the previous stages is important to stay grounded as you do this work.

This stage is also a great time to begin working one-on-one or in a group with a therapist, coach, or other practitioner, if you feel that may be beneficial for you. Someone that's professionally trained in a therapeutic modality that focuses on improving your coping strategies, working on embedded alarms, or retraining your attachment patterns can be an invaluable ally during this stage.

It's not uncommon to spend a long time working on the root causes that led to dysregulation. The time it takes to resolve your root causes of dysregulation varies significantly for different people. After a few weeks or months of establishing a routine to work on your root causes, you may feel ready to move to the next stage of the 5-Stage Plan. But even after you move on to the next stage, you can continue working on attachment, coping strategies, and embedded alarms in the background. No stage of the 5-Stage Plan is left behind when you move to the next stage—it's simply added to the previous stages while the skills of the previous stages slowly become second nature.

experiencing, and eye movement desensitization and reprocessing (EMDR). In my healing journey, I found the internal family systems modality immensely helpful for unlearning embedded alarms.

At this point in your journey, your path becomes much more personal. The most important part is not that you follow these particular practices, but that you learn how to navigate between different practices to discover what works best for you. In the next section, I show you a practical strategy informed by scientific evidence for trying different practices and discovering what works best for you.

RESILIENCE: CULTIVATING FLEXIBILITY TO OVERCOME ADVERSITY

Research tells us that most people face at least one terrible event in their life, like losing someone they love unexpectedly or being in a serious car crash. Yet, amazingly, even after going through these tough times, most people can eventually heal and move on with their lives. It's even more surprising that many kids who grow up in heart-breaking circumstances are able to overcome these hard times and end up living fulfilling lives. Ann Masten, a leading expert in the development of resilience in children, called this surprising outcome "ordinary magic."

How do so many people overcome extreme adversity? What are they doing differently? What can we learn from them? These questions have fascinated researchers and inspired them to dig deeper into understanding *resilience*.

Resilience is the ability to adapt and recover from adversity or challenges, and to grow positively through the process. Resilience doesn't mean you're tough or that you won't face struggles when dealing with adversity. Instead, resilience is about activating your nervous system's stress response in a way that helps you face challenges, get through them, and then recover.

For instance, you might experience painful feelings like guilt or shame about something you did or something that happened to you. Or, after a difficult experience, you might undergo a taxing phase in the subsequent weeks or months during which time you have heightened alertness, anxiety, and recurring or intrusive thoughts about the experience. But these symptoms don't mean there's something wrong with you, or that you lack resilience. They are normal responses to difficulty as your nervous system integrates an experience.

Being resilient means that the stress response, and any symptoms connected to the painful experience you went through, gradually recedes over a time span that's appropriate for the situation. Without the safeguard of resilience, your stress reactions and symptoms may linger longer than necessary, which can lead to a dysregulated nervous system and a range of chronic symptoms.

George Bonanno, whose research on trauma I discuss in chapter 4, is a leading researcher in the field of resilience. Bonanno's work stands out because he uncovered the nature of resilience through research rather than relying on anecdotes, theories, or unreliable methods.

One of his major findings came from studying survivors of the September 11 attacks. He observed three patterns in symptoms of New Yorkers following the extreme traumatic stress of the 9/11 attacks. Most people saw their symptoms diminish rapidly after the events. He called this pattern of how survivors moved through their symptoms the "resilient" pattern. There were others whose symptoms took much longer to fade, but they were still able to recover eventually. This pattern he called the "recovery" pattern. A small group of people didn't return to their normal selves, even after a significant period of time. This pattern of stress response was associated with people experiencing chronic symptoms after the event, and he called it the "chronic symptoms" pattern.

Various scientific teams have found that those who exhibit the resilient pattern and overcome adversity tend to employ a set of practices that you too can incorporate into your life. When you use these practices, you improve your likelihood of falling into the resilient pattern when faced with adversity. If you're currently experiencing ongoing symptoms from something that happened in the past, these practices can help guide you toward the recovery pattern.

People demonstrating the resilient pattern generally adopt specific attitudes when dealing with stress, and these ways of thinking help boost their resilience. Further, when they come across tough situations, they usually follow a special set of steps to help them adapt.

Adopting a Resilience Attitude

Although you might not have control over your immediate feelings or the occasional negativity, you do have the power to guide your mind toward holding attitudes that are more useful for responding resiliently. You probably won't always feel these attitudes and that's totally okay. Instead, just setting the intention to embrace these helpful attitudes more often, especially when times get tough, is enough.

This mindset, which I call the "resilience attitude," consists of three key elements:

1. Maintaining optimism for the future
2. Having confidence in your ability to cope
3. Viewing adversities as challenges rather than threats

Optimism is crucial because it helps you imagine a brighter future, even during tough times. Imagining a brighter future motivates you to work toward that future, reinforcing your determination to overcome whatever obstacles you encounter.

Self-confidence in your ability to handle hardships is also vital. When you believe you can handle whatever comes your way, you're more likely to try new things and take on challenges. Bonanno describes this confidence as "a self-fulfilling prophecy." How you see yourself is typically how you behave.

The third component, viewing adversities as challenges, is another vital part of the resilience attitude. During tough times, it's natural to feel threatened. But if you can shift your viewpoint to see these situations as challenges, you'll be more proactive and start to strategize about overcoming these obstacles. This perspective shift can also directly influence your body's stress response and your nervous system's state. Viewing a stressor as a challenge primes your body for action: Your heart pumps more blood, and adrenaline helps keep blood pressure in check, preparing you for a more energetic response. In contrast, focusing on the threat can lead to high blood pressure and a less effective stress response.

The integration of optimism, trust in your coping skills, and the perspective of viewing adversities as challenges creates a powerful synergy that supports resilience across the brain and body. But this resilience attitude is not designed to dismiss or minimize the real pain, sorrow, anger, or difficulties you might be experiencing. Instead, it's an approach that allows you to truly acknowledge these feelings and face your difficulties directly. There will be times when you need to yield to your pain and allow yourself to grieve or cry. After you've let yourself feel the pain, the resilience attitude gives you useful tools like hope, trust in your own strength, and the ability to see problems as challenges. These can help you face tough feelings and situations, things that may have seemed too big or frightening before.

A STRATEGY FOR COPING WITH ADVERSITIES

Although developing a resilience attitude is extremely helpful, having a specific strategy for confronting challenging situations is also critical for developing more resilience. The approach I suggest here has been found by researchers to be a common strategy among individuals demonstrating resilience. You can use this strategy for navigating any challenging or stressful situation.

Let's explore the strategy's three steps: (1) analyze your current circumstances; (2) expand your tool kit of coping strategies; and (3) monitor your results while continuing to correct course.

>> DO THIS

CULTIVATE A RESILIENCE MINDSET

1. Bring to mind a mildly challenging, difficult, or annoying situation you're currently experiencing. It's best to stick to something relatively minor while you train this skill. If you go straight for the most challenging stressors, the experience may be too overwhelming to practice shifting your attitude.
2. Optimism: On a scale of 1 to 10, with 1 being totally pessimistic that things will never improve and 10 being totally confident that things will get better, assess your current level of optimism about the situation you brought to mind: _______
   - Close your eyes and imagine what it would feel like if this situation improved. Don't worry about how that might happen, just focus on the felt sense in your body if the situation had already improved, even slightly. Would you feel more relaxed? More joyful? Relieved?
   - Come back to your level of optimism and reassess it using the same scale. You may notice that simply by imagining the possibility of an improved outcome, you feel a little more optimistic about the situation, perhaps increasing your self-assessment by one or two points.
3. Confidence in your ability to cope: On a scale of 1 to 10, with 1 being no confidence in your ability and 10 being totally confident in your ability, assess your current level of confidence in your ability to cope with the current situation: _______
   - Close your eyes and bring to mind a time when you overcame some adversity, when you met a challenge and succeeded in overcoming it. It doesn't need to be a large challenge. For example, maybe you passed a test in school that you were afraid of failing, or maybe you performed a challenging physical activity that pushed your abilities. Bring this memory to mind and invite the felt sense of that accomplishment into your body. Really feel it now for a few moments.
   - Reassess your level of confidence using the same scale. You may notice that you feel a little more confident about your ability to cope, perhaps increasing your self-assessment by one or two points.
4. Viewing adversities as challenges: On a scale of 1 to 10, with 1 being that you view the current situation entirely as a threat and 10 being that the situation feels like a challenge, assess your current level of challenge orientation toward the current situation: _______

- Now switch from dog mind to lion mind, while also imagining yourself as the powerful lion. Adopt the attitude of the powerful lion. Instead of asking yourself, "Why me?" say, "Try me!" Feel any intense sensations of stress in your body as energetic resources there to help you meet this challenge. For an extra boost, scream as loud as you can into a pillow (don't worry, pillows muffle the sound well and no one can hear you) to increase the felt sense of challenge orientation even more.
- Reassess your level of challenge orientation using the same scale. You may feel a little less threat and a little more challenge, perhaps increasing your self-assessment by one or two points.

5. Come back to the original situation. What does it feel like to approach the situation with this slightly different attitude? Do you see it differently with these shifts in your attitude? Do you *feel* it differently?

Analyze Your Current Circumstances

Step 1 involves noticing your current situation and asking yourself, "What is happening to me?" "What is the problem?" and "What do I need to do to get past it?" Recognizing the context helps you determine how to respond appropriately. You've been practicing noticing context since you started the 5-Stage Plan, beginning with stage 1, Awareness. Use your awareness to take in your current circumstances.

To apply this to an everyday challenge, pause and take the time to understand the challenge fully. Just like you're doing by reading this book to fully understand nervous system dysregulation, try to get a full picture of the challenge you're facing before taking any action.

Albert Einstein said, "If I were given one hour to save the planet, I would spend fifty-nine minutes defining the problem and one minute resolving it." Although it may seem obvious that you need to understand the situation before trying to fix it, you might be surprised when you begin to notice how often you neglect to fully take in what's really happening before trying to move forward with a solution.

A Note on Perceptions

Become aware of the difference between what you perceive and the *interpretation* you make of it. This is especially important if you're highly sensitive. If you're highly sensitive, you may already have an advantage in noticing context. Your nervous system can take in a lot of cues from the environment. But heightened sensitivity doesn't *automatically guarantee* that you accurately interpret these cues.

For example, scientific experiments have shown that people interpret facial expressions differently based on their own state of mind, personal history, and other environmental cues. If you're in the red or yellow state, you might interpret someone's facial expression as a sneer, but in the green state you might interpret it as a friendly smile.

This isn't to say you should dismiss your interpretations. Your interpretations are still valuable pieces of your current context, but hold them a little more loosely. Whenever possible, try to test your interpretations before fully relying on them, for example by asking someone how they feel and noticing what kind of attitude they respond with.

Expand Your Coping Strategies Tool Kit

Next you must consider your current coping strategies. Here, you shift from asking, "What do I need to do?" to "*What am I able to do?*" Build a list of coping strategies and emotional regulation tools that are available as options. In the Awareness and Regulation stages, you've already learned several new coping strategies, such as switching from dog mind to lion mind and using portals to gain agency over your stress response.

Outside of an immediately stressful situation, you can also work on increasing the number of strategies available to you by thinking through them or practicing them in a low-stress situation. Building a diverse set of strategies increases your options for handling a particular situation well.

For daily life challenges, brainstorm a list of current coping strategies you have available. There's no one-size-fits-all approach to coping. Different strategies may work better in specific scenarios, or for different people. Don't try to limit yourself only to the most effective coping strategies; instead, focus on applying those that serve you best in each situation. At times, you might feel shame or guilt for utilizing coping strategies considered maladaptive or harmful, like eating a lot of sweets to cope, for example. However, you're probably using them because they served an important purpose during challenging times in the past. Rather than trying to shame or control yourself into forsaking a coping strategy you know has negative side effects, like eating a lot of sweets, try to offer your nervous system an even more effective coping strategy that doesn't have the same negative side effects. Remember, there are no bad coping strategies, just those that are more or less helpful in different situations.

As you navigate this Restoration stage, think about the coping strategies available, including the tools learned in previous stages, and the exercises in this chapter. If you have financial resources, you could consider hiring professional help to process difficult emotions and expand your tool kit of coping strategies. If you have resources in the form of friendships or family, ask them if they'd talk through the situation with you so you can reach a deeper understanding. If you have resources in the form of time, you could go for long walks and do a lot of journaling during this stage. If you're good at navigating social media, connect with people online, or join the Heal Your Nervous System online community.

Monitor Results and Continue Correcting Course

The final step is to implement a coping strategy and then monitor the results you're getting. It helps you build the habit of assessing whether your chosen strategies are working. During this step, ask yourself, "Have I met the challenge?" "Is my coping strategy working?" "Do I need to adjust my response?" and "Should I try another strategy?" You never know whether a coping strategy will be effective until you try it. Rather than getting stuck waiting to find the perfect strategy, resilient people just try something they think might work and then monitor the results, adjusting course or trying a new strategy until something works.

Monitoring results gives you the information you need to adjust or change your response based on how well it's working. If a strategy isn't working, recognize that and adjust accordingly. And, if a strategy is successful, you should be aware of its success to avoid switching to a less effective approach inadvertently.

For example, if you're training your nervous system to be more securely attached, do you notice any positive differences after a few weeks or months of regular practice? Do you feel any better? Do you notice that it's easier to trust people, or do you feel less stressed? If yes, continue. If no, try doing something differently. If you take this attitude of learning from feedback, then you can't go wrong on your healing journey. There are no mistakes, just things you've tried that weren't useful for you at that time in your life.

Interoceptive awareness, the awareness of all the different sensations and subtle cues that come from inside your tissues and organs, which we started building in stages 1 and 2 of the 5-Stage Plan—Awareness and Regulation—is also extremely useful for feedback monitoring. Later in this chapter, I show you how to build your intuition with interoceptive awareness, so that monitoring can become second nature.

THE NERVOUS SYSTEM NAVIGATOR: WORKING WITH YOUR COPING STRATEGIES

It's best to develop and refine your coping strategies during everyday life when you are not overwhelmed by stressors. Studies have shown that consistently working on these strategies during less stressful times can significantly improve your ability to adapt and respond effectively when faced with challenging situations.

Researchers who study coping strategies have found that they could distill a large group of people's strategies from survey results into four broad categories: (1) seeking social support; (2) problem solving; (3) avoidance; and (4) positive thinking.

As you think about your current strategies, when they're appropriate, and which you might be able to add to your tool kit, consider examples in each of the four categories, including how you might do those focusing more on the mind pillar or more on the body pillar. For example, problem-solving strategies, such as creating pros and cons lists (mind-based) or physically sorting sticky notes of potential solutions (body-based), can be ideal when the adversity you're facing requires a practical solution. When you need to feel safe to be with uncomfortable sensations, seeking social support could be a much better strategy.

The goal of this practice is to get better at matching your coping strategy to your current situation so you recognize the variety of effective coping strategies you have in different situations.

Step 1: Create or Retrieve Your Alertness Elevator Map

If you've already done this mapping in chapter 7, refer back to it and ensure you clearly understand each state. If you haven't, reread the section and create an elevator map outlining your nervous system's different states and how they feel in your body and mind.

Step 2: Reflect on Each State

Spend about five minutes reflecting on each state on your map. Focus on the physical sensations, emotions, and thoughts you experience while in each state.

Step 3: Identify Coping Strategies

For each state on your map, brainstorm a list of coping strategies you have used in the past, or that you believe might be helpful in the future. You can use the following Nervous System Navigator Cheat Sheet as inspiration. Consider both body-based and mind-based strategies. Spend at least ten minutes on each state.

THE NERVOUS SYSTEM NAVIGATOR CHEAT SHEET

COPING STRATEGY	BODY-BASED	MIND-BASED
Seeking Social Support		
Venting	Participate in group sports	Share feelings with a friend
Emotional support	Hug or embrace someone you trust	Discuss emotions with a therapist
Instrumental support	Help with a physical task	Get practical advice
Spirituality	Perform yoga or meditation	Pray or engage in a spiritual practice
Problem Solving		
Active coping	Use physical exercise to reduce stress	Brainstorm solutions to a problem
Planning	Set up a physical space to organize tasks	Create a step-by-step action plan
Avoidance		
Disengagement	Engage in unrelated physical activities	Engage in unrelated mental activities
Self-distraction	Engage in a hobby or sport	Watch a movie or read a book
Denial	Avoid places that trigger memories	Suppress thoughts related to the issue
Self-blame	Overwork	Negative self-talk
Positive Thinking		
Humor	Engage in laughter yoga	Watch or listen to comedy
Positive reframing	Engage in physical activities that remind you of your strengths and resilience	Reframe a situation in a positive light
Acceptance	Practice deep breathing or relaxation techniques	Practice mindfulness meditation or acceptance exercises

Step 4: Rehearse Coping Strategies

Once you have identified coping strategies for each state on your map, take about fifteen minutes to rehearse using these strategies mentally and physically (if applicable) in various situations. Visualize yourself in different scenarios where you might find yourself in each state and imagine how you would apply the chosen coping strategy to navigate the situation effectively.

Step 5: Evaluate Each Coping Strategy's Effectiveness

After rehearsing each coping strategy, take about ten minutes to reflect on how effective each felt in addressing the challenges associated with each state. If a strategy doesn't seem to fit well, try a different one or modify the strategy to better suit your needs.

Step 6: Practice and Refine Your Coping Strategies in Real Life

As you encounter situations that bring you into different nervous system states, put your rehearsed coping strategies into practice, then monitor feedback. Observe how effectively they help you navigate each state and make any adjustments necessary to your approach. Regularly revisit your elevator alertness map and the coping strategies you've identified. Assess how well these strategies are serving you, and adjust or explore new strategies as needed.

BUILDING SECURE ATTACHMENT TO INCREASE NERVOUS SYSTEM FLEXIBILITY

As I discussed in chapter 4, your attachment system shapes your perception of the world and your stress responses. Numerous studies have found a significant link among secure attachment, resilience, and emotional regulation. Fostering secure attachment enhances your ability to regulate your nervous system, thereby increasing resilience and adaptability in the face of stressors.

Imagine a young child forming a strong bond with a caring, attentive adult who is in tune with the child's emotional and physical needs. The child feels safe and secure with this person, and they're supported and encouraged to explore their internal and external worlds. This is a secure attachment bond, and it lays the foundation for the child to have a well-functioning nervous system capable of handling new experiences and stressors that come with human life.

This bond acts as a safety net and creates, in the child, a background sense of well-being throughout their life. It's like having an invisible safety blanket that provides comfort and security even when they aren't aware it's there. This background sense of safety and deep okayness helps them feel more resilient and confident that they can cope with whatever life throws at them.

Much like you've been practicing using portals from stage 2, Regulation, to feel an embodied sense of safety repeatedly, the secure child experiences a felt sense of safety in their body over and over again. They cycle through their alertness elevator hundreds of thousands of times throughout childhood, always coming back to that felt sense of safety. They get activated by life's stressors, moving into a yellow or red state, and then their caregivers' presence or comforting helps them feel safe again, moving the child back to green. Cycling through these states repeatedly trains the nervous system to move flexibly through different levels of arousal, always coming back to green.

But if you didn't receive this training as a child, or if the training you received was missing some elements, you can still train your nervous system to have this same kind of flexibility now, as an adult. Training your nervous system for secure attachment is like building a strong and sturdy house. Just as a house needs a solid foundation, strong walls, and a reliable roof for stability, secure attachment requires a combination of elements that, together, create a stable, nurturing environment for emotional growth.

Five Core Needs for Attachment

Let's explore the five core needs, the "building blocks," of secure attachment. These core needs come from the book *Attachment Disturbances in Adults* by Harvard psychologists and attachment experts Daniel P. Brown and David Elliott.

1. **Foundation: safety and protection**
The foundation of a house ensures stability and support. In attachment, safety and protection are the foundation, providing a sense of security for the child. Parents and caregivers provide safety through reliability, honesty, and respecting boundaries, which helps the child feel secure in later relationships.

2. **Walls: attunement**
Walls in a house not only provide structure and support but also define the living spaces within, connecting the rooms in a meaningful way. In attachment, attunement is like the walls, enabling the child to feel seen, understood, and connected to their caregivers. Parents and caregivers attuned to their child's thoughts, feelings, and needs act like walls, creating a secure and supportive environment that allows the child to develop a strong sense of self and emotional understanding, ultimately shaping their ability to form meaningful connections with others.

3. **Roof: soothing and comfort**
A roof offers shelter and security, creating a safe place to feel cozy in a storm. Soothing and comfort are like the roof of a house, with parents and caregivers

providing soothing touch, reassurance, and emotional support to help the child feel better during challenging moments. Soothing and comfort from caregivers teaches the child's nervous system how to move back to the green state after feeling distressed.

4. **Windows: expressed delight**
Windows bring light and warmth into a house. Expressed delight is like windows, with parents and caregivers regularly expressing joy, love, and pride in their child. This helps the child develop a strong sense of self-esteem and positive emotions associated with their sense of self.

5. **Garden: support of best self-development**
A garden represents growth, beauty, and individuality. A garden symbolizes the support parents and caregivers give to help the child discover their unique strengths and develop their best self. Secure parents and caregivers encourage exploration and celebrate their child's unique qualities, fostering a strong sense of identity.

A Note for Caregivers: Aim for "Good Enough," Let Go of Perfection

If you care for a child, you know that meeting their five core needs of attachment can be a real struggle, especially if you're dealing with other challenging life circumstances. For example, it can be hard to give kids all the emotional support they need while simultaneously juggling work life, home life, and getting your own needs met. Lack of access to quality health-care, education, nutrition, or a strong social support network can also make it difficult to meet all of a child's five core needs. On top of that, your own prolonged stress and embedded alarms can put you in the red or yellow state when your children need you in the green state to help them feel safe or soothed. This can prevent them from feeling a consistent embodied sense of safety and protection. Challenges like these can make the already tough job of building a secure caregiver-child relationship and fostering emotional resilience even more difficult.

However, attachment researchers have shown that you don't need to be perfect to raise securely attached children. You only need to be "good enough." The concept of "good enough" parenting was introduced by pediatrician and psychoanalyst Donald Winnicott in the 1950s and has been widely accepted in attachment theory. A recent study shed light on what exactly it means to give the gift of "good enough" care from an attachment perspective.

Infant attachment expert Susan S. Woodhouse and colleagues studied infant-mother pairs. The researchers found that caregivers needed to "get it right" and respond appropriately to an infant's needs about 50 percent of the time to have a positive impact on the infant's attachment status. This study demonstrates that you have a lot of leeway to make mistakes and fail to meet the child's attachment needs, while still giving your children the gift of "good enough" parenting to foster secure attachment.

Woodhouse and other infant attachment researchers emphasize that "good enough" parenting does not require specific practices, like baby wearing or breastfeeding. Some popular child-rearing styles, such as "attachment parenting," advocate for very specific practices for raising infants, but using these specific practices is scientifically unrelated to secure attachment. Although these types of practices may be a great choice for your family, what matters for raising securely attached children, according to the research, is that infants feel supported in exploring their world without being interrupted, and they feel welcomed when they need comfort and protection.

You don't need to have perfect attachment behaviors all the time to be a great caregiver; simply hold the intention to meet the five conditions for your children as often as possible. Children are extremely sensitive and will pick up on your intentions. When things don't go as planned, make amends and repair it. That's enough. We will discuss repairing ruptures in more detail in chapter 10, the Connection stage of the 5-Stage Plan.

Your Attachment Status: How Your Early Childhood Attachments Affected Your Nervous System

If you've heard of attachment theory, you may have heard of different categories, or statuses, of attachment—*secure attachment, dismissing attachment, preoccupied attachment, and disorganized or fearful attachment*. Most attachment experts agree that attachment status is not completely categorical; rather, it exists on a spectrum. For example, two people could both have secure attachment status, but one has secure status with more dismissing behaviors and the other has secure status with more preoccupied behaviors. As with other self-assessments in this book, naming your attachment status can be a useful tool to learn more about yourself, but don't let the label limit you. You are much more than any label.

Secure Attachment

Adults with secure attachment have generally had all five core attachment needs met reasonably well. They can handle stress well by maintaining a healthy balance between closeness and independence. They are comfortable expressing emotions and relying on others for support as well as spending time alone. Even when faced with the inevitable difficulties and heartbreaks of life, they have a deep sense of being okay in the background, which helps them navigate different levels of alertness flexibly. In general, adults with secure attachment can:

- Effectively balance seeking support and help from others and relying on their own abilities when facing personal challenges or work deadlines
- Openly share their feelings and thoughts with loved ones during difficult times, fostering strong communication and support networks
- Confidently ask for and accept help from others in times of need, while also recognizing their own strengths and capabilities
- Enjoy spending time alone to recharge and reflect, using self-care activities to build resilience and maintain well-being
- Navigate life's challenges, such as a job loss or a relationship ending, maintaining a background sense of okayness while feeling all the difficult and painful emotions that naturally arise—drawing on both inner resources and support from others
- Set healthy boundaries in relationships, allowing for a balanced interdependence between personal space and connection with others
- In romantic relationships, trust and commit to their partner without becoming overly possessive, demonstrating a healthy mix of reliance and independence
- Adapt to new situations and cope with change by embracing personal growth and learning opportunities and seeking support when needed
- Calmly address issues during conflicts, working toward resolution by both understanding others' perspectives and asserting their own needs
- Demonstrate empathy and understanding toward others, providing support and encouragement while also valuing their own well-being and self-reliance

Dismissing Attachment

People with dismissing attachment, sometimes called avoidant attachment, tend to keep their distance in relationships and may push away intimacy. In childhood, their body learned to reduce their perceived need for emotional connection and closeness with others and, instead, found comfort in distraction or through suppressing negative emotions. For example, after a rough day at school, they might have preferred to spend hours riding their bike alone or drawing pictures in their room rather than talking to family or friends about their feelings, as playing alone often felt more comforting or secure than talking about difficult feelings with caregivers. Although playing alone didn't truly address their emotional needs, it did provide a sense of temporary relief. It also gave them a sense of agency in the situation.

In general, their caregivers may have been especially encouraging of their independence and good at the core attachment need of supporting their best self-development. But, typically, their caregivers were not very attuned to these children's needs and feelings, and may have neglected to soothe or comfort them sufficiently, especially when they were experiencing negative emotions or stress. Their nervous system learned to come down from red states by suppressing negative emotions, rather than soothing them and feeling better.

As adults, they tend to be more disconnected from their internal experience and find themselves most comfortable in relationships where they do not feel too close to the other. They often idealize loved ones, such as parents or partners, subconsciously ignoring the others' faults to avoid feeling sad or disappointed. In stressful situations, they might cope by showing off their independence, trying to "problem solve" their way out of pain, or getting absorbed in an activity that turns off their need for connection. Examples may include:

- Becoming a workaholic; obsessing over career or business
- Immersing themselves excessively in intellectual pursuits or research
- Overwhelming themselves with managing every detail of their children's lives—from scheduling extracurricular activities to handling all school-related tasks—without seeking help or delegating responsibilities
- Overexercising or engaging in extreme sports to the point of exhaustion
- Traveling nonstop or obsessively exploring new places
- Compulsively learning new skills or taking up multiple hobbies
- Overcommitting to volunteering or community work, leaving no time for themselves
- Networking or attending social events to the point of neglecting deeper personal relationships
- Dedicating all their free time to artistic or creative projects, to the exclusion of other aspects of life

Preoccupied Attachment

People with preoccupied attachment, also known as anxious attachment, often struggle with self-esteem and may feel inadequate compared to others. In childhood, their nervous system learned to increase their emotional distress to get the attention, safety, and comfort they needed from caregivers. Of the five core needs, they typically most lacked expressed delight and support of best self-development. They did get some attunement and soothing, but it was unreliable.

As adults, their nervous systems may increase feelings of anxiety or anger in response to not getting their attachment needs met. In relationships, they tend to worry about abandonment, seek extra reassurance from others, and find it hard to be alone. They often subconsciously fixate on the faults of loved ones, harboring significant anger or hurt when thinking about their unmet needs in relation to parents or long-term partners. In stressful situations, they may cope by activating strategies that keep others close to them, like becoming overly reliant on others and entangling others in their emotional world. For example, a high-functioning adult with preoccupied attachment, at work or in their relationships with family and friends, may:

- Constantly seek approval, validation, or reassurance from colleagues, supervisors, friends, family members, or romantic partners
- Become overly dependent on others for emotional support, decision-making, or help, even when it's not necessary
- Be highly sensitive to rejection, taking criticism personally and struggling to accept constructive feedback
- Tend to overshare personal issues or emotions with others in an attempt to connect, gain sympathy, or create strong bonds quickly
- Cling to relationships, including friendships and romantic partners, even when these are not healthy or beneficial because they are especially afraid of being alone
- Frequently check in with loved ones or colleagues for fear of being left out, forgotten, or abandoned
- Experience intense anxiety or anger when their need for connection isn't met, leading to overreactions and escalating conflicts
- Struggle with setting boundaries, becoming overly involved in the issues or well-being of family, friends, or coworkers
- Offer help and support, even when it was not asked for, in an attempt to maintain close relationships
- Overcommit to social events and obligations to avoid feeling alone, even when they need rest
- Feel jealous of or threatened by other people's relationships, friendships, or connections
- Struggle with delegating work tasks, fearing colleagues will not support them or will perceive them as incompetent

Disorganized or Fearful Attachment

Some people who have had especially difficult attachment experiences early in life have an attachment system that is less organized around one particular strategy and, instead, displays a mix of preoccupied and dismissing attachment strategies. Their nervous systems can fluctuate between two opposite attachment strategies—a preoccupied strategy and a dismissing strategy.

When the preoccupied strategy is activated, they become overly focused on their distress and may get anxious or upset until they receive comfort or attention. When the dismissing strategy is activated, they suppress or ignore their distress as a way of coping, usually also pushing away intimate connections.

This inconsistency can be scary and painful and make the disorganized person feel powerless and lost, with unclear goals and an unstable sense of who they are. In childhood, the five core needs may not have been met or met inconsistently, but most important, the first core need of safety and protection was not met by their caregivers. They often didn't feel safe with their caregivers. Like everyone, they desire to love and belong but have an extreme fear of being hurt or rejected by others. This may show up in several ways, including:

- Struggling with a sense of identity and goals, leading to feelings of ineffectiveness and helplessness
- Having relationships characterized by a pattern of "stable instability," making it hard for them to maintain long-lasting, healthy connections
- Oscillating between seeking reassurance and validation from others and pushing others away out of fear of rejection or abandonment
- In social settings, having difficulty finding a balance between connecting with others and maintaining emotional boundaries
- In conflicts, alternating between extremely intense emotions and withdrawing or shutting down, making it hard to find a solution
- At work or in personal relationships, struggling to express needs or emotions consistently and clearly
- Experiencing intense feelings of insecurity and fear, which can drive them to be overly cautious or guarded in relationships
- In times of stress, wavering between relying heavily on others and trying to cope entirely on their own, making it difficult to find a healthy balance

Training Attachment Security as an Adult

Your attachment status isn't set in stone. It exists along a spectrum, and no matter where you find yourself, you can always work toward healing and becoming more secure. Building more security can help you handle your emotions better and become more resilient, while also building deeper connections with others. Although being in a relationship with a secure partner can aid this process, this is not always available, or it may be challenged by both partners' attachment issues.

Various therapeutic modalities can help train secure attachment status in adults who struggle with stress, anxiety, and overwhelm. One highly effective method is the Ideal Parent Figure (IPF) protocol, developed by psychotherapy researchers and clinicians Daniel P. Brown and David Elliott. Amazingly, you don't necessarily have to have different experiences in the real world to change your attachment status. You can use your imagination to train your nervous system to manage emotions and expectations of relationships in a more secure and flexible way. The IPF protocol uses visualizations of secure attachment experiences with imaginary caregivers to shift your attachment status.

Working with the IPF protocol typically takes six months to two years of weekly sessions with an IPF therapist to transition from insecure to secure. However, even *incremental changes* in your ability to imagine having all your attachment needs met can significantly help increase your nervous system flexibility. In a study by psychologist Federico Parra and colleagues, complex post-traumatic stress disorder (PTSD) symptoms were significantly reduced in just five weeks of using the IPF protocol, even for patients who didn't change their attachment classification from insecure to secure.

Attachment security, just like nervous system regulation, is not just a mental exercise. It engages both your mind and your body. You can't train attachment security by trying to think through it; you have to engage your interoceptive awareness, or internal sensations, to train your nervous system to be more secure. The IPF protocol does this by having you imagine the embodied feelings, or felt sense, of having each of your five core attachment needs met over and over again in different situations. For example, you don't just think about what ideal parents would say to you to express delight; you imagine being a child and bring to mind what it would feel like in your body as that child for your ideal parents' eyes to sparkle with delight as they take great joy in you just as you are without wanting you to be any different.

SHARPENING INTUITION AND CALMING ANXIETY

Intuition, often perceived as a mysterious force, comes from strong interoceptive awareness, or your ability to perceive your body's internal signals, such as your heartbeat, breathing, and other internal sensations. Intuition is extremely helpful for navigating life and regulating your nervous system. It's your inner voice, or "gut

>> DO THIS

DEVELOP A SENSE OF SECURE ATTACHMENT

Although the IPF protocol requires a trained therapist, this exercise draws on elements of the protocol to start introducing characteristics of secure attachment into your nervous system. This exercise is best done in a calm and relaxed state.

Note: At any point during this practice, if you experience overwhelming sensations or emotions, pause and use a portal from the Regulation stage to come back to an embodied sense of safety. It's essential to prioritize your safety during this process. If you find it challenging to work through these feelings on your own, consider seeking the guidance of a therapist experienced in the IPF protocol.

1. Find a quiet space and time when you won't be disturbed. Have your journal or notebook and a pen nearby.

2. Take a few deep breaths—in through your nose and out through your mouth. Allow your body to settle and your mind to clear.

3. Begin by identifying what you need from a parent figure, such as feeling seen, heard, valued, safe, loved unconditionally, free to be yourself, supported in pursuing dreams, or feeling like you belong and matter. Reflect on your needs as a child and as an adult. Write down these needs in your journal.

4. Once you have a clear understanding of what you need from a parent figure, imagine ideal parent figures—not your real parents. Using your imagination helps create new possibilities. Instead of reflecting on what you did or didn't receive from your parents, focus instead on internalizing a new representation of your current needs and how they can be met.

Even if your real-life parents or caregivers were "good enough" and did the best they could, they were still human and probably didn't meet every one of your attachment needs all the time. You can train your nervous system using ideal parents who, in your imagination, can meet all your unique attachment needs every time in just the right way.

5. Create an image of what your ideal parent figures would be like. The most important thing to focus on is what it would *feel* like to be with them. You can

continued on following page

>> DO THIS *CONTINUED*

visualize them in your mind, draw them, or write about them in your journal to imagine more vividly what it would feel like to be with them. You can ask yourself:

- What do these figures look like?
- What is their energy like?
- What kind of voice do they have?
- What are their values and beliefs?
- How do they make you feel?
- What's the felt sense in your body of getting your needs met by them?

6. Once you have a clear image of your ideal parent figures, imagine them interacting with you as a child and meeting your attachment needs. Picture how they would respond to you in various situations and how they would provide the love, support, and safety you need. Go back to step 3 and imagine a scene for each of the needs you identified where your ideal parents are meeting that need in just the right way. You can shift and change the scene again and again until it feels *just right* for you. Write these interactions in your journal.

7. Spend some time each day or week visualizing and journaling about your ideal parent figures. Over time, these new images and experiences will help retrain your nervous system to manage emotions, stress, and connections with others with more and more secure attachment.

feeling," that helps you know what you want, which decisions are best for you, and when something doesn't feel right. By strengthening your intuition, you can improve your decision-making to promote more regulation, inner peace, confidence, and a stronger sense of connection with the world around you.

To strengthen your intuition, you need to work on noticing your body's signals and correctly understanding what they mean. To notice more of these signals, pay more attention more often to your internal body sensations, such as changes in your breathing patterns or heat rate. To understand these signals correctly, compare what you feel inside with what's happening around you. For example, if you notice your heart racing, assess whether it started when the room got noisier. This way, you get better at connecting your body's reactions with what triggers them in your surroundings.

Merging your awareness of your body's inner workings (interoception) with your observation of the world around you (exteroception) gives you a brilliant way to see how your nervous system responds to various situations. More importantly, it lets you see how well that response works for you. This mix of your body's internal awareness and your outer world perception is especially valuable in feedback monitoring.

Feedback monitoring is a vital part of the three steps to creating a resilience attitude introduced earlier in this chapter. It allows you to handle challenging situations more effectively by tracking how you respond to situations and how well your responses work. This gives you the ability to adjust your reactions and make changes when needed. As you understand more about your stress responses and how they align with your external circumstances, you can start trusting your intuition more. Heightened intuition makes you more capable of effectively navigating life's challenges.

Is It Intuition or Anxiety?

Anyone can develop broader and more accurate interoceptive awareness to access more intuition, but if you have a highly sensitive nervous system, you may have an increased ability for intuitive understanding because your nervous system naturally takes in and processes more information than someone with less sensitivity. However, if your nervous system is dysregulated, the voice of intuition may be drowned out by anxious thoughts and bodily symptoms of stress. Distinguishing between the voice of intuition and the voice of anxiety can become challenging. When considering a new job, a move, a partner, or spending time with a friend, it can be difficult to know whether your intuition is saying yes or no because your feeling may be anxiety-driven or intuition-inspired.

Recent research into interoception has shown that training interoceptive awareness, for example by noticing changes in your heart rate, can significantly reduce anxiety. When someone has low interoception, they're not very good at sensing what's going on inside their body or matching it to other aspects of their experience. This can cause them to have trouble understanding and regulating their feelings. They might not be able to connect their physical sensations (like a racing heart) with their emotions (like feeling scared). Without being able to make these connections, it can be hard for them to manage their emotions and feelings.

Imagine you're at work, and you're assigned a challenging task with a tight deadline. As you start working, you begin to experience self-doubt and anxious thoughts. You're thinking things like "I'm not good enough," "I'm not sure I can finish this on time," and "What if I fail?"

Instead of being drawn into this cycle of rumination, you switch from dog mind to lion mind and consciously decide to focus on your physical sensations and activate your interoception. You become aware that your breathing is shallow and your shoulders are tense. You take notice of your racing heartbeat, sweaty palms, and upset stomach. This is your interoception at work, making you aware of the stress response you're experiencing internally.

Instead of getting lost, though, in these internal sensations, you recognize the importance of connecting your interoceptive awareness with your external environment. You take a moment to observe your surroundings and consider how they might be contributing to your stress. You realize that your office space is cluttered, and there's a lot of noise from nearby colleagues having a conversation. Acknowledging these external factors allows you to address the stressors that are within your control. You tidy up your workspace, put on noise-canceling headphones, and remind yourself of the resources and support available to you, such as your helpful teammates and your past experiences tackling similar challenges.

After taking these actions, you observe your body's response. Your breathing becomes deeper and more relaxed, your shoulders loosen, and tension dissipates throughout your body. A sensation of warmth and relaxation spreads, and your mind settles into a state of ease, ready to tackle the challenge. This awareness of your body's response completes the feedback loop, verifying the effectiveness of your actions in addressing the situation. Integrating interoception and exteroception in this way allows you to recognize and address both your internal stress response and the external circumstances that contribute to or mitigate it.

Experiencing these positive changes not only helps you feel more regulated but also teaches your nervous system that you can help it feel safe and soothed. Your nervous system learns that you possess the ability to influence your circumstances in a positive way. This sense of agency fosters resilience, equipping you to tackle future challenges confidently.

Up until this point, from building the underlying structure to support nervous system regulation through the first three stages, you've been focusing primarily on the mind and the body pillars in the 4 Pillars of Nervous System Health. Like putting on your own oxygen mask before helping others, focusing primarily on just your mind and body is necessary to regulate your nervous system before including the complexities of other people's nervous systems in your healing journey. But it's crucial not to limit your focus solely to your own nervous system. Once your nervous system is more regulated, establishing deep connections with the people and world around you will further increase your regulation and offer a rich source of meaning. In the next chapter, stage 4, Connection, you'll learn how to integrate your nervous system regulation into connections with other people, nature, beauty, and purpose.

>> DO THIS

DEEPEN YOUR INTEROCEPTION AWARENESS

Heartbeat Awareness

This exercise helps improve your interoception by increasing your awareness of how your heartbeat changes in response to various levels of physical activity. Throughout the practice, take note of how your heartbeat changes with each level of activity.

1. Find a quiet and comfortable place to perform this exercise.
2. At rest, locate your pulse on your wrist or neck, and focus on your heartbeat for thirty seconds.
3. Engage in thirty seconds of minimal physical activity, such as slow walking or gentle stretching.
4. After the activity, locate your pulse again and observe your heartbeat for thirty seconds.
5. Perform one minute of moderate physical activity, such as brisk walking or light jogging.
6. Locate your pulse once more and observe your heartbeat for thirty seconds.
7. Finally, engage in two minutes of intense physical activity, like running, jumping jacks, or burpees.
8. Locate your pulse and observe your heartbeat for thirty seconds.
9. Repeat this exercise regularly to enhance your interoceptive awareness and your understanding of your body's response to different activities.

Breathing Awareness

This exercise helps improve your interoception by increasing your awareness of how your breathing changes in response to various levels of physical activity. Throughout the practice, take note of how your breathing changes with each level of activity, including the rhythm, depth, and any other sensations you may feel.

1. Find a quiet and comfortable place to perform this exercise.
2. At rest, close your eyes and focus on your breathing for thirty seconds. Notice the rhythm, depth, and any other sensations associated with your breath.
3. Engage in thirty seconds of minimal physical activity, such as slow walking or gentle stretching.

continued on following page

>> DO THIS *CONTINUED*

4. After the activity, close your eyes and observe your breathing for thirty seconds.
5. Perform one minute of moderate physical activity, such as brisk walking or light jogging.
6. After the activity, close your eyes and observe your breathing for thirty seconds.
7. Finally, engage in two minutes of intense physical activity, like running, jumping jacks, or burpees.
8. After the activity, close your eyes and observe your breathing for thirty seconds.
9. Repeat this exercise regularly to enhance your interoceptive awareness and your understanding of your body's response to different activities.

Integrating Interoception and Exteroception

This practice helps you develop the ability to switch between interoception—focusing on internal bodily sensations—and exteroception—focusing on the external environment. Integrating these two types of awareness can improve your decision-making, regulation, and overall well-being.

PART 1: INTEROCEPTIVE AWARENESS

1. Find a quiet place where you can sit comfortably for a few minutes without being disturbed.
2. Close your eyes and take a deep breath in through your nose, filling your lungs with air.
3. As you exhale through your mouth, bring your attention inward, focusing on the sensations within your body.
4. Start at the top of your head and slowly scan down your body, noticing any sensations you feel. Use the table of sensations (see Identifying Interoceptive Sensations, chapter 8) as a reference, and try to identify three to five sensations in each body part.
5. As you notice these sensations, simply acknowledge them without judgment or interpretation. Just observe and name the sensation, and then move on to the next part of your body.
6. Take your time as you scan your body, and try to stay present and focused on the sensations you feel. If your mind begins to wander, simply bring your attention back to your body and continue the scan.

7. Once you've scanned your whole body, take a few more deep breaths and then slowly open your eyes.

PART 2: EXTEROCEPTIVE AWARENESS

1. With your eyes open, find a point of focus in your external environment, such as a candle flame, a plant, or a picture on the wall.
2. Allow your gaze to rest on the object, and begin to expand your awareness to include the sounds, smells, and sensations around you.
3. Take a deep breath in and notice any smells or fragrances in the air. What scents do you detect?
4. Continue to expand your awareness to include the sounds around you. What do you hear? Can you identify specific sounds?
5. Finally, shift your focus to the physical sensations in your body that arise as you take in these external cues. Do you feel any tension or relaxation? Any warmth or coolness?
6. Allow yourself to stay present and aware of your external environment, while still remaining connected to the internal sensations within your body.
7. Take a few more deep breaths and then slowly return your attention to your normal activities.

By alternating between interoceptive and exteroceptive awareness, you're practicing the ability to stay present and connected to both your internal and your external environments. This practice can help you develop a more finely tuned awareness of your body and the world around you, which can improve your ability to regulate your emotions and make decisions that align with your needs and values.

10

Stage 4: Connection—Repairing Bonds and Cultivating Kinship

IMAGINE YOUR HEALING JOURNEY is like a tree. In stage 1, Awareness, you learned how to recognize the rain and sunlight that will sustain your growth. In stage 2, Regulation, you learned how to produce individual leaves. In the Restoration stage, stage 3, you began to grow roots to stabilize your foundation so that even when a storm comes, you remain solidly connected to the ground.

This stage, stage 4, Connection, is like building a network of roots connected to the other trees in the forest. Trees may seem like they exist on their own, but they are actually deeply intertwined with the entire ecosystem around them, which helps sustain them. In fact, many species of trees have root systems that are directly connected to one another. When one tree is struggling, the others will feed it nutrients through its root system. Similarly, at this stage of the healing journey, you're learning to connect your roots to other trees, which will lead to an even deeper sense of nervous system regulation, an increasing sense of trust—not just in yourself but in the whole unfolding of life—and a growing sense of meaning and purpose.

The journey until now, from structure to restoration, has focused primarily on the first two pillars of the 4 Pillars of Nervous System Health, mind and body. In this chapter, we turn our attention to the third pillar, connection. At this stage, you might notice a growing appreciation for how important others are in your life and how much you have to offer others in return. The more nutrients you have from building a strong tree with lots of leaves and a solid root network, the more capacity you have to offer others healing nutrients without compromising your boundaries or giving more than you have to offer.

BUILDING MOMENTUM

SHARE WITH OTHERS

While everyone needs connection, the flavors of connection you need at any given time might look very different from the ones that other people need. Likewise, the best practices that will lead you into that sense of connection and reciprocal support with the people and the world around you might be different for you than for others.

In this stage, I emphasize four different pathways into connection: (1) higher purpose; (2) other people; (3) the natural world; and (4) beauty or creativity. All are fundamental needs for your nervous system to be fully integrated with life, but you may find one or more of them more relevant for you right now—that's okay. Focus on what resonates with you now and come back to other aspects of connection as you feel called to them.

Sharing with others during this stage is even more important than in the previous stages. For some, connection might feel easier in some spaces than in others. Many people find it easier to practice building connections in online spaces or facilitated groups, and much more challenging in intimate relationships or with family. Whatever the case is for you, if you feel brave enough, I encourage you to connect with others who can understand the journey you're on. Find a loved one, an in-person group, or an online community where you can spend at least five to ten minutes per week checking in about your journey and listening to others. You're always welcome to join the online Heal Your Nervous System community to connect with like-minded people, especially if you don't have people currently in your life or local community who are available for this type of connection with you.

CULTIVATING AN ATTITUDE OF KINSHIP

Imagine the power of a single drop of water as it cascades into a still pond. The ripples it creates reverberate, affecting every part of the water, transforming the stillness into a dance of movement and energy. In the same way, our lives are deeply interconnected with the people and the world around us. Our bodily states, thoughts, and emotions have the power to create far-reaching ripples, impacting the broader tapestry of existence.

Spiritual leader Thích Nhất Hạnh, also known as the father of modern mindfulness, called this interconnectedness "interbeing," underscoring its essential role in fostering health, peace, and harmony within us and the world. The bonds we form with one another, and our environment, have always been essential for supporting our ability to thrive under stressors and adapt to changing circumstances.

Interconnectedness is not just a philosophical or spiritual idea but a fundamental aspect of our biological makeup. The biological need for connectedness, encoded in our DNA, has been passed down through generations, shaping our instincts, behaviors, and even our biochemistry.

At this stage of your journey, the mission is to strengthen your bonds, repair ruptured relationships, and cultivate *kinship* with the world around you. Just as the ripples in the pond transform the water, your individual efforts to regulate your nervous system resonate into the world around you. Just as a magnet pulls metal toward it, your work on regulating your nervous system will also have a pull. It will create a ripple effect. You'll notice that the positive changes you've made don't just benefit you, but they also reach the people around you. And these ripples of influence won't stop there: They'll spread, touching many more lives in the process.

Kinship encompasses not only the connections shared with others and the world around you but also the idea of reciprocity—the give and take that sustains these relationships and keeps them vibrant and alive. When you approach your connections with a spirit of reciprocity, you acknowledge that your actions and the attitudes you bring to your interactions can have a profound impact on others, just as they, in turn, have an impact on you. This continuous exchange of energy and support forms the basis of true kinship and interconnectedness.

CONNECTION TO A PURPOSE

One of the essential aspects of building strong connections and fostering kinship is connecting to a *sense of purpose* in life. Robert Emmons, a prominent researcher in the field of positive psychology, offered valuable insights on how purpose can significantly impact your mind-body health in his book *The Psychology of Ultimate Concerns*. According to Emmons, throughout life, you may have various personal goals and aspirations, which often contradict one another, causing internal conflict and reducing overall life satisfaction. Emmons introduced the concept of an "ultimate concern," which is a higher order goal that guides your life and provides a strong sense of purpose and clarity. By focusing on your ultimate concern, you're likely to experience less conflict and enjoy a greater sense of fulfillment.

Cultivating an ultimate concern allows you to hold a broader perspective that encompasses all your specific action plans and goals. This perspective helps organize your goals around your larger sense of purpose, enhancing your resilience in the face of stress and deepening your sense of purpose in life.

Developing an ultimate concern is not about making radical life changes. Rather, it's about recognizing your core values and incorporating them into your daily life. Aligning your personal goals with your ultimate concern enables you to make decisions that reflect your values and priorities. Moreover, a significant body of research has shown that connecting to a purpose in life improves mind and body health. By focusing on an ultimate concern, you not only enhance your health but also create more meaningful relationships and cultivate a stronger sense of kinship with others.

Getting Real About Purpose: A Perspective Shift

In *The Top Five Regrets of the Dying*, Bronnie Ware, a nurse specializing in end-of-life care, shares the common regrets she frequently encountered when talking with her patients nearing the end of their lives. These recurring themes included living to meet others' expectations rather than their own, overworking at the expense of quality time with loved ones, insufficient expression of emotions, losing connection with friends, and not letting themselves be happier.

Just like the people Ware cared for, it's all too common to become buried in day-to-day tasks, losing sight of what's truly important. Yet, there's no need to wait until life's end to refocus on your key priorities. By identifying and prioritizing what genuinely matters to you right now, you can build a deeper connection with your life's purpose, making every day count. One practice that can help you remember and stay connected with the things that matter most to you is the Buddhist practice of maraṇasati, which involves contemplating death.

Recognizing your own mortality can be difficult, as your mind often shields you from this awareness. However, becoming more comfortable with the idea of death can have a profound effect on your relationship to life. Developing this awareness can help you stay mindful of your core purpose, appreciate the moment, and live each day with a greater sense of earnestness and presence. Contemplating your death can make your goals and actions clearer, ensuring they align with your values. This awareness promotes living with a purpose beyond immediate self-interest, which has been shown to positively impact long-term happiness.

>> DO THIS

JOURNALING EXERCISE: UNCOVER YOUR CORE PURPOSE

To start, locate a calm and peaceful spot where you won't be interrupted. Choose a prompt that resonates with you from the four I provide here. Set a timer for ten to fifteen minutes—this will be your dedicated writing time. Then, using the prompt you've chosen as your starting point, open your journal and begin writing, allowing your thoughts to flow freely onto the page. Keep your pen moving for the whole duration of the time, even if you feel stuck or unsure of what to express. If you're struggling, it's perfectly fine to write "I don't know" as many times as you need to—just keep writing. The goal is to maintain a continuous stream of writing. This can help you get past any internal roadblocks and allow deeper insights to surface.

Prompt 1: Identify your core purpose.

In your journal, write a sentence or two about the main value or belief that drives your actions and gives your life meaning. What gives your actions their deepest meaning? This could be a spiritual belief, a desire to help others, or something else entirely.

Prompt 2: Connect the dots.

Think about the moments and activities that are most important to you. Write about how your core purpose is present in these experiences. Look for a common thread that connects these moments to your central guiding principle.

Prompt 3: Imagine your guiding principle in action.

Describe a specific situation in which your core purpose is more clearly in your awareness while you're doing something. How does this awareness affect your experience? How does it make you feel? Why do you think this is?

Prompt 4: Apply your guiding principle to daily life.

Reflect on how you can keep your central guiding principle in mind as you go about your daily activities. Write about the ways this awareness might affect your sense of presence, engagement, and satisfaction in various aspects of your life.

>> DO THIS

SIMPLE MARAṆASATI *PRACTICE: REFLECT ON MORTALITY*

Before starting, ensure you're in a safe environment and check with your intuition to see whether you're ready for a potentially challenging practice like this. You can practice checking with your intuition by switching from dog mind to lion mind, and then noticing your interoceptive sensations, especially in your heart and gut. Signs indicating that you're ready for this practice include feeling calm, excited, interested, or a sense of challenge. It's normal to feel some trepidation before reflecting on your mortality, but if you feel significant anxiety, panic, or anger, those signs indicate you're not yet ready for this. It's totally okay to put this exercise aside for now and come back to it a different time. If you start to feel significant anxiety at any point in the process, take a break and return to it later.

1. **Find a comfortable space.** Choose a place where you feel safe, like your home, and consider having a loved one nearby for support.

2. **Reflect on different time frames and complete the following sentences in your journal or on this page:**

   - If I had one year left to live, I would ____________

   - If I had one month left to live, I would ____________

   - If I had one week left to live, I would ____________

3. **Check in with your body.** As you work through the exercise, observe any physical sensations that arise. Notice these sensations and bring gentleness toward yourself. If anxiety or other difficult feelings surface, take a break.

4. **Review your responses.** Once you've completed the exercise, read your responses and consider:

   - How did your priorities and activities change as the time you had left decreased?

   - What stayed consistently important to you across different time spans?

   - What do you do in your everyday life that didn't seem worth including?

5. **Unwind and share.** Take some time to relax and, if you feel comfortable, share your thoughts and experiences with others. Remember, this practice aims to train your mind gently to embrace your sense of mortality. Always prioritize your well-being and approach the exercise with self-compassion.

CONNECTION TO OTHERS

After all the work you've done on releasing the alarms at the body level, creating safety, and restoring your nervous system's flexibility, you're now in a great spot to look at your relationships with fresh eyes and a healthier perspective.

It's normal to experience some shifts in your relationships as you become more self-aware and regulated. By understanding your needs better, you can choose how much to work on existing relationships and when to find new ones that fit your new way of thinking and feeling. Paying attention to your body and emotions can help you figure out which relationships provide the support and love you need.

Your bodily state serves as a powerful tool for evaluating relationships. It can guide you toward making connections that meet your needs for regulation and love—and away from those that don't. By tuning in to your body and observing how you feel in the presence of others, you recognize the level of safety and support each relationship provides. If you can understand and rely on your bodily responses and nervous system cues, you can choose to be with people who regulate with you in a reciprocal way. This can enhance resilience and regulation for both people in the relationship.

To make this happen, it's crucial to learn and practice fostering connections that feel safe to you. However, you may face challenges along the way. In the next section, I discuss some common struggles in achieving safe and supportive connections and how to overcome them.

From Empathy to Compassion

If you have higher sensitivity, you possess a unique capacity to understand or feel what other people are experiencing. The world needs caring and empathetic individuals like you. However, being attuned to others can also come with an immense amount of struggle. Continually picking up on others' emotions can take a lasting toll on your nervous system. Not only can you feel the positive emotions of others, but you also pick up on negative emotions, which can affect your well-being.

You may even have difficulty distinguishing which emotions are yours and which belong to someone else. This can lead to struggles with emotional dysregulation, anxiety, and difficulty separating your emotional state from others'. Your sensitive nervous system might often be hyperaware, continuously scanning the environment for cues of other people's emotional and nervous system states.

Empathy is your natural ability to connect with and feel others' emotions, whether they're reassuring or distressing. It's a key skill and has an important place in connection with others. However, when you become overwhelmed by the suffering of others, you can experience "empath burnout," "empath shutdown," or "compassion fatigue," terms that highlight the result of experiencing what researchers call "empathic distress." If you find yourself experiencing signs of emotional overwhelm and exhaustion, as well as disconnection, cynicism, and detachment, you'll feel the need to withdraw to protect yourself from those negative emotions. You can benefit significantly from practicing the skill of switching from empathic distress to compassion, where you feel love and care for others while they are suffering rather than feeling their suffering with them.

Compassion is the ability to hold a safe space for other people's emotions while experiencing feelings of warmth, concern, and care. When you feel compassion, you do not want people to suffer and you feel motivated to improve their well-being. Unlike empathy, which researchers describe as a self-related emotion, compassion is relating to others and characterized by feelings such as love and kindness. Developing compassion is essential for a healthy, connected, and regulated nervous system, especially for sensitive people.

"Compassion" can be defined as a process with five critical elements related to both self-compassion and compassion for others:

1. Recognizing when others are suffering
2. Appreciating that everyone suffers—even the most fortunate people are still susceptible to sickness and aging, and will eventually die
3. Feeling attuned to the person suffering
4. Staying open in the face of their suffering, even when they're experiencing extremely uncomfortable feelings such as anger or fear
5. Feeling motivated to act whenever possible to ease someone's suffering

Research has shown that you can train your brain to develop compassion, even when faced with others' distress. Just a few days of compassion training can lead to increased positive feelings and brain activity. This training not only promotes your connection with others but also boosts feelings of joy and fulfillment, and increases resilience, helping you cope better with stress.

All the work you've already done to regulate your nervous system can also help move you from empathy to compassion. By staying flexible and returning to a calm state under stress, you can remain regulated when those around you are not, which makes you a lot more helpful to others in stressful situations than if you also were dysregulated.

Shame, Self-Criticism, and the Quest for Compassion

In my work with sensitive people, I often find that they are extremely empathetic, but struggle with compassion, especially self-compassion. Why is it that we don't naturally gravitate toward developing more kindness and compassion toward ourselves and others?

While compassion toward others and toward yourself might feel disconnected, it turns out that you can't be compassionate toward others if you are not compassionate toward yourself first. In scientific studies on self-compassion, people who score high in self-compassion tend to live healthier, more fulfilling, authentic lives. When you apply compassion to yourself, you can reap its wonderful benefits both as a giver and as a receiver.

It's hard to open your heart to compassion if you have never experienced this sense of safety, connection, and unconditional acceptance from others. Most people are much more familiar with self-criticism than self-compassion, tending toward coldness toward themselves, or even believing they are unworthy of compassion. These feelings are rooted in shame.

If you carry this baggage of shame, it can be hard to open your heart to kindness, compassion, and love for yourself. Our culture and upbringing are filled with messages of shame. But shame is often also part of our childhood experience. If you grew up feeling neglected, unseen, or your unique sense of self wasn't delighted in and celebrated by your caregivers, it's almost impossible not to internalize a sense of shame.

When a child's attachment needs are not sufficiently met by their caregivers, especially the need for attunement and expressed delight, they subconsciously assume there must be something wrong with them, and they must be undeserving of compassion. What's more, this can happen to just certain "parts" of yourself, meaning that your primary sense of self might not have internalized much shame, but some of your innate desires and behaviors, such as your desire for power, your need for emotional connection, or your sexuality, might feel deeply ashamed and unworthy.

To heal from the grip of shame, you need to learn that your needs matter, that it was not your fault that your needs were not met in the past, and that you can hold yourself and others in this space of kindness and compassion. You need to internalize the feeling that you are worthy of being loved fully and unconditionally.

Self-compassion means actively moving toward these painful feelings of shame and being in the moment with them, even when they're uncomfortable. It's putting your head completely into the mouth of the demon, like Milarepa, and saying, "Eat me, if you wish." Right here, in this body of yours, in this moment, you can allow yourself to feel all your unmet needs that have been shut down. You don't need to linger in your personal suffering, but, instead, open yourself to the reality that everyone suffers and is connected in this place of suffering.

Using Boundaries to Overcome Enmeshed Relationships

Growing up, you may have internalized the idea that setting boundaries isn't acceptable or fair to others. You might have learned that saying "no" to your caregivers could

>> DO THIS

CULTIVATE COMPASSION THROUGH EMPATHETIC REFLECTION

1. **Become aware.** Become aware of your internal voice and notice when you engage in self-talk, particularly if it's negative or self-critical.
2. **Pause.** When you find yourself in the act of negative self-talk, gently pause and take a deep breath to create a space for reflection.
3. **Imagine a loved one.** Visualize someone you care deeply about, like a friend, family member, or pet. Bring their image to mind and feel the love and care you have for them.
4. **Change perspective.** Imagine that the situation or circumstance you're experiencing is happening to your loved one instead of you. How would you speak to them in this situation?
5. **Write it down.** Write down the supportive and compassionate words you would say to your loved one in this circumstance. Pay attention to the tone, language, and encouragement you offer.
6. **Apply it to yourself.** Read the words you've written and imagine saying these compassionate and supportive words to yourself. Allow yourself to receive the kindness and empathy you would extend to a loved one.
7. **Practice regularly.** Incorporate this practice into your daily life. The more you practice, the more natural it will become to treat yourself with the same kindness and understanding you show others.

Remember, it takes time and consistent effort to shift your internal dialogue toward a more compassionate and supportive tone. Be patient with yourself and celebrate the progress you make as you cultivate a kinder, more empathetic inner voice.

reduce their ability or desire to care for you. A family dynamic with blurred emotional boundaries, where saying "no" feels uncomfortable or unsafe, is called "enmeshment." Enmeshed family dynamics often stem from caregivers' own unmet emotional needs and heavy reliance on their children for emotional support. For the child, the blurred boundaries of an enmeshed relationship with their caregiver can lead to a lack of autonomy, personal identity, and emotional independence.

The belief you may have learned in childhood, that having boundaries in a relationship is bad, wrong, or even dangerous, can become deeply ingrained. It's very easily carried into adult relationships, such as friendships, work relationships, and especially romantic relationships. It takes hard work to become aware of this belief, feel the fear in your body of setting a boundary, and reassure yourself that, now that you're an adult, it's actually okay to set boundaries. But to cultivate relationships in adulthood that support your long-term nervous system regulation, you need to relearn that having boundaries in relationships that are respected by both parties is safe and healthy.

Setting boundaries for the first time with people in your life can be incredibly challenging. A deeply ingrained part of you was programmed by evolution for millions of years to fear abandonment, and setting boundaries can reignite that primal fear of being abandoned. Setting healthy boundaries will require you to reassure that part of you that fears abandonment, and hold it with love and compassion. It takes courage, firmness, and lots of forgiveness for yourself and others to navigate relationships based on boundaries. If you're in connections with others who are enmeshed, they may initially also react negatively when you set boundaries, so it's important to stay strong and patient. With time, practice, and self-compassion, you can become skilled at setting boundaries and having them respected.

One of my mentors, Jerry Colonna, taught me a simple yet powerful seven-word phrase that helps me confront the fear of saying no: "I wish I could, but I can't." By using this phrase when necessary, you can start to build relationships based on genuine connection between two separate and unique individuals, rather than a merging of two individuals into one undifferentiated system.

Here are some guidelines for setting effective boundaries:

1. Always back up boundary setting with action and consequences. For example, if you say that you have only five minutes to talk on the phone, take action to end the conversation after five minutes.
2. Be direct, firm, and gracious.
3. Don't debate, defend, or overexplain your boundaries.
4. Have support readily available, especially in the beginning.
5. Stay strong, and don't give in.

Remember, setting healthy boundaries is essential for your emotional well-being and the quality of your relationships.

Rupture and Repair

We start learning to decipher human faces and expressions as soon as we're born. Even in infancy, one of your brain's top priorities was to figure out how to form connections with others and mend them when they break. Infants' and children's nervous systems use their caregivers' facial expressions as one way to know whether they can relax into a safe connection where they'll be cared for, or whether they need to be vigilant and keep trying to get their needs met. When the caregiver's and baby's facial expressions match, that signals to the infant that they are safe, connected, and can rest into the green state.

You might think that a healthy caregiver and their infant would mostly match each other's facial expressions when they looked at each other, but mismatched facial expressions are, in fact, very important for the baby to develop a regulated nervous system. Developmental psychologist Edward Tronick performed a well-known experiment called the "still face experiment," which demonstrated how babies learn from interactions with their mothers' facial expressions to regulate their nervous systems. Tronick found that in the healthy mother-child relationships that he measured, the mother and child were in sync only about 30 percent of the time. The rest of the time was spent as a dance of rupture, where the mother's and the child's facial expressions didn't match, and repair, where one or both individuals found a way to rematch the other. Practicing this kind of rupture and repair interaction over and over equips a child with a flexible nervous system. Their nervous system learns how to come into synchrony with another person's nervous system, and that the synchrony can lead them back to the green state.

Ruptures in relationships, like misunderstandings, disagreements, or conflicts, are an inevitable part of being in connection with another human. Partners in thriving relationships don't avoid ruptures; instead, they're experts at repairing the connection after a rupture happens.

If your caregivers didn't model the skill of repair effectively during your early development, navigating interpersonal conflicts later in life can be much more challenging. The art of repair is like a blueprint we carry within us. It guides us in mending those moments of rupture—from tiny misunderstandings to big arguments. If this blueprint is missing or incomplete, conflict can feel like a maze with no exit.

Let's explore some examples of parental styles that don't lead to repair:

- **The avoidant parent:** This parent tends to shy away from conflict at all costs. When a disagreement arises, they might change the subject, crack a joke, or leave

>> DO THIS

BOUNDARY SETTING 101: A PRACTICAL APPROACH

1. **Identify the situation.** Identify a specific situation for which you want to establish a boundary, for example, with a friend who constantly asks you for advice on their personal issues, which leaves you feeling drained.
2. **Use first person language.** Begin your statement using "I," "my," or "mine." This centers the conversation on your feelings and needs, reducing the chances of the other person getting defensive. For example, "I've noticed that our conversations often revolve around your personal issues."
3. **State your feelings.** Describe your emotional and physical sensations regarding the situation. This can help create an empathetic connection with the other person. For example, "When this happens, I feel drained and overwhelmed."
4. **State your needs.** Clearly express what you want in the situation, focusing on the positive. For example, "I need our conversations to be more balanced, which will help me enjoy our connection more."
5. **Describe your desired outcome.** Explain what your boundary looks like in practice. For example, "What that might look like is us taking turns to share and discuss our personal issues."
6. **Practice.** Prepare yourself to express this boundary in real life. Practice saying it out loud or write it down several times to make sure you're comfortable with the phrasing.
7. **Implement.** When you feel ready, have the conversation with the person involved. Remember to stay firm, emphasizing the importance of this boundary for your well-being.

So your final statement might be: "I've noticed that our conversations often revolve around your personal issues. When this happens, I feel drained and overwhelmed. What I need is for our conversations to be more balanced. What that might look like is us taking turns to share and discuss our personal issues."

the room. The child, observing this behavior, never witnesses how a conflict can be addressed and resolved healthily.

- **The volatile parent:** This parent's emotions can be explosive and unpredictable. They might overreact to minor disagreements, escalating them into major conflicts. The child learns to tread carefully to avoid triggering these explosions, which doesn't teach them how to face and resolve conflicts in a calm, measured way.
- **The silent treatment parent:** When this parent is upset, they might retreat into cold silence, refusing to discuss the problem or engage in resolution. The child learns that conflicts lead to emotional abandonment, rather than being opportunities for growth and understanding.
- **The placating parent:** This parent always aims to keep the peace, often at their own expense. They might say they agree with the other person, even when they don't feel in agreement, just to avoid conflict. The child learns to suppress their feelings and needs in conflict situations, rather than expressing them openly and working toward a compromise.
- **The defensive parent:** This parent immediately becomes defensive in the face of conflict, turning the blame onto others rather than accepting responsibility for their part in the disagreement. The child learns to deflect or deny responsibility in conflicts, which hampers the process of understanding, reconciliation, and repair.

In each example, the child doesn't learn the healthy sequence of rupture and repair. Without learning that repair is possible, and even easy most of the time in a collaborative relationship, they learn to fear or avoid ruptures at all costs, or to handle them in noncollaborative ways, like dominating the other person, to get their needs met.

If you didn't learn how to repair ruptures as a child, then as an adult in conflict, you might just feel lost, scared, angry, or defensive. You might go to great lengths to avoid these uncomfortable situations altogether because you don't have a strategy to handle them.

But it's never too late to learn. Just as you can learn a new language or a new skill, you can learn to face conflict in a healthy way instead of avoiding it. One especially beautiful thing about learning to repair connections is that it helps you build much stronger, deeper relationships. Every time you repair a rupture, you're also saying, "Our connection matters to me, and I'm willing to work for it."

Navigating Rupture: A Practical Example of Relationship Repair

After a demanding day at work, Mia walks into the house. Her shoulders are sagging, her steps slow and heavy. She glances toward the kitchen sink and finds it piled with dirty dishes. Alex, her partner, had promised to wash them, but he hadn't. Mia's frustration surges and she snaps, "Why can't you ever do what you say you're going to do?" The rupture started when Alex neglected his commitment to Mia to clean the dishes, and Mia's sudden outburst intensified the rupture.

Alex, caught off guard, feels a knee-jerk defensiveness well up. He retorts, "Well, I was busy, too, you know!" The temperature in the room rises a few degrees as the rupture escalates.

However, after a few moments of uncomfortable silence, Alex starts to reflect. He realizes that their connection and mutual respect are far more important than defending his inaction. This realization sets the stage for the repair process, which they navigate together through several steps:

1. **Acknowledgment:** Alex breaks the silence, "Mia, I see you're upset, and I can understand why." He's acknowledging Mia's feelings, which is a crucial first step. "And you're right," he continues, "I promised to do the dishes, and I didn't. That was wrong and you probably felt disrespected when I didn't stick to my agreement." By doing so, he admits his mistake, contributing to the acknowledgment process.

   Mia, feeling heard and validated, feels safe to acknowledge her part in escalating the rupture. She says, "I got reflexively mad at you as soon as I saw the dirty dishes. I've had a stressful day, and I took it out on you, which wasn't fair." Here, Mia is also taking responsibility for her part in the conflict, another crucial element in the repair process.

2. **Intention:** Alex then clarifies his intention, saying, "It wasn't my aim to make you feel disregarded, Mia, I just lost track of time. I should've prioritized better."

3. **Apology:** Next comes the apology. Alex looks at Mia and says sincerely, "I regret not keeping my promise, and I'm sorry for causing you frustration." This apology is specific, and Alex takes full responsibility for his actions without trying to shift blame or justify his behavior. Mia also apologizes for snapping at Alex.

4. **Learning:** Alex then shares what he will do differently next time, saying, "I wasn't taking into account the way coming home to these dirty dishes that I committed to do would make you feel. Your feelings matter to me, so next time I'll manage my time better to make sure I can keep my commitments to you."

5. **Amend:** As a final step, Alex amends the situation by committing to do the dishes as soon as their conversation is over. He also makes a friendly joke about how good Mia is at sticking to commitments, which helps her feel seen and

respected again. They finish the repair feeling connected and loving toward each other again.

Alex does the dishes, and they decide to sit down and talk about how they can manage household chores better in the future to balance both of their needs. This conversation signifies the repair process, with both of them working together to prevent similar ruptures.

The key aspects of this story are the couple's commitment to their connection, willingness to admit mistakes, readiness to apologize, and efforts to prevent future ruptures. These elements combined create a healthy cycle of rupture and repair, reinforcing their bond and teaching them to navigate future conflicts effectively.

How Changing Perspective Can Improve Social Connections

Imagine you're wearing a pair of glasses that makes everything look less friendly or more challenging. You might start to feel uncomfortable or agitated by social connections. When you're around groups of people, you might feel as though you're on the outside looking in, like you're not totally safe and don't quite belong. This further exacerbates feelings of loneliness and disconnection, even when people surround you.

The lens through which you view your social interactions can significantly shape the outcomes of your interactions. Sometimes your lens becomes a self-fulfilling prophecy; for example, holding a distorted view that nobody likes you might cause you to act defensively toward others and make them less likely to enjoy your company. Scientific studies have shown that by adjusting your social lens from a threat-oriented perspective, where people are out to get you, to a more collaborative one, where others are seen as potential friends or cooperative partners, you can reduce your sense of loneliness.

When you're aware of your perspective and make conscious efforts to change it, you can start to feel more connected and less isolated. This change in outlook can make a huge difference in improving social connections and enhancing overall health, nervous system regulation, and happiness.

Breaking Free from the Comparison Trap

Comparison is an innate human experience. It's something we all do, often without even realizing it. We compare ourselves to others to better understand our place in the world and our identity. However, the act of comparing can sometimes lead us down a path of self-doubt and isolation because we tend to overestimate others' happiness and underestimate their struggles, making us feel alone in our own challenges.

The way you compare yourself to others can significantly affect your attitude, behavior, health, motivation, and overall well-being. It can put you within a hierarchy where you're constantly striving to climb higher, often at the expense of your peace of mind. But it doesn't have to be this way. By understanding how comparison affects you, you can navigate the natural tendency to compare yourself to others in a healthier way.

When your mind starts to compare yourself to others, imagine it's like getting on a circular balance board. You could come down in many directions. In some of these directions you'll find yourself in a comparison trap and in it you feel threatened and unsafe. The comparison trap triggers your fight-or-flight response and clouds your judgment. One outcome of the comparison trap is landing in a direction where you adopt a competitive stance, in which you feel superior to others and see people as "beneath you." Another direction of the trap has you perceiving yourself as "not measuring up" or unworthy, and here you might feel anger, fear, or shame.

Alternatively, you could come down from the balancing board in the direction of curiosity. Since the Awareness stage, you've been practicing curiosity and compassion. Curiosity allows you to observe and understand yourself and the world around you without judgment. It enables you to acknowledge thoughts, emotions, and physical sensations with an open mind. As you navigate the experience of comparison, curiosity can guide you toward compassion for yourself and others, promoting a sense of acceptance and cooperation.

Just as learning to balance on a balance board means falling and then getting back up, you can notice whenever you've fallen into the comparison trap and shift to curiosity. When you find yourself in the midst of comparison, take a moment to shift from dog mind to lion mind. Ask yourself, "What am I feeling right now?" If you notice yourself feeling unsafe or uncomfortable, you can use the portals from the Regulation stage to invite in a sense of safety.

Once you no longer feel overwhelmed by uncomfortable feelings, you can get curious about the reasons that comparison might be coming up. For example, comparison can stem from an admiration or desire for qualities or achievements, such as status, recognition, financial stability, self-assuredness, social attention, or a spirit of adventure. It's possible that within your upbringing or cultural background, these aspirations were subtly discouraged or not valued. However, such human needs and desires are common and natural. Noticing this, you might shift from a negative comparison where you feel envious of others to seeing their success in one of these areas as a gift that shows you more about what you want.

Another common reason our minds compare us to others is simply to understand our strengths and see how we fit into society. If you've cultivated enough background self-esteem to avoid the comparison trap, it can be extremely valuable to evaluate yourself and your strengths in comparison to others. Scientifically validated personality tests, like the Big Five Personality Test, are one way you can better understand yourself and how you compare to others in a nonjudgmental manner. But if you find yourself sliding into a negative self-evaluation or start feeling bad in your body, that may be a sign that you need to cultivate more background self-esteem before social comparison will be helpful. Returning to the attachment practices in the Restoration stage, especially the core attachment need of expressed delight, is one of the most powerful ways to cultivate self-esteem.

Comparison is a normal human social behavior and it's not inherently bad, but without a solid background of self-esteem, you can fall into the comparison trap. Getting stuck in the comparison trap can lead to unhealthy social interactions and less nervous system regulation.

To shift out of the comparison trap, continue to cultivate self-esteem from the Restoration stage practices. And, in the moment your mind starts comparing, switch to a curious lion mind instead of a threatened dog mind. With self-esteem and curiosity, comparison can be a healthy, even enjoyable, activity that lets you discover more about your desires, needs, and personality.

The Loneliness Cure: Personal Action and Societal Change

Feeling lonely can take a big toll on our health. Some research shows that not having enough social interactions might raise your chances of an early death by a hefty 50 percent. Loneliness significantly increases your stress levels and plays a major role in the pinball effect that contributes to nervous system dysregulation. But there's a lot we can do to deal with loneliness.

Think of it like a two-step dance: Step one is about us as individuals. It involves taking all the steps I have described so far in this book. Step two is about getting connected with others—join group activities, become part of support groups, or take part in community efforts like shared meals, gardening projects, or classes. And in today's digital age, we can even use online programs to connect to a like-minded community.

Although addressing loneliness at the individual level is important, many of our social policies and cultural habits affect how likely you are to be lonely. Local governments can implement policies that address social isolation, such as funding for mind-body health resources or initiatives to promote community participation. They can change zoning laws to encourage more "third places," or comfortable locations outside of home and work where people can gather socially with the intent to spend time together rather than consume goods. Public spaces that facilitate social interaction, like parks, community centers, and libraries, are some examples of third places that can help bring people together. Medical professionals could also integrate questions about social connection into routine health checkups. By identifying people who

PRACTICAL STRATEGIES TO INCREASE SOCIAL CONNECTEDNESS

Collective Activation	Shared Experiences
• Attending a music festival or concert	• Joining peer support groups
• Participating in a religious or spiritual event	• Organizing or attending shared meals
• Going to sports events	• Engaging in community gardening
• Engaging in activism and political action	• Taking part in book clubs
• Enrolling in group exercise classes	• Joining hobby or interest groups
• Attending cultural events or art exhibitions	• Volunteering for local organizations
• Participating in community theater or performance art	• Attending workshops or classes
• Going to social dance events	• Hosting or joining game nights
• Attending local community festivals	• Participating in neighborhood cleanups
• Joining group travel or adventure trips	• Engaging in skill-sharing sessions
• Participating in group meditation or yoga sessions	• Organizing or attending potluck dinners
• Attending comedy shows or open mic nights	• Joining local sports or recreational teams
• Going to trivia nights at local venues	• Participating in community art projects
• Joining a community choir or musical ensemble	• Engaging in collaborative DIY projects
• Participating in themed social events or parties	• Attending caregiving groups
• Visiting outdoor art installations or sculpture parks	• Taking part in nature photography outings
• Attending outdoor concerts or live music events	• Joining an *en plein air* painting group
• Participating in nature walks or forest bathing	• Organizing or attending outdoor film nights
• Going on group bird-watching or wildlife tours	• Engaging in creative writing groups
• Taking part in outdoor art or music workshops	• Attending or organizing group poetry readings

may be experiencing loneliness, they could help facilitate connection as part of someone's overall health plan. Companies can set up programs to foster social connections among employees, such as team-building activities, mentorship programs, or communal spaces for breaks. They can also provide health resources and foster a culture that supports work-life balance.

While we can all contribute to social policies and culture that increase social connections and reduce loneliness through our actions, conversations, advocacy, and votes, to help reduce your loneliness you need practical strategies you can implement right now to find more of a sense of social connection that feels fulfilling and meaningful to you. I've put together a list of examples of practical strategies to get your juices flowing. Use this list for ideas of the kinds of experiences you might enjoy to increase your sense of social connectedness. The experiences include both collective activations, or events, where you can feel part of a bigger group, and shared experiences, where you can connect in a more intimate context that could facilitate building individual or group friendships.

CONNECTION WITH NATURE

When I was growing up in Italy, one of the milestones for every kid, including me, was learning Italian poems by heart. It was our introduction, our rite of passage, into the rich tradition and literature of our homeland. Despite my aversion to memorization, learning St. Francis's famous poem, "Canticle of the Creatures," has become a cherished memory of my childhood. I remember drawing St. Francis, his humble figure etched against the backdrop of vast forests, chatting away with the birds, wolves, and sheep.

St. Francis of Assisi was a beloved Italian friar who lived in the thirteenth century. His profound connection with nature was so intrinsic to his worldview that he considered all creation to be part of his family. Here's what he wrote in "Canticle of the Creatures" that had such an impact on me as a child:

> Be praised, my Lord, through all your creatures,
> especially through my lord Brother Sun,
> who brings the day; and you give light through him.
> And he is beautiful and radiant in all his splendor!
>
> Of you, Most High, he bears the likeness.
> Praised be You, my Lord, through Sister Moon and the stars,
> in heaven you formed them clear and precious and beautiful.

Praised be You, my Lord, through Brother Wind,
and through the air, cloudy and serene,
and every kind of weather through which you give sustenance to Your creatures.

Praised be You, my Lord, through Sister Water,
which is very useful and humble and precious and chaste.

Praised be You, my Lord, through Brother Fire,
through whom you light the night and he is beautiful
and playful and robust and strong.

Praised be You, my Lord, through Sister Mother Earth,
who sustains us and governs us and who produces
varied fruits with colored flowers and herbs.

This poem isn't just a prayer or a poem: It is a lesson in love, respect, and harmony. It's a lesson that has stayed with me all these years.

St. Francis saw "Sister Mother Earth" as a nurturing mother, a figure that sustains and governs. Seeing Earth as a "sister" and a "mother" illustrates St. Francis's profound comprehension of our connection to the natural world. He recognized that we are not separate from nature; all of the creatures on earth are children of the same mother, sharing the same resources she provides. He referred to the sun as "Brother Sun," the moon as "Sister Moon," and so on, illustrating his deep sense of connection and, importantly, *equality* with all elements of nature. This relationship wasn't one of domination or exploitation but of mutual respect and appreciation.

Scientific investigation into the effects of our relationship with nature is beginning to echo the ancient wisdom—that connection with nature matters for our nervous system health. One theory of nature's effects on the nervous system, called the stress reduction theory, comes from a famous 1984 study in which researcher Roger Ulrich observed that hospital patients with a window looking out at a natural setting recovered faster and with less pain after surgery than patients without a nature view. Since then, significant additional evidence has corroborated and expanded the theory. Studies have shown that people who spend time in natural settings are less stressed, have a more positive outlook, and generally feel better about life than those who spend most of their time in man-made environments.

Another acclaimed model to explain nature's profound impact on our nervous system is University of Michigan psychologists Stephen Kaplan and Rachel Kaplan's attention restoration theory. The Kaplans collected considerable data showing how nature can help us recover from the mental fatigue that comes with our fast-paced, modern lives. According to the Kaplans' theory, nature can provide our busy attention systems with a gentle distraction that allows us to relax and recharge. Nature, with its tranquil sights and sounds, captures our attention in a soft and subtle way. This "soft fascination," as scientists call it, doesn't demand any mental effort. It simply allows your overworked mind to take a breather, so you can come back refreshed and ready to tackle tasks with renewed focus and energy.

Imagine walking in a forest, your senses fully engaged. You hear the rustling leaves underfoot, the distant call of a bird, the wind brushing past the trees. You see the vibrant hues of green in the foliage, the play of light and shadow. You smell the earthy scent of soil, the crisp freshness of leaves, the subtle fragrance of wildflowers. You feel the texture of bark under your fingers, the cool breeze on your skin, the uneven ground beneath your feet. And if you're lucky, you might taste the sweet tartness of a wild berry or the freshness of spring water.

As we open our senses to the natural world, we begin to notice things we might have previously overlooked: the intricate pattern of a leaf's veins, the soft cooing of a dove, the way the sunlight filters through the forest's canopy. Over time, we will become more aware of nature's rhythms and cycles, and our place within them. This deepening connection with nature fosters a sense of peace and tranquility. It can feel like coming home. This sense of coming home to our place within the natural world, rather than feeling separate from it, is the *essence* of connection with nature.

CONNECTION TO BEAUTY AND CREATIVITY

In the rugged peaks of Tibet, a seven-year-old and a twelve-year-old are making their mark, pressing tiny hands and bare feet onto soft limestone, their giggles echoing through the mountains. Unbeknownst to them, their playful mosaic will survive two hundred thousand years, their innocent act bearing a deeper, symbolic message about the meaning of their existence. This mosaic, described in a study recently published by David D. Zhang and his team, is a testament to the primal nature of art. Other studies have also revealed forms of prehistoric art from Indonesia and Europe dating back forty thousand years. Together these discoveries remind us that creativity and the creation and appreciation of beauty are ancient human instincts to bridge our nervous systems out beyond ourselves. They can help connect our deepest nature with the world around us, and even beyond that, to the great mysteries life, the universe, and existence itself.

>> DO THIS

TAKE A SENSORY FOREST BATH

This practice is inspired by Lyanda Lynn Haupt's "Staying Dirty During a Forest Bath" in her book *Rooted*. You can use a sensory forest bath to calm your nervous system and shift it from red or yellow to green. You might be surprised at how quickly and easily your nervous system shifts down to green with just this short and simple practice.

If you do this practice consistently, you might start to notice a much more significant shift in your relationship with the natural world. The earth can become another foundation into which your nervous system is grounded or rooted. Like a loving mother, it's always there, ready to support you, comfort you, and hold all your tension or worries. By regularly doing sensory forest baths, you can strengthen this connection with the natural world.

Strolling through the forest isn't just about stretching your legs or filling your lungs with fresh air. It's about letting your senses take the reins and fully experiencing what the forest has to offer.

- Start by letting your feet guide you. Feel the rough texture of the forest floor beneath your shoes, the crunch of leaves, the snap of twigs. Let the sensation of mossy patches surprise you, like a secret invitation to stray from the path.

- Don't shy away from the bushes that brush against your arms as you pass. Their leaves create a gentle tickle, like nature whispering, "Hello." Maybe you're lucky enough to have a delicate butterfly perch on your hand for a moment, a fleeting feeling, like a secret handshake with the forest.

- Let your nose lead you too. Inhale the rich scent of damp earth, the tangy fragrance of pine, and the sweet perfume of wildflowers. Each breath is like a conversation with the forest; each scent tells you a different story.

- Listen to the forest's soundtrack. The rustling leaves, the distant birdcalls, the soft murmur of a nearby stream—these are the forest's lullabies. They're the forest's way of sharing its secrets with you, if you're willing to listen.

- Keep your eyes wide open—take in the mosaic of green hues, the dappled sunlight filtering through the leaves, the sudden flash of a squirrel darting up a tree. Each sight is a gift from the forest, a glimpse into its heart.

continued on following page

>> DO THIS *CONTINUED*

- And taste? Yes, taste the forest too. The slightly tangy taste of the air after a rain, or the sweet berry you plucked from a bush—the forest has a flavor all its own.

- During this time, guide your mind to truly engage with the forest around you. Take time to focus on the minutiae, the tiny details that make the forest a living, breathing entity. You're not just standing amid the trees. You're intertwined with the woodland, syncing with its pulse, its vitality, its core. Allow your mind to be gently captivated by the subtleties—this is the essence of soft fascination.

- By the end of your forest bath, you may feel like a part of the forest has seeped into your being, leaving you feeling more grounded, connected, and alive. Anyone who sees you will wonder where you've been and feel a longing to follow in your footsteps.

The impact of art on the nervous system is the subject of considerable recent research in neuroaesthetics, a new field of scientific research that combines neuroscience, art history, and psychology to understand the relationship between art and our brains. Many activities of creating or appreciating beauty have been scientifically demonstrated to have positive benefits to the nervous system. Drawing or coloring, for instance, is a simple activity that can help dial down anxiety levels. Studies show that these activities can calm minds and even slow heart rates. It's not just for kids either. One study showed that mandala coloring helped reduce anxiety in older adults.

Mindfulness-based art therapy, which combines meditation practices with tactile art experiences, also has measurable benefits. It can improve sleep, reduce symptoms of anxiety and stress, and even lower blood pressure.

Engaging in poetry, whether by reading or writing it, fires up unique parts of our brain. The rhythm and sound patterns in poetry stimulate different areas of the brain than regular speech or writing do.

Visual art, such as drawing, painting, or sculpting clay, has a real and positive impact on the brain. Any form of visual creative expression, including activities as varied as cake decorating and scrapbooking, can activate the brain's reward pathway. One study even showed that creating art for forty-five minutes could significantly lower stress hormone levels, and this was true for both experienced and novice artists.

Then there's dance, an art form that involves the whole body. Research shows that dancers are more sensitive to emotions expressed through body movements. So whether you're a professional ballet dancer or just cutting a rug in your living room, dance can help you connect with your emotions and those of others.

Even the sound frequency of music can affect us, with research showing that music at 528 Hz can reduce stress and anxiety.

So whether you're painting a picture, writing a poem, or dancing to your favorite song, your nervous system can benefit from indulging in creative self-expression. Creativity and beauty can improve your regulation in the moment, making it easier to come back to a green state. And over time, engaging with beauty and doing creative activities can build another link that keeps your nervous system rooted and connected to the world around you.

Creative expression is a fundamental aspect of being human. By connecting with your innate creative instincts to make art, express yourself, or appreciate beauty, you open up your nervous system to deeper levels of connection between your most intimate self and the vibrant world around you, improving your overall regulation, flexibility, and resilience for the long term.

By the conclusion of the Connection stage, you'll find your nervous system significantly more flexible and regulated than it was at the beginning of the 5-Stage Plan. You might even be noticing that much of the damage your body accumulated from having a dysregulated nervous system for so long is starting to reverse. Don't get discouraged if you're not noticing a dramatic reduction in long-term symptoms. It took a long time for your body to accumulate this damage and reversing it isn't going to happen overnight. But now that your nervous system is regulated and connected to the world around you, it can finally repair itself and the other bodily systems that stopped functioning optimally, allowing your chronic symptoms to ease. As you start to feel better in your daily life, you have the opportunity to enter the final stage: Expansion.

The Expansion stage is not appropriate for your nervous system until it's relatively regulated on a daily basis. (You can always go back to chapter 1 and retest your current level of nervous system regulation.) One common mistake people make when they're not following a structured plan, like the 5-Stage Plan, is to do expansion practices, such as physical resilience enhancers and mindset practices, to expand their nervous system's capacity before it's fully regulated.

>> DO THIS

EXPRESS YOURSELF

Expressing yourself artistically can be a powerful way to cultivate a sense of connection and further increase your nervous system regulation. Here are some suggestions to help you engage with beauty and creative self-expression:

- **Explore various art forms:** There's no hierarchy in art. All forms, be it painting, sketching, dancing, writing, or music, have their unique charms and benefits. The key is to explore and experiment. For example, today you might resonate more with watercolor painting, capturing the vibrant colors of a sunset. Tomorrow, you might feel drawn to expressing yourself through poetry or immersing yourself in the rhythm of dance. The beauty of art is in its diversity, so don't restrict yourself.
- **Engage your senses:** Art is a multisensory experience. When painting, feel the brushstrokes on the canvas, notice the blend of colors, smell the paint, and listen to the ambient sounds around you. If you're dancing, pay attention to the feel of the floor beneath your feet, the rhythm of the music, and the way your body moves. By using all your senses, you deepen your connection to the activity and the world around you.
- **No expertise needed:** Don't worry if you're not an expert or a professional artist. You don't need to be. Art is a personal journey and it's the process of creation that matters, not just the results. So whether you're doodling on a notepad, strumming an unplugged guitar, or molding clay with your hands, remember it's about expression, not perfection.
- **Seek professional guidance:** If needed, consider seeking guidance from a professional art therapist who can provide a safe space for expression and help you explore how art can contribute to your well-being.
- **Make art a habit:** Consistency can enhance the benefits of art. Consider setting aside specific "art time" each week. This could be anything from an hour of drawing every Saturday morning to a five-minute daily doodling break.
- **Switch to lion mind:** Try to be present in the moment while creating. If you're writing a story, immerse yourself in the narrative. If you're dancing, let the movement and music guide you.
- **Express emotions through art:** Art can be an effective outlet for expressing emotions. For instance, if you're feeling stressed, you might want to create an intense, abstract painting with bold colors. If you're feeling calm and peaceful, you might prefer sketching a serene landscape.

- **Group art activities:** Consider participating in group activities such as a dance class, a community mural project, or a book club. It can foster a sense of community, stimulate new ideas, and add a social aspect to your art experience.

Remember, the aim is to enjoy the process of creating and to connect more deeply with yourself and the world around you. So pick up that paintbrush or coloring book, lace up those dancing shoes, or start writing in that notebook, and let your creativity flow.

Engaging in these practices too early can backfire, potentially hindering the healing process. However, when performed at the right time—once your nervous system is more regulated—these expansion practices can significantly increase the strength of the 4 Pillars of Nervous System Health, greatly enhancing your journey toward better health.

This is also the stage where I'll show you how to incorporate the fourth pillar, spirituality, or the connection to something larger than yourself. The practices I'll introduce in the Expansion stage will lead to more energy and vitality, and cultivate calmer mental states across all aspects of your life.

11

Stage 5: Expansion—Growing Your Capacity

WE'RE FINALLY HERE: the last stop on our journey toward healing nervous system dysregulation. Before we dive in, let's do a quick recap.

Before you started the 5-Stage Plan to Reverse Nervous System Dysregulation, you established a foundational set of daily habits and routines. These practices form a supportive structure, acting as your bedrock, particularly during challenging times in your healing journey.

The 5-Stage Plan started with *Awareness*, which focuses on becoming fully accepting of your physical and emotional pains—not rushing to fix them. By switching from dog mind to lion mind and maintaining an open and compassionate attitude, you practice understanding and accepting your pains for what they are. This stage in the plan is like pressing the "slow-motion" button on your reactions, providing the space to just be with them.

From Awareness, the plan adds *Regulation*. This is when you shift to start trusting your body again. Through somatic practices and emotional regulation, you face your triggers with less fear, less anxiety, and more curiosity, eventually gaining more agency over your thoughts, emotions, and physical sensations. This stage helps you learn to ride the waves of stressors without feeling powerless.

Next you add *Restoration*, where you face your deepest wounds and old coping strategies. It's a delicate process that requires a slow, careful approach. Yet, with patience, you're able to regenerate nervous system flexibility by reevaluating your coping strategies, training your nervous system in the regulation patterns you missed during childhood, addressing your embedded alarms, and getting back in touch with your intuition.

The fourth stage in the plan—*Connection*—is where you begin to experience a newfound sense of your own autonomy and individuality in relationships. This stage is all about getting along better with others and the world around you. You learn to keep emotions in check while still being compassionate. You get better at setting boundaries and find that you can be around people without feeling drained. Plus you experience the power of aligning with the natural world and your unique creative self-expression, strengthening your sense of interconnectedness with all of life.

And now, the final stage in the 5-Stage Plan to Reverse Nervous System Dysregulation, *Expansion*. This is where you push boundaries and see just how far you can go. It's about taking your strengths and using them to face life's unfolding with a sense of curiosity and courage. In this stage, you'll learn some of the best techniques available to expand your nervous system's capacity by pushing the boundaries of your mind, harnessing physical stress in the body to increase your nervous system health even further, and reveling in experiences of awe. Awe experiences are an excellent path to start cultivating the fourth pillar of nervous system health, spirituality, or connection with something greater than yourself. In this stage, your focus is on reinforcing all 4 Pillars of Nervous System Health. As these pillars grow stronger, they increasingly support your nervous system, enabling you to navigate the demands and challenges of living a fulfilling life more effectively.

THE JOURNEY TO EXPANDED CAPACITY

In chapter 4, I introduced the image of a cup filled with marbles and water, representing your capacity to handle stress flexibly without getting dysregulated. The water represents the current load of stress on your nervous system, and the number of marbles represents your sensitivity. If the water overflows the cup, your nervous system becomes dysregulated, and you'll eventually develop painful physical and mental symptoms.

Throughout the previous stages, your nervous system has been learning how to manage the amount of water in your cup. You've learned to recognize the amount of water in your cup (Awareness); how to pour water out of your cup (Regulation); how to manage the flow of new water coming into your cup (Restoration); and how to work with flows of water in the broader ecosystem with purpose, people, creativity, and nature (Connection). But in this final stage, you turn your attention to a different dimension of keeping your nervous system regulated: the size of your cup.

Imagine taking your cup full of marbles and pouring everything into a larger container, like a jug. This jug can hold all those beautiful marbles—those vivid

BUILDING MOMENTUM

KEEP PRACTICING WHAT YOU HAVE LEARNED

The journey of improving your nervous system health doesn't have a finish line, and the five stages aren't a to-do list on which you just tick off boxes. As you move through each stage, you don't leave the previous ones behind. Instead, you deepen your understanding and your skills. So while progressing from Awareness to Regulation, Restoration, Connection, and finally, Expansion, you'll continue to develop and deepen those previous stages. They remain part of you, unfolding and evolving as you grow and change.

Once you have gradually developed the capacity to self-regulate and connect with others confidently, the world is your oyster. You feel ready to venture outside of your comfort zone and thrive. I recommend slowly experimenting with the practices in this chapter as you feel called to them. Each will help you continue to expand your capacity to show up more fully in the world, in relationships, and in doing the activities that feel most meaningful to you. But give yourself plenty of grace along the way too.

Even once your nervous system has achieved a high level of flexibility, there will be times when you feel overwhelmed, or have difficulty coming back to the green state after being in yellow and red. So much of the modern world expects a linear pathway to success, but this simply isn't accurate. Just like breathing, a natural process of expansion and contraction is always happening in your nervous system's capacity, and it's only over the course of many cycles of expansion and contraction that your overall capacity grows. As you work with the practices in this Expansion stage, enjoy the waves of expansion and contraction. Instead of struggling against them, strive to navigate the waves like a ship that maintains its forward momentum, gracefully rising and falling with the ebb and flow of the seas.

characteristics of sensitivity—and still have room for even more liquid. By expanding your nervous system's capacity, you can hold on to all the beautiful facets of your sensitivity and still manage to handle stressors without your nervous system spilling over.

There are two strategies to expand your nervous system's capacity and increase the size of your cup: (1) focus on your body and enhance your physical adaptability; or (2) focus on your mind and boost your brain's ability to manage higher levels of stress without becoming overwhelmed. Both are extremely useful, and you can work on both at the same time.

First, I'll show you the body path—how to harness a moderate amount of temporary physical stress to expand your capacity.

HARNESSING STRESS FOR NERVOUS SYSTEM CAPACITY

When you experience a moderate level of stress for a relatively short period of time, and then come back down to the green state on your alertness elevator, your body will adapt by becoming stronger and more resilient to stress in the future. Your body has a built-in mechanism to adapt to stress called "hormesis," a process in which small doses of a harmful substance can actually be beneficial. Although stress is harmful in doses that are too high, such as when your nervous system is dysregulated, in the right doses, stress is actually very helpful for your nervous system health.

The key to hormesis is finding that optimal level of stress. Not too little stress, because your body needs some stress to stimulate growth and resilience, and not too much for too long, because excessive stress can lead to nervous system dysregulation and its associated health problems. Achieving this optimal level can help slow the aging process, stimulate the development of new neural pathways, and keep your nervous system healthy and thriving.

Scientific research on stress has shown that, with optimal levels of stress, your capacity to handle stress *can* improve significantly over time. As your body develops stronger adaptability to stress, you'll likely find that you're also growing in other areas of your life—increasing your sense of mastery, finding greater purpose, and boosting self-esteem. And these personal developments, in turn, further enhance your ability to handle future stressors.

HORMESIS: THE CATALYST FOR BODY ADAPTABILITY

Hormesis is the process by which our bodies become stronger and healthier in response to optimal levels of stress. Historically, our ancestors were exposed to multiple stressors, including extreme weather, physical exertion, and occasional food scarcity. This exposure to temporary, moderate stress led to the development of survival mechanisms over millions of years of evolution. Our modern lifestyles, however, lack many of these same challenges, which is one of the factors that contributes to weaker immune and metabolic systems. Hormesis interventions help rekindle these dormant survival mechanisms, enhancing your flexibility and resilience by bolstering your body's stress response systems. The controlled exposure to mild stress through these practices trains the nervous system to handle more intense, more substantial stressors.

Just as your muscles grow stronger through regular exercise, your resilience can be enhanced through regular exposure to controlled stressors. Before I show you some practical hormetic interventions and how they can be applied in your daily life to improve your nervous system's flexibility and resilience, let's look more closely at the science of how hormetic stressors increase nervous system health and when they're beneficial to introduce into your healing journey.

The Ripple Effect on the Body's Systems

Hormetic stressors activate a cascade of physiological responses: Your body responds to hormetic stress by strengthening cellular structures, enhancing metabolic processes to produce more energy in your cells, and bolstering your immune response. This equips your cells to handle the next stressful situation you encounter even more effectively.

In 2017, a group of scientists conducted an interesting experiment. They wanted to see whether exposing people to conditions similar to what our ancient ancestors experienced would have any effect on their health. So they took fifty-five healthy people on a ten-day journey through the Pyrenees Mountains. This wasn't a typical vacation, though. The participants had to walk about 9 miles (14 km) every day, carrying backpacks that weighed nearly 18 pounds (8 kg). They ate food they prepared themselves from wild, raw ingredients based on ancestral diets, such as berries, fruit, and animals they killed themselves. They drank water from natural sources, like local streams and waterholes. At night, they slept outdoors where temperatures could be anywhere from 53°F to 108°F (12°C to 42°C). By doing this, the researchers mimicked conditions our hunter-gatherer ancestors faced: exposure to physical exercise from walking, experiencing thirst and hunger, and adapting to different weather conditions. These are also examples of moderate hormetic stressors.

After the ten-day trip, the researchers checked the participants' health, paying special attention to metabolic functioning, or how well their bodies converted food into energy. Metabolic function is one of the major factors in the pinball effect that leads to a dysregulated nervous system.

Given the intensity and sheer physical challenge of the ten-day journey, you might expect that the participants' health would have declined and that they would need time back in the comforts of modern society to recover. But instead, the researchers found that the participants' health had improved. This experiment illustrates that exposing your body to moderate stressors, like our ancestors did, can actually improve your health and the functioning of your nervous system.

When Hormesis Practices Are Appropriate

Although the benefits of hormesis practices are undeniable, it's important to consider timing and strategy when incorporating them into your life. One of the most common mistakes I see people make in their healing journey is hearing about some new hormetic practice that's supposed to help them feel better, and them implementing it before regulating their nervous system, which could actually make symptoms worse.

These practices are not quick fixes or bypasses to avoid addressing deeper issues in your healing journey. That's why I introduce them in this final stage of the 5-Stage Plan, once you've done the hard work to regulate your nervous system. It's only once you've regulated your nervous system and can respond flexibly to stress that you should explore hormetic practices. If you're still in the early stages of healing and haven't yet established strong nervous system regulation, these stressors could easily be overwhelming and counterproductive.

Harnessing Hormesis in Everyday Life

Moving the body has been a fundamental aspect of your healing journey from the start, emphasized first in structure (chapter 6) and then in the use of portals (chapter 8). Muscles play a vital role in organizing and regulating your nervous system. As you progress and achieve greater regulation, the nature of your exercise regimen will evolve. Initially, the focus is on gentle activation and de-contraction of your body. However, as your symptoms become more manageable, the intensity of your exercises will increase. In this advanced stage, exercise serves less as a regulating mechanism and more as a form of hermetic stressor to further challenge and enhance your nervous system's resilience—expanding its capacity.

Vigorous physical exercise is the quintessential hormetic stressor. During exercise, cells in the cardiovascular and musculoskeletal systems are stressed as the demand on them increases. The cells respond by preparing to handle stress even more effectively in the future, enhancing overall resilience. Studies have shown that regular exercise can increase the odds of healthy aging by 39 percent.

Aim to incorporate vigorous exercise into your lifestyle, including both endurance activities, such as jogging or cycling, and strength-training exercises, such as lifting weights. Start with moderate exercise and increase the intensity gradually as your fitness improves.

High-Intensity Interval Training (HIIT)

High-intensity interval training is a type of exercise regimen that alternates between short periods of intense exercise and less intense recovery periods. The intense activity causes your cells to temporarily consume extra oxygen and produce more by-products, called "reactive oxygen species," which, in higher amounts, can damage cells. At moderate levels, however, reactive oxygen species activate a hormetic response and cause your cells to get cleaner and stronger. For example, moderate amounts of reactive oxygen species trigger the release of antioxidant enzymes and other protective mechanisms that neutralize harmful substances in your cells and make your cells more resilient to future stressors.

You can incorporate high-intensity interval training into your workouts by alternating short bursts of intense exercise (thirty seconds to two minutes) with less intense recovery periods (the same or double the amount of time you spent in the high-intensity burst). These workouts can be done with many types of exercise, including running, cycling, and bodyweight exercises.

Heat Therapy

Regular sauna usage can help the body cool down for proper sleep. Heat exposure activates DNA repair pathways, increases the activation of heat shock proteins, and lowers cortisol levels, contributing to an improved stress response and overall health. One of the simplest ways to gain the benefits of deliberate heat exposure is to use a sauna for a total of one hour per week, split into two or three sessions.

Cold Therapy

Brief exposure to cold temperatures, like taking cold showers or immersing yourself in the cold water of a lake or river, can improve immune function, metabolism, mood, and nervous system relaxation. It's especially beneficial in the morning to stimulate the body's natural warming process, which can help regulate your circadian rhythm.

Cold therapy also stimulates mitochondrial growth and replication, leading to more efficient energy production, and promotes the formation of heat shock proteins, protecting cells from stress-induced damage.

Wim Hof Method

This practice combines specific breathing techniques, cold exposure, and meditation. Wim Hof, also known as "the Iceman," teaches cycles of deep breaths followed by breath holds, which lead to temporary hypoxia, or a state of low oxygen, which causes a mild stress reaction. Much like exercise, the mild stress reaction of hypoxia stimulates a hormetic stress response. Wim Hof combines hypoxia with cold exposure, using regular cold showers or ice baths. The exposure to cold induces a stress response that boosts the immune system, improves circulation, and enhances mental focus. Finally, meditation is used to integrate the physiological and psychological responses to these stressors and practice feeling a sense of calmness and agency in the face of stress.

Hormetic Stress through Diet

Your diet is another way to stimulate your hormetic stress response. Plant-based foods, such as fruits, vegetables, beans, and grains, contain phytochemicals, compounds that plants produce to protect themselves from bacteria and fungi. Foods containing these phytochemicals cause a mild hormetic stress response in the body, which leads to increased resilience and longevity. For example, resveratrol, found in red wine and grapes, and sulforaphane, found in broccoli, are phytochemicals that stimulate a cellular stress response, leading to various health benefits.

Another way to use diet to stimulate a hormetic stress response is through temporarily reducing caloric intake or practicing intermittent fasting. These dietary practices trigger a type of mild metabolic stress that can improve metabolic efficiency, enhance cellular repair processes, and increase life-span.

To implement hormesis through diet, aim to consume a variety of plant-based foods, particularly those rich in beneficial phytochemicals, such as berries, dark chocolate, green tea, and olive oil. Consider incorporating practices like intermittent fasting or caloric restriction into your routine, but always consult with a health-care professional to adapt them to your needs.

CULTIVATING A SUPPORTIVE MINDSET

We've discussed how your body responds to stress and how to leverage hormesis to increase its capacity, but what about your mind? According to research, your understanding of stress also affects your ability to handle it, and can be another gateway to expanding your nervous system's capacity.

The idea of cultivating a "positive mindset" or doing "positive affirmations" has been thrown around loosely in popular culture, and is often associated with quick fixes or oversimplified solutions. Some influential figures use the idea of a positive mindset to imply that merely changing your attitude or outlook can magically erase deep-seated physiological problems. Consequently, this has led to a somewhat tarnished reputation for the concept of "mindset" in the context of healing a dysregulated nervous system.

As I've shown throughout this book, nervous system dysregulation is a complex issue that cannot be fixed simply by thinking positively. Nonetheless, once you've regulated your nervous system, working on your mindset can significantly help increase your nervous system's capacity.

So what exactly is a "mindset"? At its core, a mindset refers to the beliefs or assumptions you hold about different areas of life. Mindsets are like lenses through which you view the world, coloring your perceptions and experiences. They are shaped by various influences, including your upbringing, culture, media, influential people in your life, and even your conscious choices.

Dr. Alia Crum, an American psychologist who leads the Stanford Mind and Body Lab, describes mindset as "a portal between conscious and subconscious processes." Your mindset, she says, is like a "default setting of the mind." This means your mindset doesn't just affect how you consciously think about things, but it can also impact your subconscious reactions and behaviors.

Here's where it gets interesting. The beliefs you hold as part of your mindset can have real, tangible effects on the outcomes of your actions. For example, what you believe about stress can actually influence the way that stress impacts the physiological systems in your body. Clearing up misunderstandings about stress can improve your mindset, which, according to the research, has direct positive physiological impacts on your nervous system.

The Widespread Misunderstanding about Stress

Somewhere along the way, you've probably heard that stress is the enemy, something to be avoided at all costs—something that can only do harm. But that's a misunderstanding about stress. In fact, there's nothing wrong with experiencing stress. It's a natural response to challenges and adversity, and it's designed to prime your body for action.

Understanding that stress is a normal reaction that helps your nervous system meet the demands of life can shift your view of difficult events. Instead of seeing hard situations that cause you to feel stress as threats, you can begin to see them as challenges—with your stress response giving you more energy to meet those challenges. Your stress response helps prepare you for action, allowing you to process information faster, and your body to release hormones that help you grow muscle and learn. Simply recognizing that your stress response is trying to help you, rather than work against you, leads to measurable physiological benefits in your body.

The positive impact that understanding stress can have on your body isn't just wishful thinking. Research has shown that people who view stress as an opportunity for growth have better health outcomes, increased well-being, and higher overall performance. I'm not saying you should start celebrating every difficult situation you might experience, but you can recognize that your nervous system's stress response can be part of the solution and lead to better outcomes than if you had no stress response.

If you have a highly sensitive nervous system, redefining stress is especially important for you because your experience of stress is likely magnified. A project or task that might cause a moderate amount of stress in someone else could cause significant stress for you. You may have struggled a lot with stress in the past and you might even habitually avoid situations that put you in the yellow or red state.

The more you regulate your nervous system, however, the more you're able to reap the benefits of stress. By using the 5-Stage Plan, you've been building a tool kit of practices to come back to green after experiencing stress, so stressful situations no longer cause you to feel so scared or out of control. With a highly sensitive nervous system, just as the challenges of stress affect you more, you are also more responsive to the benefits of stress.

Once your nervous system is regulated, stress can be a great benefit. Stress is an indication that something about a situation matters to you, that you deeply care. Especially if you're highly sensitive, the right amount of stress can lead to more growth, more depth of processing, and more beauty, precision, or creativity in your work.

Some of the people I've seen make the most dramatic shifts in their lives by regulating their nervous systems and then redefining stress as additional energy that helps them face challenges include creatives, entrepreneurs, parents, people who volunteer, heads of nonprofits, and leaders of all kinds. When you're deeply engaged with people or projects that matter to you, the opportunities for stress are high, but so too are the opportunities for making a positive impact from the extra energy that stress can provide.

Making Stress Meaningful

Stanford health psychologist Kelly McGonigal says, "A meaningful life is a stressful life." This idea may seem counterintuitive, but think about the things that matter most to you. For many, it's our role as parents, partners, friends, or professionals. Now consider this: Don't these roles bring stress along with joy and satisfaction? Stress is not just an unavoidable negative part of life but it can also be a sign that we're living a life filled with purpose.

Take parenthood, for example. Raising a child comes with its fair share of stress. Yet it's also linked to a lot of smiling, laughing, and rich, meaningful experiences. But it's also incredibly challenging, demanding, and often a source of worry. This is the stress paradox—where the source of stress is also the source of joy.

We often believe we'd be happier if we were less stressed or less busy, but research indicates the opposite. People are generally happier when they're busy, even if they're juggling more tasks than they'd ideally like. A sudden decrease in busyness, like retirement, can even lead to an increased risk of depression.

Of course, not every stressful event brings meaning to your life, but you may be surprised to notice just how often you get stressed because you deeply care about a

>> DO THIS

WRITE DOWN YOUR VALUES

Psychologists Geoffrey Cohen and David Sherman analyzed more than fifteen years' worth of research and found that writing down your values can profoundly shift your capacity to handle stress. When you encounter a stressful situation, reminding yourself of your core values can be a powerful coping strategy.

In one study at the University of Waterloo, participants were given bracelets inscribed with "Remember your values." The results were remarkable—just wearing the bracelets helped them manage stress more effectively.

Here's a simple activity that can help you realize or remember the value these stressors bring to your life. To do this, get out a pencil and paper, or your journal, and find a quiet space where you can think without being disturbed. Set a timer for ten to fifteen minutes and put your phone on silent to help you stay focused on the task without getting distracted.

1. Think of a stressful role or event in your life.
2. Write about why this role or event is important to you. You might ask yourself, "What important things in life would be missing if I didn't take on these kinds of roles or participate in these types of events?"
3. From what you've just written, isolate one or more things that stood out to you. Examples of things that might stand out include values like compassion, taking care of your health, your children, connection, joy and excitement, or commitment to something greater than yourself.
4. Consider pinning a note on your laptop, changing the background screen or your phone, or taping an index card to your fridge or front door with the short reminder of these values. Alternatively, you could find objects that represent these values and put them around your house as a reminder of what matters to you.

Kelly McGonigal says that "remembering your values can help transform stress from something that is happening against your will and outside your control to something that invites you to honor and deepen your priorities." Stress can be a sign that you're living a life rich with meaning and purpose. By remembering your values when stressors arise, you can turn challenges into opportunities for personal growth and increase the overall capacity of your nervous system to handle intensity.

role you're taking on or an event you're participating in. Research shows that noticing and remembering why you're stressed, and how that connects to your values, can expand your capacity to handle that stress gracefully without becoming overwhelmed.

Living with the Unchangeable: Radical Acceptance

There are stressors in life that you didn't ask for, wish weren't there, and simply cannot be removed. For example, the stress of managing chronic illness cannot simply be removed or wished away.

One practical approach to these difficult situations is a practice called "radical acceptance." Radical acceptance is about fully acknowledging that something awful or life-altering has occurred. It's a mindset that willingly admits the truth: You can't rewrite what has happened. By embracing radical acceptance, you can soften the impact of distressing feelings, like guilt, shame, sorrow, and anger, that are tied to the difficult situation, allowing yourself to let go of the struggle against it. This frees up mental and emotional space and helps your nervous system adjust to your new reality.

Radical acceptance doesn't mean you condone or approve of what happened. Just because you accept something doesn't mean you morally endorse it or that you want it in your life. It just means you acknowledge reality as it is right now.

Let's say you had a tough childhood with an absent parent, a situation that caused you pain and is something you wish didn't happen. As an adult, those feelings of abandonment still affect you. Radical acceptance, in this case, isn't about forgiving or justifying what happened. Instead, it's about acknowledging the truth: Your parent wasn't there for you as a child, and that hurt. By acknowledging this, you're not saying the situation was right or fair. You're simply recognizing the reality of what happened. This act of recognition can help you process your emotions, heal, and move forward.

A 2019 review by psychologist Ekin Secinti and colleagues of the scientific research on acceptance practices for patients with cancer diagnoses found that patients who incorporated radical acceptance practices or similar activities into their daily life experienced less distress related to their condition.

Radical acceptance is different from resignation or having a "fighting spirit." Resignation is a passive response, where you believe there's nothing you can do about your situation, so you give up on ever improving your life. Having a "fighting spirit," on the other hand, is an active response to the situation and you keep trying to change it. Both engage with the future, predicting or trying to influence how the future might turn out. Unlike resignation or having a "fighting spirit," radical acceptance is about acknowledging what happened and what's true right now, before making any assessments about how the future might turn out.

Here are some practical life situations where radical acceptance may be helpful:

- **Stress of caregiving:** If you're caring for a loved one, the stress can be immense. Radical acceptance of your loved one's situation and your role now as their caregiver can help you acknowledge the difficulties without judgment and focus on the things you can control.
- **Chronic illness:** Whether you or a loved one is diagnosed with a chronic illness, radical acceptance can help with acknowledging the reality of the situation, letting go of "what ifs," and, instead, focusing on the best ways to manage the condition.
- **Loss of a loved one:** Experiencing the loss of someone dear is painful and difficult. Radical acceptance doesn't diminish this pain but allows you to accept the reality of the loss, helping you move through the grieving process.
- **End of a relationship:** Whether it's a romantic relationship, a friendship, or even a professional relationship, endings can be hard. Radical acceptance can assist you in acknowledging the end and moving forward.
- **Job loss or career change**: These events can be unexpected and challenging, particularly if they're not by choice. Radical acceptance allows you to accept the situation as it is and helps you focus on next steps.
- **Aging:** Growing older is a fact of life that many struggle with. Radical acceptance can help you embrace the changes that come with aging, rather than resist them.

A well-known proverb in Buddhist and addiction recovery communities is that pain is inevitable, but suffering is optional. There are painful aspects of your circumstances that you cannot change, but you can significantly reduce the overall stress and suffering they cause by choosing to radically accept reality, acknowledging the way things are right now rather than fighting against it. Practicing radical acceptance in the face of unavoidable pain can powerfully expand your nervous system's capacity to confront even the most difficult situations.

AWE: THE ULTIMATE PATHWAY TO EXPANDING CAPACITY

Have you ever looked out across a mountain range and felt amazed by how big it is compared to you? Or have you been so absorbed in a piece of music that it feels like it's part of you? Perhaps you've been immersed in a spiritual practice or even embarked on a psychedelic journey that took you beyond the confines of yourself. These experiences, though vastly different, share a common thread—the feeling of *awe*.

Awe is an emotional and physical response to experiences that are vast, grand, or in some way take you beyond your usual understanding. These experiences can inspire you to reevaluate your perception of the world. You might feel wonder, amazement, or a sense of humility as part of the experience of awe.

The feeling of awe has fascinated humanity for centuries, but it's only recently that we've begun to study it from a scientific perspective. Research suggests that experiencing awe can have positive effects on well-being, creativity, and empathy because it often leads individuals to feel more connected to something greater than themselves. Experiences of awe can have a profound effect on your nervous system, expanding your capacity to handle even the most intense stressors flexibly without getting dysregulated.

Having a well-regulated nervous system does not mean it's stuck in the green state all the time; rather, it moves flexibly between different arousal states in a way that matches the demands of the current situation. Just like a muscle tightens over time when you don't use it, your nervous system can become less flexible when your existing mental structures are never stretched. Awe experiences can loosen your nervous system, just like stretching muscles. They can improve your nervous system's flexibility, which expands your capacity to handle stressors.

According to awe researchers, a hallmark of awe is that something about your experience doesn't fit into your mental structures. You can't quite grasp or contain the vastness of the experience that causes you to feel awe. Think about the unimaginable enormity of the cosmos, for example. Even if you could travel at the speed of light, it would take twenty-six thousand years to get to the other side of our galaxy, the Milky Way. That's more than twice as long as humans have been farming, and over five hundred times as long as you've been able to buy a tomato out of season at your local grocery store. Now consider that the Hubble telescope has allowed astronomers to document over one hundred billion galaxies in the universe, and most astronomers estimate there are far more. There's something about this amount of vastness that we simply can't wrap our minds around. Touching that sense of something beyond your ability to comprehend expands the nervous system, increasing your capacity and leading to a variety of documented health benefits.

Whether awe originates in your experience of looking up at the stars, a science lab, a temple, a forest, or an art gallery, it seems to act as a kind of "superfood" for our nervous system's capacity. In 2023, researchers Maria Monroy and Dacher Keltner at the University of California, Berkeley, published a study that found awe leads to a wide variety of measurable changes. In the body, awe can slow heart rate, reduce inflammation, and even decrease the risk of some physical diseases. In the mind, awe can improve mood and lower levels of anxiety and depression. It can also increase your sense of meaningfulness. At the social level, it can increase feelings of connectedness and belonging, and give you a more cooperative attitude toward others. And at the level of spirituality, awe can transform your relationship with yourself, reducing the tendency to be overly self-focused. Each of these experiences leads to direct benefits to your nervous system, making it more flexible and resilient.

Five Flavors of Awe

According to psychologists Dacher Keltner and Jonathan Haidt, awe is not one standard experience, but, rather, a nuanced mix of various flavors, or types, of awe: threat, beauty, ability, virtue, and supernatural causality.

- **Threat:** This type of awe is a mix of fear and amazement. It happens when you encounter something powerful or intimidating, like a fast-approaching storm or a strong leader. It's the kind of awe that makes your heart race, reminding you that there are forces in the world bigger and more powerful than you.
- **Beauty:** This flavor of awe arises from witnessing exceptional beauty. It could be a breathtaking landscape, a stunning sunset, a piece of art that moves you, or anything else that strikes you with its aesthetic appeal. It's a serene and peaceful type of awe, filling you with an appreciation for the beauty in the world.
- **Ability:** This is the awe you feel when you see someone display remarkable skill or talent. It could be an athlete performing an extraordinary feat, a musician playing a complicated piece flawlessly, or any demonstration of exceptional ability. This kind of awe leaves you amazed at what humans can achieve with practice and dedication.
- **Virtue:** This flavor of awe comes from witnessing strength of character, moral goodness, or extraordinary kindness. It might be inspired by stories of saints or by everyday heroes who demonstrate extraordinary virtue in their lives. This type of awe leaves you inspired and might even motivate you to become a better person.
- **Supernatural causality:** This awe is triggered by experiences that seem supernatural or unexplainable. Seeing an apparition, witnessing a miracle, or having an uncanny coincidence happen might trigger this type of awe. It's a mysterious and intriguing form of awe, challenging your understanding of reality and opening you up to the possibility of the unknown.

Researchers have found that when awe is based on fear or danger, as in the case of the *threat-flavored* awe, like being caught in a natural disaster, feeling judged by a very powerful God, or being involved in a violent protest, it usually doesn't elicit the same powerful positive effects on your nervous system that the other flavors of awe can produce. Instead, these kinds of experiences are more often associated with chronic

>> DO THIS

DISCOVERING AWE IN YOUR LIFE: A SELF-ASSESSMENT

If you're wondering how often you experience awe in your life, this self-assessment can help you. The Dispositional Positive Emotion Scale, developed by awe researchers in 2006, measures how prone you are to feel certain positive emotions, including awe. The assessment has a specific section, or subscale, focusing on awe, which I present to you here.

Read the following six statements and give each a rating from 1 to 7—if you **strongly disagree** with a statement, give it a **1**; if you **strongly agree**, give it a **7**. The key is to be honest with yourself and not overanalyze your answers.

1. I often feel awe. ________
2. I see beauty all around me. ________
3. I feel wonder almost every day. ________
4. I often look for patterns in the objects around me. ________
5. I have many opportunities to see the beauty of nature. ________
6. I seek out experiences that challenge my understanding of the world. ________

Once you rate each statement, add up your ratings. The total score will give you an idea of how much awe you typically experience. Higher scores, between 24 and 42, mean you feel awe on a more regular basis, whereas lower scores, between 6 and 23, mean awe is a less frequent visitor in your life.

This self-assessment isn't meant to diagnose anything. It's a tool to help you reflect on your experiences and emotions. Give it a try and see how much awe is present in your life.

stress and nervous system dysregulation. As we explore ways to cultivate experiences of awe, focus on the beauty, ability, virtue, and supernatural causality flavors of awe for the best benefits to expanding your nervous system's capacity.

Four Practical Strategies to Enhance Awe in Everyday Life

1. **Nature:** Spending time in nature is one of the easiest ways to inspire awe. This could be as simple as taking a walk in a local park or as grand as going on a camping trip in the mountains. Immerse yourself in the natural world and allow yourself to be amazed by its beauty and complexity. You may find that you can access awe more easily by doing something active in nature, like hiking, biking, or rafting.
2. **Spirituality and religiosity:** If you're spiritual or religious, participating in rituals, ceremonies, or prayer can be a source of awe. Even if you're not religious, you can still find awe in spiritual practices, such as meditation or chanting. The key is to find a practice that connects you to something bigger than yourself, whether that's a higher power, the universe, or just the larger human community.
3. **Collective experiences:** Participating in group activities such as music, dance, and singing can also create feelings of awe. This could mean joining a choir, going to a concert, participating in a dance class, or attending a cultural festival. The sense of unity and shared experience in these activities can be a powerful source of awe.
4. **Psychedelics:** Emerging research suggests that psychedelics can induce intense feelings of awe when used in a safe setting. If you're interested in this topic, it's crucial to engage safely and legally, under the supervision of a health-care provider or in a clinical research setting.

Remember, the key to awe is that the experience makes you feel connected to something bigger than yourself, whether that's nature, community, the divine, or the universe as a whole.

A Path to Spirituality

Experiencing awe can lead to a profound sense of belonging and purpose, connecting you not only to your immediate surroundings but also more broadly to the whole of existence. The sensation of connection to something beyond yourself often brings a feeling of humbleness. You might notice a felt sense of your smallness within the grand scheme of things, while simultaneously feeling that you are a meaningful part of a greater whole. This paradoxical experience is the essence of spirituality, the fourth pillar of nervous system health.

Spirituality is a sense of connection to something larger than ourselves, a higher power, a divine entity, or simply the vast expanse of the universe. It's a recognition of the interconnectedness of all things and the mysterious forces that drive life. Spirituality can bring a much greater sense of purpose, direction, and meaning to our lives, completing the connection between mind, body, and spirit.

Awe-inspiring experiences can deepen your spiritual connection. Whether it's standing at the edge of a deep canyon, gazing at the stars, or being part of a moving ritual, awe offers you a glimpse of the sublime, the truly extraordinary, and the deeply meaningful aspects of existence.

Experiencing awe, then, is not just about thrill or excitement; it's about opening yourself up to life, embracing its mysteries, and acknowledging your place within it. It's about feeling connected, alive, and part of something greater than yourself. Recognizing and appreciating your connection to something bigger than yourself has a powerful effect on expanding your nervous system's capacity. As you deepen your understanding of your place within this larger context, your nervous system gains more flexibility, allowing it to respond to new demands or challenges with even more grace, dignity, humility, and compassion.

As you learn to incorporate practices from this final stage of the 5-Stage Plan—expanding your nervous system's capacity—you're on the threshold of a new chapter in your life that could very well signal the start of your journey to reversing nervous system dysregulation. Alternatively, you might already have integrated all five stages into your nervous system, and now you're prepared to shift your focus toward other projects and adventures. For me, once I no longer needed to focus so much attention on regulating my nervous system, I was inspired to start a family and guide others on their journey toward healing their nervous systems. This new sense of peace and openness allowed me to connect the dots of my life's events, making sense of things I previously couldn't fully comprehend and building a coherent narrative of my life. This is an ongoing process, but the groundwork we've laid together in this journey may give you the necessary tools to embark on your own exploration sooner. In the upcoming chapter, I'll share my personal journey with you and introduce a final practice that I found immensely useful in my path of growth, healing, and self-discovery: connecting with my ancestors.

12

Connecting the Dots: The Ongoing Practice of Building a Coherent Life Narrative

AS I STOOD that gray winter day on the desolate pedestrian bridge, I stared at the message on my phone's screen about Milarepa, the Buddhist master who learned to face his demons instead of chasing them away. The story resonated strongly in my body, and reading it suddenly shifted something deep within me. It felt like I was at a turning point in my life.

From the outside, my life looked great, even enviable. I was a successful surgeon, the CEO of a growing digital health start-up, and active in charity work. I had gained recognition and visibility in the public sphere as an innovator in Italy's digital health and start-up scene, even presenting at an event with the Italian president. It seemed like I had everything under control. But inside, I was struggling. I was collecting relationships with emotionally unavailable people, playing out old wounds I hadn't yet learned to recognize, let alone heal. I found myself constantly drawn to those who, like me, were successful, high functioning, and hardworking. But I hadn't yet understood that, just like me, underneath their high functioning was an emotional unavailability that left my heart feeling unsafe and my needs unmet on a fundamental level.

I also had never learned how to assert clear and healthy boundaries. Without clear boundaries at work, I internalized every issue, every setback. The lines between my professional and personal life blurred, causing the weight of my responsibilities to feel overwhelming. Even as I was leading a life that appeared successful and privileged, I was wracked with chronic stress and anxiety.

Over time, the symptoms of my chronic stress began to manifest more strongly in both my physical and my emotional health. I developed a persistent skin rash—rosacea. Being hit with rosacea was like a sucker punch to my self-esteem. The red, angry patches on my face weren't just annoying, they were deeply embarrassing. They felt like a physical mark of my inner turmoil, visible for everyone to see. I'd always felt confident in my skin—literally and figuratively. But with rosacea, that confidence started to crumble. I found myself constantly worried about how I looked, paranoid that people were staring at my skin.

With my skin flaring and my self-esteem on the decline, I started retreating from the public sphere, pulling back from the recognition and visibility I had earned as an innovator in Italy's digital health and start-up scene. Gradually, I began to withdraw from social events, distancing myself not just from the media, but also from friends and loved ones.

As I hid away, both my emotional distress and my physical symptoms of rosacea escalated, intensifying my need for isolation. It was a brutal cycle. The more stressed I became about my skin, the worse my rosacea seemed to get. And the worse my rosacea got, the more it fueled my stress and anxiety.

The rash was just the first sign of my body's distress. I also experienced a constant gnawing gut pain that would later be diagnosed as irritable bowel syndrome (IBS). The pain was persistent and exhausting, leaving me feeling drained as I pushed myself to keep up with my daily responsibilities.

The day my IBS really hit home I had just stepped out of a networking event in Atlanta. Instead of soaking in the vibrant culture or networking with colleagues, I found myself doubled over in pain, my insides feeling like they were being twisted and pulled. Initially, I tried to shrug it off, but the pain intensified. It was sharp, relentless, and completely overwhelming.

Suddenly, I was hit with the realization that this was not a passing discomfort. The pain was unrelenting, and its intensity provoked a sense of acute danger in me. I was scared for my life, and I asked the staff to call an ambulance. Soon enough, I found myself being whisked away in the back of the vehicle, the city lights melting into a blur as I was sped off to the hospital. There, the doctors thought I had pancreatitis—a condition that can be severe and lead to lifelong complications. All I wanted was for the pain to stop. But it didn't. Instead, it dragged on for hours in the stark hospital room.

Further tests revealed it wasn't pancreatitis, but what they referred to as "just" irritable bowel syndrome. Yet there was nothing "just" about it for me. I still felt thrown off balance even after the intense pain subsided. I was upset, and not just because of the physical discomfort, but also because of the lack of a clear explanation.

Not knowing why left me feeling disoriented and somehow at fault. The dismissive tone used by the doctors made it seem as though the agony I'd experienced was in my head, as if I had conjured up the pain and distress, causing all this commotion over nothing. This sense of confusion and self-blame added a new layer of frustration to the already challenging situation.

It wasn't only my body that was in chaos. My emotional state was also in free fall. I had been the poster child for high-functioning anxiety. To my friends, colleagues, and patients, I still appeared to be a competent and successful professional. But behind closed doors, my mind was like a hamster on a wheel, thoughts constantly racing and spiraling into worst-case scenarios, stuck on repeat about past slipups or future "what ifs." This mental noise was exhausting, and it only made the physical symptoms of my chronic stress, IBS, and rosacea worse.

I didn't understand this at the time, but my nervous system was extremely dysregulated. I was caught in the pinball effect—mental symptoms leading to physical, and physical to mental, all contributing to my nervous system getting stuck in the yellow and red states. What had led to this point of extreme dysregulation, where my life was a paradox of external success and internal turmoil?

There were demons lurking in the shadows of my cave, and until that moment on the bridge, reading the story of Milarepa, I had not truly acknowledged their existence. And now they weren't just whispering, they were roaring. Some of these demons, or harsh internal voices, kept saying that I wasn't good enough, that I didn't matter. These callous voices felt like a constant reminder of all the doubts and insecurities I had. I was about to learn that my journey to healing wasn't just about silencing the voices and their accompanying symptoms—it was also about facing the demons, understanding them, and bowing to them.

I wish I could tell you that the epiphany I had on that pedestrian bridge—that I needed to go all in on facing my demons honestly—was a simple turning point where my physical and emotional symptoms suddenly started getting better. That my pathway to healing was a straightforward and ascending one. But I wouldn't be telling you the truth. In fact, in the beginning, as I began to confront my demons, things seemed to get worse.

But in the middle of this physical storm, I started to feel a strange sense of peace and acceptance. This peace emerged as I began to let go of the image I thought I needed to maintain of myself to be accepted by others. Yes, my demons were still present, but they weren't as terrifying or as overwhelming as before. I began to approach them with curiosity and acceptance. Just like Milarepa, I accepted that my demons and I would be spending time together, so I made a choice to observe them, not as foes to be defeated, but as parts of myself that deserved understanding.

I committed to giving myself the unconditional support and understanding I had often denied myself, replacing the harsh voice that insisted nothing was ever good enough with a kinder, more compassionate one. I released my unrealistic expectations, and in doing so, I diminished the power my demons held over me.

Through this newfound self-compassion, curiosity, and radical self-acceptance, things started to improve. The change wasn't immediate or even linear, but I was finally on a path leading me away from relentless self-criticism and toward genuine self-understanding and care.

FINDING MY GUIDES ON THE HEALING PATH

In 2012, as I embarked on my journey toward healing, I was largely alone. At the time, conversations about mental health were scarcely happening, quite unlike today's open dialogue and growing awareness. Similarly, concepts like the mind-body connection or understanding how our bodies react to stress were still on the fringes, not yet embraced by the mainstream. The scientific literature on stress was sparse, and social media barely touched upon the topic.

There were times I felt like I was lost at sea. I wasn't sure whether I was getting better or just wandering aimlessly. During those times, I felt confused and unsure of myself. In those moments of confusion and self-doubt, I learned the importance of having guides—mentors, therapists, and teachers. In the absence of a supportive community, these guides became my compass. They helped me find my way through the confusing process of healing my nervous system, offering a compassionate ear, a guiding hand, and a reassuring presence. They showed me I was not alone.

It was crucial that I found a refuge where I could practice and strengthen my budding sense of radical honesty and unconditional self-acceptance. This safe haven was offered through the fresh connections I forged with my guides. It was also essential for me to learn how to let others help me. I had always been fiercely independent, scared of relying on someone else for love and acceptance. As I opened myself up to the idea of accepting help and support from others, I was, unknowingly, working on healing my dismissive attachment tendencies.

Josh Korda, a respected Buddhist teacher and pastoral counselor, played a pivotal role in my healing journey. His New Yorker spirit, Jewish roots, and punk ethos brought a refreshing authenticity to our interactions. More than a teacher, Josh provided a safe space for me, a place where I could practice self-acceptance, honesty, and self-compassion. His consistent and unconditional support helped me confront my fears of dependency, gradually supporting me to heal my deeply ingrained defensive tendencies. He remains a steady and caring guide in my life, even today.

Josh's unique teaching approach, which integrates neuroscience, somatic-based therapies, and ancient Buddhist wisdom, also sparked a profound transformation in my understanding of the mind-body connection. He encouraged me to learn, explore, and widen my perspective on the relationship between my emotional state, the physical manifestations in my body, and my spiritual connection. This was a completely novel idea for me, with my background in traditional Western medicine. The fusion of mind, body, and spirituality not only opened my eyes but also eventually reshaped my professional path. My curiosity was ignited. Books became my companions, imparting wisdom and diverse viewpoints when I felt disoriented.

Not long after I began working with Josh, he suggested I reach out to Jerry Colonna. Jerry, a highly recognized venture capitalist turned executive coach, had written the blog post that sparked the seismic shift in my perspective on that pivotal day on the pedestrian bridge. I could never have afforded Jerry's high-end coaching services, but Josh encouraged me to reach out to him as a friend and mentor, which filled me with apprehension. However, my deep-seated sense of unworthiness, this nagging belief that made me constantly question my own value, left me doubting whether someone like Jerry, whom I looked up to, would even bother responding to my email, let alone form any connection with me. But I took a deep breath and sent him an email.

I poured my heart into that message, explaining how his words had ignited a profound shift in my perspective. To my surprise, Jerry responded: His reply was warm and welcoming, far removed from the dismissive reaction I had feared. It marked the inception of a long-lasting friendship that has shaped my life in unimaginable ways. Our shared Italian heritage created an immediate connection. Jerry became a mentor and guide, providing invaluable advice and support through various professional struggles and personal challenges. His role as a mentor was incredibly important to me. He saw and affirmed my potential as a leader and an entrepreneur, a validation I had long yearned for yet struggled to receive at the time.

Jerry's support, blended with his unfiltered honesty and his consistent encouragement to face the truth—or "radical self-inquiry," as he calls it—provided a sense of safety and worthiness. At the same time, it presented a challenge, a push to confront and deal with the realities of my journey. This delicate balance of reassurance and challenge made our mentor-mentee relationship a powerful catalyst in my journey of self-healing and self-acceptance.

THE TURNING POINT IN MY HEALING JOURNEY

Jerry's belief in me as a leader and an entrepreneur became an essential counterpoint to the narrative I'd been telling myself for years—the narrative that painted me as small and insignificant. Although Jerry's encouragement provided the external validation I craved, it also finally led me to confront the truth about my internal struggle. I was always in motion, constantly driven to make a difference in the world, but never pausing to reflect on why.

I had completed my studies in oral medicine eleven years before, with a two-year clinical research project on the oral effects of bone marrow transplantation. The work required me to interact with patients who lived in isolation for months, only able to see their loved ones through a sheet of glass. Several didn't survive the transplant and spent the last precious moments of their life in those isolation rooms. The sense of helplessness and sorrow this induced in me was crushing, making any effort seem pointless. I felt embarrassed and utterly inadequate to witness their pain, let alone be of any help.

Despite my five years of specialized medical training and research, I found myself wrestling with feelings of inadequacy and unworthiness. I was merely an oral specialist, a surgeon who dealt with a small, specific aspect of the human body. Within me, there was a persistent voice whispering that maybe I should have chosen a more "worthy" specialty, though I couldn't quite articulate which that would be. How could I be making a substantial difference when I was only scratching the surface of a much broader, complex landscape of human health? Although my job brought me financial stability and independence, it left me thirsting for a deeper, more encompassing sense of purpose.

I started seeking this purpose outside my day job. I threw myself into volunteering. I traveled to Brazil and Africa, where I worked in local hospitals ran by nongovernmental organizations. I engaged in political and human rights advocacy and environmental activism. You name it, I was there. But no matter how many people I helped, how many causes I championed, it always felt like a small drop in a vast ocean.

One memory that sticks with me is a time I was on a mission in a remote village in northern Kenya, an area where Maasai and Samburu peoples still roamed the lands. The village was a stark contrast of ancient traditions and brutal modern realities. The people there were living under the constant threat of AIDS. One afternoon I found myself in the local hospital, tasked with extracting a tooth from a young boy. He was about eight or nine years old, already an AIDS orphan, and now battling AIDS himself. The volunteers with him told me he was seriously ill, and they didn't expect him to live much longer.

I remember looking at him, his eyes filled with fear and confusion, knowing the pain he was already in, and about to cause him more with the extraction. It was a feeling of helplessness I'd never felt before. My heart was breaking for this little child who had already experienced more pain and suffering in his short life than I could imagine.

I did my job, as gently as I could. But after, as he was led away, still crying softly, I sat there, full of tears and anger. The magnitude of his immense suffering made me feel small and insignificant. Every accomplishment, every goal, every good deed I had ever done felt trivial.

Despite the magnitude of this experience, I continued on relentlessly, for many more years, taking on more responsibility and more action.

Many years later, as I worked with Jerry to understand why I felt so much drive to go change the world but never paused to look into myself, I understood that the reason I felt so small in the face of that boy's immense suffering was because some deep part of me felt unworthy of existing without proving myself.

My relentless drive to make a difference, to bring some relief to others, stemmed from an unfulfilled need within myself. I was so busy trying to save the world, I never stopped to look within. I was bypassing the real issue, ignoring the hard work of understanding myself.

I had thought that my feelings of being small were due to the magnitude of the world's pain, but I began to see that the origin of this sense of smallness was not in the world but within me. It was a reflection of my unfulfilled internal needs—for acceptance, for worthiness, for self-love.

This realization marked a significant turning point in my journey. Instead of looking outward, I turned my gaze inward. I started to understand that healing others was not merely about rushing into the world to put out fires; it was equally about tending to the inner flames of my self-doubt and self-denial that had long been neglected.

No longer did I need to save the world to know I was worthy of being in it; instead, I needed to dive into the depth of my being, to acknowledge my fears and insecurities, and to embrace them with compassion and understanding. This was not about shrinking back from the world, but about expanding my inner capacity for acceptance and self-love.

Finally, I understood that I could not genuinely help others heal until I healed myself.

This insight loosened the chains of my relentless pursuit of validation through external accomplishments and set me on a path of self-discovery and self-acceptance. It gave me the courage to stop running and to start looking within. It was a monumental shift, one that would reshape my approach to healing and redefine my sense of purpose. From that point onward I knew the key to healing the world began with healing myself.

HONORING MY BODY

With my newfound understanding that I needed to heal myself from within, my journey took on a new, personal direction. It was no longer just about my interest in the mechanics of health and disease. Instead, it became a journey of deep self-discovery and understanding.

As I started tackling the root causes of my dysregulation in my work with Josh, root causes like attachment patterns, coping strategies, and embedded alarms, I found that my nervous system began to settle down. And I noticed the first significant improvement: My digestion started to get better. My gut health, for so long compromised by the continual state of high-alert stress, started to rebuild itself. I no longer experienced the bloating, gas, and discomfort that used to be commonplace. My gut began to better absorb nutrients from the food I was consuming, and as a result, my energy levels started to rise.

My rosacea, however, was another story. Despite the significant improvements in other aspects of my health, the rosacea held its ground, seemingly resistant to the new changes in my life. I sought the opinions of various dermatologists, each echoing a similar sentiment: My skin condition was incurable, something I had to live with. Then, I met Dr. Mauro Barbareschi.

Dr. Barbareschi was different. The way he spoke to me made me feel calm and reassured. And unlike the other doctors, he didn't view me as a walking skin condition; he saw me as a person, grappling with an issue that ran deeper than the skin's surface.

With his years of experience and a gift for seeing the whole picture, Dr. Barbareschi told me something that no one else had: He said my skin, like every other part of my body, was closely connected to my emotional and psychological well-being. He explained that my rosacea was not merely a stand-alone issue but was intrinsically linked to my body's stress response.

Although his medical knowledge could certainly help manage the symptoms, he admitted that he couldn't do it all. The crucial part of the healing process, he said, was in my hands. He stressed that I had to dive deeper, to the very root of my stress, and confront it. Only then, he promised, would my rosacea permanently recede.

His words were like a light bulb moment for me. Here was a seasoned medical professional reaffirming what I had already begun to suspect during my medical training and from conversations with Josh: My mind and body weren't separate entities; they were part of a complex, interconnected system. I was taken aback, not just by his honesty, but also by the enormity of the task ahead.

I walked out of his office that day feeling hopeful and empowered, something I hadn't felt in a long time. His belief in my ability to recover made all the difference. My physical healing wasn't just about treating a skin condition anymore. It was about reigniting hope and sparking a sense of control over my own health.

Years later, I'm free from rosacea and can still feel Dr. Barbareschi's influence: He helped me see that I had the power to heal myself. His approach to my rosacea wasn't just about treatment. It was about helping me understand that the real work was inside me. It was about learning to listen to and trust my body.

Growing up in Western culture, with its celebration of the logical mind and devaluation of the wisdom of the body, I held a deep-seated belief that the mind and body were separate. I had learned to highly value my mind's reason and willpower, and didn't realize that my body was constantly speaking to me too. With the help of Dr. Barbareschi, Josh, and others, I slowly learned to hear the signals that my body was sending me. I learned that my body is full of wisdom, and to heal my body, I needed to honor and respect its wisdom above all.

This journey of understanding required a radical shift in perspective and a willingness to step away from prevalent norms. Yet in doing so, I found a path to healing that was not just about treating individual symptoms, but also about nurturing and restoring the connection between my mind and my body. The pain and confusion I went through, while immensely challenging, were instrumental in guiding me toward this new approach to health and well-being.

A HEALING BOND

My healing journey brought me face-to-face with my body's truth and taught me how to sit with my discomfort, to learn from it, and to befriend it. The knowledge that my skin condition was intrinsically tied to my internal emotions led me to examine and address the very roots of those emotions—the relationship patterns that had formed the foundation of my unstable sense of self-worth. Understanding my body and its inherent healing power helped me connect to another crucial aspect of my life—my relationships.

My previous relationships were like a battleground, marred by avoidance and emotional tugs-of-war. The arrival of Alessio in my life marked a stark departure from that pattern. With Alessio, I could be myself. No pretenses, no masks, no need to be anyone but who I am. I could be completely and honestly me. This was a new feeling, a sense of security I had never known in a relationship before.

What made this relationship different? Unlike my previous relationships, I approached this relationship without the usual weight of expectations. There were no checklists, no impossible standards. I was not looking to build the perfect relationship with the perfect partner. Instead, I decided to honor the present, to "be with what is," as I had learned to do with my body.

I committed to trusting my body's intuition, to listen to its signals without any preconceived notions or plans, and it opened up space for a connection that I had never experienced before. It was different from what I had always sought or imagined, but it was exactly what I needed.

Alessio's acceptance of me, in my most vulnerable moments, played a significant role. He stood by me even during the worst of my rosacea experiences. His love and patience were proof that I didn't need to be perfect or achieve anything extraordinary to be worthy of love. I started to understand that what truly mattered to me in a relationship wasn't how many boxes the other person checked, but how much value we placed on our connection and the willingness to work and repair any ruptures that arose.

In Alessio, I experienced an unconditional form of love that was new to me, a love that asked for no pretenses or façades. This became a mirror reflecting my own capacity for such love. I realized that I was also capable of giving that same unconditional acceptance and love, not just to an idealized image of a person, but to the real, authentic individual in front of me.

Our relationship wasn't perfect—in fact, even to this day, it has its ups and downs. But then, it never needed to be perfect. The understanding that I was enough, just as I was, allowed me to approach our relationship from a place of honesty, trust, and acceptance.

As I embraced our imperfections, I learned that a critical part of committing to a relationship is doing the constant work of repairing. Instead of viewing conflicts as signs of failure, I began to see them as inevitable aspects of our shared journey. Each rupture was an opportunity to understand each other better, to communicate more deeply, and to reinforce our bond.

As this new perspective settled within me—this understanding of love as an ongoing process of repair and growth—I realized that this process of repairing relationships was not only relevant to my relationship with Alessio, but also to all relationships in my life.

HEALING MYSELF, HEALING MY LINEAGE

Learning to accept myself and my body, and practicing unconditional love in my relationship with Alessio, were massive leaps in my personal journey toward healing. But one more step on my healing journey, understanding my ancestral history, stands out as critical to the peace and integration I enjoy today.

Storytelling was a skill that was passed down through our family, from my great-grandmother to my grandmother and then to my mother. They all wielded this skill beautifully, but it wasn't until my mother, a renowned author in Italy, wrote a book about one of our female ancestors that I fully grasped the profound healing power that storytelling, and making sense of our pain through these stories, could hold.

My mother's book, *L'acquaiola*, or *The Water Carrier* in English, tells the story of my great-great-grandmother Maria, a woman of remarkable resilience. During that era, societal norms painted women as dependents of men and considered them less worthy, even if they were hardworking and self-reliant. Maria, for instance, faced strenuous physical labor every day as she carried water from the fountain to the villa of the local affluent family. Despite the difficulties she endured, she found clever ways to express herself and lead a meaningful life. Her resilience is inspiring, but the book also shows the high cost of her survival. It uncovers the personal sacrifices Maria made, the effects on her relationships, and the toll it took on her life.

The story breathed life back into my ancestors—their hopes, their dreams, their struggles. These women, full of life, love, and plenty of drama, left a strong impression on me as I read through this book. Unraveling Maria's story resurfaced memories of my grandmother, Maria's granddaughter.

My grandmother Nandina, or Nonna Nanda as I called her, was the very definition of love, strength, and resilience for me. She was born into a middle-class family, the eldest of five kids, in the Southern Italian region of Molise. As a bright, highly sensitive, and curious girl, she loved going to school and learning new things. But all that was about to change.

It was July 16, 1943, a few days after she had celebrated her sixteenth birthday, that my Nonna Nanda's life was irreversibly altered. She was sitting in an exam hall in the heart of Rome, where her family lived at the time, surrounded by dozens of other girls, all intently focused on their end-of-year high school exams. The air was thick with anticipation and an undercurrent of nervous energy. Nandina's eyes were firmly set on the paper in front of her, her hand moving diligently as she was deeply engrossed in composing her responses. But at precisely 11:03, the peace of the morning was violently ruptured. Sirens began wailing, their chilling echo reverberating through the classroom's stone walls and the hearts of the young students.

More than four thousand Allied bombs rained down on Rome that day, taking three thousand lives and injuring eleven thousand people. In a flash, the world as Nandina knew it was over. The exams that she had been so nervously preparing for were forgotten as a terrifying test of survival had begun. It was a test she never signed up for, and it had a profound impact on her, tearing away her adolescence and forcing her to grow up in the span of just a few months.

Her father had been taken hostage by Mussolini's fascists, his fate unknown. In a bid for survival, she and her family immediately fled to their ancestral village in Molise. There, they found themselves trapped in a horrifying deadlock between the retreating German forces and the advancing Allies. Hiding in the woods with her young siblings and her heavily pregnant mother, Nandina was thrown into the role of protector and provider. Lack of food pushed them to extreme measures, and they sometimes relied on roots for sustenance, a memory Nonna Nanda would share with me many years later.

She went from being a bright student, dreaming of a future filled with opportunities, to a young girl lost in the brutal realities of war, her dreams shattered. Yet, even in the midst of such immense chaos and fear, she held on with a strength that was beyond her years, a strength that would continue to shape her throughout her life.

After the war, Nonna Nanda found her family's financial stability in ruins. Her father, once a strong provider, was left physically crippled by the fascists, incapable of supporting them as he once had. She couldn't pursue her education and the opportunities that would have opened. Amid these struggles, Nonna Nanda managed to build a family of her own with my grandfather, who was in the navy during the war and who had since become a police officer.

They worked tirelessly to forge a new life, moving to Northern Italy, to Milan, to raise their three children amid the city's opportunities and challenges. Their story was characterized by relentless effort, hard work, and countless sacrifices. Her nervous system was likely dysregulated her entire life, always battling the embedded alarms instilled in her during the traumatic experiences she went through during the war.

However, she had little time or resources to address her own suffering. Instead, she had to focus on her immediate responsibilities—securing basic necessities, providing for her family, and raising her children. The harsh realities of life had propelled her into survival mode, and there was little room for anything else.

As I delved deeper into these stories, I began to see common threads weaving a familiar pattern. I recognized my struggles—the feeling of never being enough, the relentless urge to prove myself, the never-ending hurry—mirrored in the lives of these women. I finally started connecting the dots. I realized these weren't merely personal challenges I had been grappling with; they were patterns passed down through generations.

These patterns stemmed from a time when survival was constantly under threat and life was full of hardships. My ancestors lived through eras of intense adversity, where a sense of urgency was a necessary survival mechanism.

The women of my lineage didn't have the luxury of complacency. Their worlds demanded constant vigilance and the ability to quickly adapt to changing circumstances. Over time, this urgency hardened into a form of self-discipline, an ingrained belief they had to be tough on themselves to survive and protect their families.

This sense of urgency, this need to be relentless and unforgiving toward oneself, was what was passed down along with the stories. The compelling urge to "be enough," to "do enough," to be perpetually prepared for the worst-case scenario, was a survival mechanism that had transformed into a stringent internal rulebook over the generations. Understanding how I had inherited the idea that I needed to incessantly demand perfection from myself to be deserving of love gave me new insight into why I held myself to such impossibly high standards. It wasn't a flaw in me but a legacy of survival that had outlived its usefulness.

As I navigated through this new understanding of my ancestors, I started to extend to each individual in my lineage the same compassion I had learned to offer myself. I realized that each one of them, for better or worse, had done their best with what they had been given.

And with this newfound understanding, I saw an opportunity. An opportunity to heal this generational wound, to break the cycle of suffering that had been passed down through our lineage. It was up to me to decide what to pass on and what ends with me. My four children could inherit the beautiful gifts that ran in our family—the sensitivity and empathy for others, the art of storytelling, the love for knowledge, the burning passion, the relentless resilience—without the steep price attached to them. They could carry on the legacy of our ancestors without the burden.

The power to make this change is in my hands now. It was a profound realization: I was not just the recipient of this legacy, but I also had the power to shape it, to redefine it. I had the power to heal.

CREATING "HEAL YOUR NERVOUS SYSTEM"

My journey of self-discovery and healing, begun over a decade ago, initiated a profound transformation within me, reshaping how I perceived myself and my role in service to others. Gone was the compulsive need to fill an inner void. In its place grew a fulfilling sense of wholeness, joy, and a desire to give back to others.

I have finally grasped the reality that I cannot erase suffering in the world. But I can support people in their struggle with pain, making them feel stronger and more capable. I want to contribute to building a world where my children can grow up feeling secure and at peace.

This desire led me to start Heal Your Nervous System, a space where I've brought together a team of clinicians, researchers, and coaches to offer people a simpler way to navigate the complexities of healing a dysregulated nervous system.

The 5-Stage Plan to Reverse Nervous System Dysregulation is never complete, but the stages become more and more integrated into life. My personal journey of healing and growth continues. With each new insight, each step forward, my aim remains to simplify the path for others. The challenges, the confusion, and the isolation I once faced now shape the framework of support we offer at Heal Your Nervous System, and that I've laid out in this book.

In the world I want to help create, no one needs to feel lost or alone in their journey to heal their nervous system.

CONNECTING WITH YOUR ANCESTORS

Imagine yourself standing in a boundless landscape. As you glance over one shoulder, you see an unending line of women. These are your mothers, a long chain of maternal ancestors stretching back through time. You inherited DNA inside your mitochondria, your cells' powerhouses that play such a big role in the pinball effect, directly from your mother, without any influence from your father. She inherited it directly from her mother, and so on, all the way back through time.

Mitochondrial DNA does change or mutate over time, so you don't have the exact same mitochondrial DNA as your great-great-great-grandmother, but it doesn't mix and recombine with every generation like most of the rest of the DNA you inherited from your parents. Using mitochondrial DNA analysis, scientists have found that all humans who are currently alive share at least one maternal ancestor. They've called her "Mitochondrial Eve" and estimate she lived between 150,000 and 200,000 years ago. As you imagine looking back at this vast line of mothers who helped create you, eventually you'll see Mitochondrial Eve. You're a part of this magnificent, unbroken chain that extends back thousands of generations, all the way to our very great-grandmother.

Now, look over the other shoulder. There you see a continuous line of men, your fathers. Just like mitochondrial DNA is passed only from your mother, the Y chromosome that determined your father's sex has been passed down directly from father to son like a baton in a relay race. Your paternal lineage also includes at least one ancestor that all humans share—scientists call him "Y-chromosomal Adam" and estimate he lived 180,000 to 300,000 years ago.

We are all interconnected, bound by threads of shared ancestry. It's a humbling reminder of our common humanity and the enduring journey of our species. These countless generations of men and women loved, played, and toiled to survive and have children. Their legacy now includes you.

Remember, you carry within you not only the echoes of past challenges, but also the strength, resilience, and healing of your ancestors. The spirit that allowed your ancestors to prosper in times of plenty and to endure even through the immense suffering that marks our human history is part of your story now. It's part of who you are today. May this spirit of resilience thrive in your nervous system. May you always remember that you stand on the shoulders of countless generations who, against all odds, made it all the way to now.

As you deepen your connection to your ancestral lineage and to yourself, you simultaneously boost your ability to empathetically connect with others in your daily life. The resilience of your ancestors fuels your strength, infusing your present interactions with compassion and understanding.

>> DO THIS

JOURNEY THROUGH YOUR ANCESTRAL LINEAGE

A few years ago, I took part in a practice led by Nir Esterman, a respected teacher and facilitator on family constellations and intergenerational trauma. The experience resonated deeply, inspiring me to mold the lessons I learned into a practice of my own. This practice can have a profound healing effect on your nervous system, allowing you to call in resilience from your ancestral lines while letting go of some of the deepest roots of your dysregulation.

As you prepare to begin this practice, please remain aware that you should not force yourself to confront distressing memories. Maintain a gentle, compassionate approach toward yourself. Always remember, you are in control of your journey, and it's perfectly okay to step back if things become overwhelming.

1. Close your eyes and imagine yourself standing tall, aware of your surroundings. Tune in to the sensations in your body: your physical presence, the emotions you might be experiencing, and the ebb and flow of your thoughts. Take note of where your attention drifts. Whatever you experience, let it be.

2. Allow your mind to guide you toward a deeply challenging event that took place in the lives of one of your ancestors. This event may have been a traumatic stressor or a monumental challenge they faced. Assign this past occurrence a place in the space behind you, wherever it feels right. However, do not engage with it—just recognize its existence and its influence. Check in with your body once again. Note how recognizing this past event shapes your current state. The image in your mind can take any form that feels comfortable. Just remember, it's not about immersing yourself in the specifics of the event, but staying focused on your body's response and maintaining mindful breathing.

3. In your lineage, visualize the ancestor who endured this difficulty. They were the one who truly experienced it, not you. Their trials might have left an imprint on you, but you were not there when these events unfolded. Notice how including your ancestor in your awareness affects your body. Take a breath.

4. Prepare to delve deeper into your ancestral line. Gaze farther back through the line, beyond the ancestor who experienced this challenging event, back to someone who existed before them, maybe just one generation prior, or even farther back. Travel back through the generations until you find one ancestor who was not affected by this challenging event. You may not know anything about them, but trust that there once was a human being in your lineage who did not suffer from this particular challenge.

continued on following page

>> DO THIS *CONTINUED*

5. Take a deep breath and imagine the ancestor who experienced this challenge saying to you, "You are my child, and this challenge was mine. I endured it. It is enough that I suffered from it." Imagine them telling you they can now manage their own challenges and you don't need to bear their burdens anymore.
6. Check in with your body again. How has imagining this affected your body? By imagining and connecting to your ancestral past, you can shift your lineage's story to be not just a source of hardships but also of health and healing. As you imagine your ancestor, supported by their strong ancestors, gaining enough strength and courage to take back the full burden of what they went through, you regain your autonomy. You gain control over the contents of the bag of gifts and burdens inherited from your forebears. You can choose to graciously accept the gifts while completing the cycle of healing that your ancestors couldn't, returning the burdens to the past where they belong.

As you near the end of this practice, take a deep breath. Gently bring your awareness back to the present moment, feeling the weight of your body on the chair or your feet on the floor. Allow your body to stir, stretch if you need to, and feel the space around you. Let your journey through your ancestral lineage settle within you, taking with it all the resilience and strength that you've touched.

13

Flourishing Like the Fern: Adapting Amid Challenges and Inspiring Others

IT WAS JULY 2019 and my partner, children, and I were visiting family in Italy in the midst of a sweltering heat wave. I had been on a journey of healing, full of ups and downs, for several years while also juggling the challenges of parenting small kids, maintaining a long-term relationship, and handling work.

I lay sweating and sticky in bed from the heat, six months pregnant with our fourth child, when I came across a book that floored me. I already felt a strong bond with nature and a keen interest in environmental matters, but Jem Bendell's book, *Deep Adaptation*, challenged me to confront the emotional toll of a looming climate disaster. The prospect of this crisis drove me into a deep, crushing sense of grief and anxiety for the future of my children, the likes of which I had never experienced.

Before healing my dysregulation, I don't think I could have squarely faced the anxiety of the destruction of our environment. But having navigated my own healing journey, I realized I could confront this topic with a clear mind and an open heart. The profound shock I felt served as a wake-up call and fueled my drive to delve deeper into the issue. It made me more determined than ever to understand how I could leverage my personal strengths to be part of the solution. Despite the initial feelings of grief and confusion, I was able to bounce back, armed with renewed motivation to address the crisis.

As I connected with like-minded others who shared my concerns, I uncovered a surprising pattern: Many of these individuals were, like me, very sensitive and deeply caring. Our shared sensitivity helped us go beyond just understanding the environmental crisis *intellectually*: We deeply felt its gravity and its existential threat in our bodies. This sensitivity transformed our concern into a shared sense of urgency and responsibility. It was as if our collective empathy had tuned in to the planet's distress signal and heard a call to action we were compelled to answer.

This experience led me to the profound insight that personal healing and collective resilience are deeply intertwined.

Just as our individual nervous systems can reorganize and heal after traumatic stressors, so too can our local and global communities heal and reorganize. And as we heal individually, we inspire change within our wider community, ultimately contributing to a collective emergence of a more resilient and engaged society.

Confronting pain, grief, and fear is not just personal work—it's sacred work that recognizes the interconnectedness of life. Every hardship we face, every fear we confront, and every loss we endure *shapes us*. These experiences can open our hearts to the struggles that all of life faces. They mold us into beacons of sanity and compassion amid all the chaos and suffering in our world. As we journey from surviving to thriving, we inspire a ripple effect of responsibility toward our society and our environment. We're not merely healing ourselves—we're contributing to the healing of our world.

Seeing this interconnectedness, and how important each person's nervous system regulation and sensitivity is to the world, inspired me to create the Heal Your Nervous System community. Our community is a vibrant global network of people healing their nervous systems, supported by a dedicated team of professionals. We are a compassionate space where individuals can better comprehend their bodies and minds, and find support as they navigate their unique path toward healing. But the mission of the Heal Your Nervous System community goes beyond individual healing. Our greater purpose is that all the personal growth and healing people do individually will fuel collective resilience in our local and global communities, and our relationship with the planet. The strength of the community is amplified by the healing journeys of each member, inspiring us all to navigate and positively influence the broader challenges of our time.

As your nervous system becomes more regulated, you might begin to feel yourself more and more, not just as one separate nervous system, but as part of a much broader nervous system spanning the entire planet. It's as if a long, long time ago our ancestors collectively forgot that we are intimately intertwined with all life, and now, one nervous system at a time, we're slowly remembering that we are not, in fact, separate after all. This realization can move your heart deeply. There's a profound sense of relief in realizing you were never disconnected from life, but your innate connectedness was only a forgotten truth, buried by time and generations.

This healing realization often comes with a dose of tears. You may feel intense grief to recognize the pain and suffering you went through by believing you were isolated and detached for all those years, particularly when you see that many others still grapple with this sense of isolation.

Over time, as you increasingly see our collective interconnectedness, it's natural to feel a pull toward helping others. In many ways, the skills you've honed to regulate your nervous system are applicable to the larger nervous systems of your families, communities, societies, and the entire planet. Just as healing your nervous system fosters safety, connection, meaning, and resilience in your life, you can channel this into collective regulation, fostering these same qualities in our wider world.

At the beginning of this book, I introduced the fern as an analogy for a regulated nervous system. Just as a fern can bend under stress and quickly recover, so too can a regulated nervous system. But the analogy of a fern goes deeper.

Climate scientist Jacquelyn Gill wrote in "The Asteroid and the Fern" that after significant extinction events in the history of earth, like the "Great Dying" 252 million years ago, species like the fern helped restore life to the planet. The fern's resilience is an example of how, despite the odds, life persists and can even flourish in the aftermath of disaster.

Our nervous systems are resilient, just like a fern. Even after horrific events, your nervous system has the capacity to bring life back into your body, and this time, with even more wisdom and compassion.

Likewise, our interconnected nervous systems, at the level of family, community, society, and planet, can bounce back even from the most dire of circumstances. Our current crises can be viewed not just as threats, but as challenges—chances to reimagine and reshape our world for the better.

We're living through a chapter in human history that's unlike anything that's come before. If you are a sensitive person, you might feel overwhelmed by the gravity of these problems. You might be wondering, *How much change can I bring to a situation so much larger and more complex than myself?*

As a highly sensitive person, you hold a gift that the world desperately needs. You are uniquely equipped with a depth of empathy and perceptiveness. Your nervous system is fine-tuned to pick up on subtle changes in the environment, process information deeply, and feel emotions intensely. These characteristics allow you to perceive the urgency of our most pressing challenges more acutely. You may feel a deep sense of social and environmental responsibility.

However, these same traits that lead to a higher responsivity to the world's suffering can make you more susceptible to stress and emotional overwhelm. Just like the ferns that flourished in the aftermath of the Great Dying, a highly sensitive person with a flexible nervous system can overcome adversities. You can channel your deep empathy and emotional awareness into meaningful action, turning your concern for the world into a catalyst for change. You can harness your unique qualities not just to survive our biggest crises but also to take them as a challenge and contribute to something better. Your role, much like the fern, can become one of regrowth, renewal, and reimagining the world for the better.

The path to achieving a regulated nervous system, and then extending that regulation to the broader levels of our interconnected world, can be filled with obstacles, setbacks, and uncertainty. Debbie Chachra, a professor at Olin College of Engineering and the author of the newsletter *Metafoundry*, uses a brilliant analogy of mountain biking to demonstrate how you can confront this uncertainty. If you're familiar with mountain biking, then you know that the trail can often appear daunting, filled with rocks, roots, and unpredictable twists. The key to navigating this challenging path is to fix your eyes on "the line"—the desired route you want to follow—not the boulders that lie in your path. The moment you focus on the boulders, you're likely to run into them.

It's so easy to fixate on the seemingly insurmountable obstacles in your path, paralyzing you with fear and uncertainty. That's how I felt in the first few months after reading Jim Bendell's book. A sense of hopeless nihilism threatened to engulf me, tempting me to disengage entirely. But my previous work on healing my nervous system became my lifeline. After the initial shock to my body of taking in the emotional pain of the climate crisis, I set my eyes on "the line" and practiced keeping my attention there. I knew that, no matter how challenging and unpredictable the path ahead is, if I just stayed focused on the path forward and avoided focusing on the various dystopian futures, I could contribute to being part of shaping this new world.

In Chachra's words, "We can, together, learn to look at the line. Because there absolutely is a path through to a better future for everyone, one that's sustainable and resilient, and equitable. But we have to learn to see it, to stay focused on it."

Stay focused on it. As you develop focus through healing your nervous system, you build the internal tools you need to face adversity with compassion and wisdom. Your regulation, combined with your sensitivity to others, positions you to help lead the way. You're not just capable of seeing "the line," but you also have the ability to inspire others to recognize and follow it too.

Each person has unique gifts that they can offer others. Your special qualities are desperately needed by the world, but finding your unique role isn't always straightforward. It's not something you can conjure in your head. Instead, it unfolds as you follow "the line." It emerges as you immerse yourself in life while staying open and attentive to your surroundings.

Naturalist Lyanda Lynn Haupt wrote in *Rooted* that our unique power "cannot be prescribed, proscribed, or even thought up in our head. It can, however, be listened for—a rooted, ongoing, reciprocal conversation with the wild earth—a spiral of inward, receptive stillness, and outward, creative action."

Haupt's words point to the unlimited ways we can engage—from artistic expressions, like painting, singing, or writing, to more direct forms of contributing to our collective healing, like environmental activism, seeking justice, and raising resilient children. From caring for the people and the environment directly around us through activities like gardening, farming, or mentoring to caring for big communities of interconnected people through politics or contributing to a meaningful business. No two paths are identical. Each person's contribution can be as diverse and unique as life itself.

Healing our nervous systems allows us to face life's challenges resiliently, and this resilience is our key to contributing to larger healing in our families, communities, societies, and planet.

Always remember, as a sensitive person, your deep empathy and keen perception make you a potent force for change. Your sensitivity isn't a liability—it's a strength. Harness it with courage and conviction as you navigate these challenging times.

>> DO THIS

LEADING CHANGE: THE SENSITIVE PERSON'S OPPORTUNITY

1. **Accept the existential crisis:** As a sensitive person, you might feel the weight of existential threats more deeply. That's okay. Harness your unique intensity to spark hope, awe, and resilience. Remember, every crisis is an opportunity for growth.

2. **Respond proactively:** As a sensitive person, you have a deep-rooted sense of social, moral, and environmental responsibility. Channel this into actions, small or large, that counteract harm and promote healing both for yourself and for your community.

3. **Engage with your grief and fear:** These are natural reactions to loss. You might feel them strongly. The practices I shared in this book will help regulate your nervous system and ground you in times of stress. Keep them handy.

4. **Stand up to stereotypes:** Society may sometimes view sensitivity as a weakness. Don't buy into this narrative. Your sensitivity is a strength. Seek out supportive communities, like the Heal Your Nervous System community, where your deep empathy and perceptiveness are valued.

5. **Welcome transformation:** As a sensitive person, your capacity for profound change is tremendous. Embrace the healing process as an opportunity to recalibrate your emotional responses and build resilience.

6. **Go beyond survival:** Thriving isn't just about weathering storms—it's about learning to dance in the rain. Use your challenges as fuel to grow and create deeper, more courageous connections with life.

7. **Revel in interconnectedness:** Celebrate the sacred interconnectedness of all life. Your emotional depth is a testament to this interconnectedness. Use this profound understanding to catalyze healing, resilience, and meaningful change.

Epilogue

WE'VE COVERED A LOT OF GROUND together in this book. We've delved deep into the world of nervous system health and focused on people who feel everything a little bit more, who pick up on things that others might not. And while this sensitivity might sometimes feel like a burden, I believe it's one of your greatest strengths.

After pouring over studies, reflecting on personal experiences, and taking in the wisdom of experts in various fields—alongside the shared experiences from our Heal Your Nervous System community—I've come to believe that sensitivity, despite its potential biological costs, has been preserved through generations because it is fundamental to our survival.

I know, it's a big claim. Let me explain.

From an evolutionary standpoint, our highly sensitive ancestors' heightened awareness could have helped them spot danger or changes in their environment before anyone else—the rustle of a predator in the underbrush, the scent of a storm on the wind, the barely perceptible change in a plant that signals it's ready to eat. This not only increased their survival chances but also helped protect their entire community.

Sensitivity is more than just a survival tool; it's also an instrument of connection. Sensitive individuals, with their heightened empathetic abilities, create deeper bonds and strengthen community cohesion and resilience. They contribute to social harmony, often acting as peacemakers and mediators. Their ability to understand others' feelings and perspectives is invaluable in fostering empathy, understanding, and cooperation within a group—all vital for societal survival and advancement.

Evolution has allowed sensitive people to survive and pass on this trait to future generations for good reason. But in addition to simple survival, I believe sensitivity serves an even higher purpose.

In our efficiency-driven modern society, we're forever chasing "health optimization" or "health hacking." But real health isn't a linear measure of productivity or a perfect combination of diet and exercise. It's a state of wholeness and connection, a sense of *belonging* to an expansive web of life that transcends individuality.

Life is about connection—from the neural networks firing in our brains to the social bonds that bring love, meaning, and depth to our lives. Beyond these tangible links, there's a deeper connection, an interconnectedness that ties together every living and nonliving thing and permeates all of existence. This connection isn't a philosophical concept but a fundamental reality that has profound implications for our well-being and health.

To grasp this concept, think about the overview effect—the profound cognitive and emotional shift astronauts experience when they see earth from space. They often describe an overwhelming sense of unity, a profound understanding that we're all on this tiny blue planet together, connected in profound ways. Their sense of self is transformed, and they see the world in a whole new light as a unified, interconnected whole.

As part of the overview effect, astronauts sometimes speak of a captivating visual. As the sun sets over earth, it illuminates a thin blue airglow line above the planet—earth's precious atmosphere, our planet's life-protecting shield. From space, it appears as a slender blue band hugging the earth's curvature against the backdrop of the infinite expanse of space.

Every life, every story, every event that has ever occurred in human history has been contained within the confines of this narrow strip of atmosphere. This delicate boundary holds our collective past and future, symbolizing both our vulnerabilities and our inherent resilience.

Astronauts, upon viewing this line, often experience an intense sense of awe, vulnerability, and protectiveness. The blue airglow line they see is not just a line; it's also a testimony to our existence, a fragile sanctuary preserving life amid the unimaginable vastness and emptiness of the cosmos.

As a sensitive individual, you have an innate ability to grasp this sense of shared experience, vulnerability, and belonging. You don't need a spaceship to sense that interconnectedness. Your sensitivity provides you with an intuitive understanding of this truth. And it serves as a bridge, a connector, guiding others toward an understanding of our interconnectedness.

In leadership roles, your empathy and intuition become valuable tools that help you understand collective needs. You can lead with a vision that values the connectivity of your team above individualistic pursuits. As a parent, your sensitivity nurtures empathy and awareness in your children, fostering a generation that understands and values our interconnected existence. Your sensitivity can be a catalyst for change, drawing attention to critical issues in areas such as advocacy, politics, nongovernmental organizations, or local communities. In creative domains, your unique perspective could birth art that illuminates the interconnectedness of our experiences. In spiritual communities, your sensitivity can foster unity, deepening our collective understanding of our place within the grand tapestry of existence.

Your sensitivity isn't just about you, it's about all of us. It's about not letting humanity lose sight of what truly matters—our interconnectedness, our shared home within the thin blue airglow line of our atmosphere, and our shared responsibility to safeguard it.

Take up the challenges that come with this gift. Continue to create, connect, and inspire in all aspects of your life. Remember, your sensitivity is a bridge to a more connected world.

Embrace it.

Nurture it.

Celebrate it.

About the Author

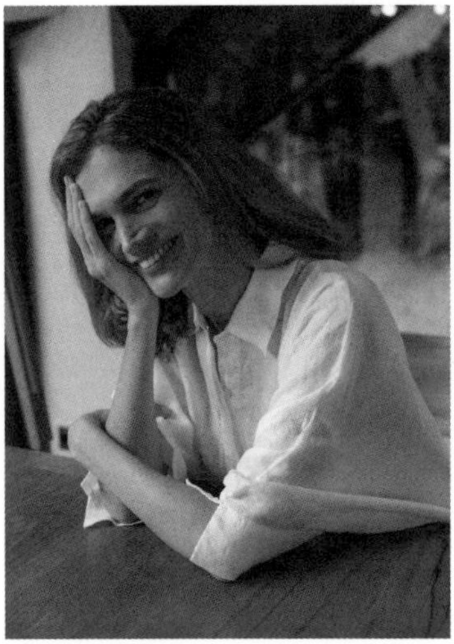

Dr. Linnea Passaler is the founder and CEO of Heal Your Nervous System, a community that connects thousands of people globally, offering them tools to nurture a well-regulated mind and body. Leveraging scientific research, a bespoke digital platform, and backed by a dedicated team of clinicians, researchers, and coaches, Heal Your Nervous System is on a mission to help people reverse anxiety, burnout, and other chronic physical and psychological symptoms of a dysregulated nervous system.

With a degree in oral medicine from the prestigious Università degli Studi in Milan, Dr. Linnea has more than twenty-five years of experience in health care, serving patients as an oral surgeon, a health educator, a scientific researcher, and a health-care entrepreneur. Through her professional life and personal journey to heal her own dysregulated nervous system, she has developed a unique understanding and deep respect for the connection between the body, mind, and spirit.

Dr. Linnea has been widely recognized for founding Pazienti.it, a digital health start-up, which, under her leadership, quickly evolved into one of Italy's most trusted online medical platforms. The Italian press referred to her as "the symbolic face" of Italy's innovation and she's spoken at events alongside the Italian president.

She splits her time between Bali and Italy, alongside her partner, Alessio, and their four children, Anais, Lelia, Amal, and Ariel.

Acknowledgments

Now that I stand on the other side of writing a book, I've come to deeply understand those acknowledgments where authors say it took a village to bring their work to life. Like a forest, this book has grown from the seeds of many contributions, though only my name appears on the cover.

To my partner and anchor, Alessio, your unwavering love and support have been the bedrock upon which this book was built. Time and time again, you've demonstrated your commitment in actions that speak louder than any words could. You've shouldered extra responsibilities, looking after our children and being endlessly patient with me, especially during those long months when I had to work extra to write this book. I've learned that writing a book drains almost all your energy, leaving very little for those around you. Thank you for being patient. Thank you for being an amazing dad to our children, the best I could ever hope for. I love you.

To Anais, Lelia, Amal, and Ariel, each of your arrivals in the world marked a beautiful, exciting new chapter in my life. I came to understand how my sense of safety was woven together with yours—a realization that shook me to my core. You've become my guiding stars, shaping my decisions, actions, and life's purpose from the day you were born.

Becoming your mom also meant diving into the world of sensory processing sensitivity, which showed up in your behaviors. This was a big challenge with all four of you arriving in less than five years! I was fortunate to have the guidance of experts like occupational therapist Georgina Ahrens, for whom I'm deeply grateful. Discovering sensory processing sensitivity in you wasn't just a parenting lesson. It was like looking in a mirror. It gave me a new perspective on my own body and nervous system, giving me insights into myself in ways I'd never imagined.

To my mom and dad, your constant support and encouragement always pushed me forward. Your influence nurtured my curiosity and passion for exploration and knowledge. For this, and for all the love you've given me, I am truly grateful. Thank you.

To my sister, Gaia, my cousin Marina, my uncle Ettore, and all the other members of our family, including our wonderful nannies Mira and Wayan, your unwavering love and the bond we share has always warmed my heart. Thank you for being there and for making our family what it is.

A special note of gratitude to Alessio's family, who have embraced me as one of their own.

To my grandparents Nonna Nanda, Nonno Pino, Nonna Teresa, Nonno Giovanni, and all my ancestors who have walked this earth before me, you have laid the foundation for me to stand tall today. *Grazie per avermi dato ali per volare, radici per tornare, e motivi per rimanere*. Thank you for giving me wings to fly, roots to come back, and reasons to stay.

Your legacy lives on in these pages and in my heart.

To my mentors and guides who've made a profound impact on my journey:

Josh Korda, your steadfast support, candid honesty, and warm affection have been my guiding light. Thank you for always being present in my life.

Jerry Colonna, your friendship is a treasure, and your caring nature has made a significant impact on my life. Thank you for your profound kindness and compassion.

Roberto Bonanzinga, your mentorship and the authenticity of our friendship have been pillars in my personal and entrepreneurial journey. Your unwavering support hasn't just been a game changer—it's given me a sense of confidence that is rare and precious. Thank you.

Salvo Mizzi, your early belief and support in me, when I was just starting my professional journey, was the catalyst I needed. Thank you for your faith in me.

Adriano Pala, you've stood by me through challenging circumstances, providing the assurance that I am not alone. Thank you for your steadfast support.

Ali Schultz, Kathy Cherry, and Cara Dinley, your leadership as strong women has been an inspiration. Your friendship and mentorship have provided a much-needed support system. I am lucky to have you as friends. Thank you.

To my cherished friends: Matilde Angelucci, Elena Morollo, Anita Schimdeg, Ron Elba, Mercedes Hurtado, Marina Trifogli, Paola Regina, Marco Castelnuovo, Alberto Picci, Tejpaul Bathia, Alessandro Colombo, Rudy Ricchizzi, Luca Babini, Morten Lauknes, and so many others—your presence in my life has been a sanctuary. You've given me a space where I could simply be myself, surrounded by peace, safety, nurturing, and unconditional support. Through the ups and downs, you've stood by me, and for that I am ever grateful. Thank you.

There are many more mentors and friends who have significantly impacted my life with their support. Although I haven't named each of you here, please know you are deeply cherished. Your influence remains with me, and I hold you close to my heart, brimming with gratitude.

To the dynamic, inspiring community at Heal Your Nervous System spread all around the globe, I am constantly awed by your dedication to personal healing and the transformative journeys that each of you undertakes. Your shared passion fuels not just our community but also sparks a global movement. Thank you for walking this path with me.

To the exceptional team behind Heal Your Nervous System: Gina Johnson, our head of operations, your dedication and capability are nothing short of extraordinary. I'm eager to see where our shared journey takes us.

Elizabeth Stratton, Daniel Suciu, Lara Hemeryck, Maryanne Taylor, Morgan de Klerk, Fabricio Yutaka, Ryan Bentley, Federica Tucci, and everyone on our team: you've infused our mission with your unique talents, passion, and spirit, and it shows. Mercedes Hurtado, your exceptional creativity in translating our ideas into compelling visuals has been instrumental in conveying our message. I'm grateful to Daniela Schrittenlocher for her invaluable guidance and expertise in all matters related to social media. My deepest gratitude to our incredible coaches: Cara Dinley, Kathy Cherry, and Josh Kelly. Your dedication to our community is visible every single day. Your unwavering support, especially during the writing of this book, has been invaluable. Thank you.

And a big, heartfelt thank you goes to my book team, starting with my friend and collaborator, Josh Kelly. Josh, your understanding of my ideas and your help in shaping them has been invaluable. Your touch is on every page, not just as an extraordinary editor but often as a coach, pushing me to deliver my best. The book is vastly improved because of your involvement—I consider myself lucky to have you on board. And your role wasn't limited to just editing. Your contribution to the research for this book, along with Lara Hemeryck, has been immense. You and Lara have worked tirelessly to gather, scrutinize, and analyze every piece of data, mirroring my own passion for scientific accuracy. For this, I am deeply thankful.

A hearty thank you to Jill Alexander. You planted the seed of this book in my mind when I least expected it, persistently nurturing it until I was ready to let it bloom. Your faith in this project, even before I fully committed, has been a guiding light.

A sincere thank you to Stephanie Tade, my agent. Stephanie, your trust in me, a newcomer to this writing world, meant more than I can express. Your speedy commitment, solid expertise, and robust support made this daunting project feel possible. Knowing you were on my team instilled the confidence I needed. Thank you for standing beside me on this journey.

To Mary Cassells, for her determined and relentless efforts in editing this manuscript. Mary, your insight, diligence, and linguistic skills have truly honed this book.

I also want to thank my publisher, Erik Gilg. Your constant belief in the potential of this book and your support have played a huge role in its creation. Thank you for being part of this incredible journey. A huge shout-out to the entire team at Quarto, including Giuliana Caranante and Todd Conly, and to everyone else working behind the scenes. Your tireless efforts have turned this book from an idea into a reality. Your hard work hasn't gone unnoticed and is truly appreciated. Thank you all.

Lastly, I want to extend a big thank you to all the hardworking scientists, doctors, and researchers around the world. You have inspired my love for science and medicine since I was a kid. I've made every effort to honor your work within this book. Thank you for being our compass in this vast universe.

References

Chapter 1: The Missing Piece of Your Healing Journey: A Dysregulated Nervous System

W. Thomas Boyce and Bruce J. Ellis, "Biological Sensitivity to Context: I. An Evolutionary–Developmental Theory of the Origins and Functions of Stress Reactivity," *Development and Psychopathology* 17, no. 2 (May 12, 2005), https://doi.org/10.1017/s0954579405050145.

Corina U. Greven et al., "Sensory Processing Sensitivity in the Context of Environmental Sensitivity: A Critical Review and Development of Research Agenda," *Neuroscience & Biobehavioral Reviews* 98 (March 1, 2019): 287–305, https://doi.org/10.1016/j.neubiorev.2019.01.009.

Roberto Guidotti et al., "Neuroplasticity within and between Functional Brain Networks in Mental Training Based on Long-Term Meditation," *Brain Sciences* 11, no. 8 (August 18, 2021): 1086, https://pubmed.ncbi.nlm.nih.gov/34439705/.

Ruth F. McCann and David Ross, "So Happy Together: The Storied Marriage Between Mitochondria and the Mind," *Biological Psychiatry* 83, no. 9 (May 1, 2018), https://doi.org/10.1016/j.biopsych.2018.03.006.

National Institute of Environmental Health Sciences. "Inflammation." *National Institute of Environmental Health Sciences*, (April 28, 2021), https://www.niehs.nih.gov/health/topics/conditions/inflammation/index.cfm.

Pedro Norat et al., "Mitochondrial Dysfunction in Neurological Disorders: Exploring Mitochondrial Transplantation," *NPJ Regenerative Medicine* 5, no. 22 (November 23, 2020), https://doi.org/10.1038/s41536-020-00107-x.

Liming Pei and Douglas C. Wallace, "Mitochondrial Etiology of Neuropsychiatric Disorders," *Biological Psychiatry* 83, no. 9 (May 1, 2018): 722–30, https://doi.org/10.1016/j.biopsych.2017.11.018.

Martin Picard et al., "A Mitochondrial Health Index Sensitive to Mood and Caregiving Stress," *Biological Psychiatry* 84, no. 1 (July 1, 2018): 9–17, https://doi.org/10.1016/j.biopsych.2018.01.012.

Kathy Smolewska, Scott McCabe, and Erik Z. Woody, "A Psychometric Evaluation of the Highly Sensitive Person Scale: The Components of Sensory-Processing Sensitivity and Their Relation to the BIS/BAS and 'Big Five,'" *Personality and Individual Differences* 40, no. 6 (April 1, 2006): 1269–79, https://www.sciencedirect.com/science/article/abs/pii/S0191886905003909.

Chapter 2: Transitioning from Quick Fix to Long-Term Solution: The 4 Pillars of Nervous System Health

Aliya Alimujiang et al., "Association Between Life Purpose and Mortality Among US Adults Older Than 50 Years," *JAMA Network Open* 2, no. 5 (May 3, 2019): e194270, https://pubmed.ncbi.nlm.nih.gov/31125099/.

Derek Bolton and Grant Gillett, *The Biopsychosocial Model of Health and Disease*, Springer eBooks, 2019, https://doi.org/10.1007/978-3-030-11899-0.

Randy Cohen, Chirag Bavishi, and Alan Rozanski, "Purpose in Life and Its Relationship to All-Cause Mortality and Cardiovascular Events," *Psychosomatic Medicine* 78, no. 2 (February–March, 2016): 122–33, https://doi.org/10.1097/psy.0000000000000274.

George L. Engel, "The Biopsychosocial Model and the Education of Health Professionals," *Annals of the New York Academy of Sciences* 310, no. 1 (June 1, 1978): 169–81, https://doi.org/10.1111/j.1749-6632.1978.tb22070.x.

George L. Engel, "The Care of the Patient: Art or Science?" *Johns Hopkins Medical Journal* (May 1, 1977): 222–32, https://pubmed.ncbi.nlm.nih.gov/859230.

George L. Engel, "The Clinical Application of the Biopsychosocial Model," *American Journal of Psychiatry* 137, no. 5 (May 1, 1980): 535–44, https://doi.org/10.1176/ajp.137.5.535.

George L. Engel, "Correspondence," *Psychosomatic Medicine* 23, no. 5 (September 1961): 427–29, https://journals.lww.com/psychosomaticmedicine/Citation/1961/09000/Correspondence.10.aspx.

George L. Engel, "The Need for a New Medical Model: A Challenge for Biomedicine," *Science* 196, no. 4286 (April 8, 1977): 129–36, https://doi.org/10.1126/science.847460.

George L. Engel, "A Unified Concept of Health and Disease," *Perspectives in Biology and Medicine* 3, no. 4 (June 1, 1960): 459–85, https://doi.org/10.1353/pbm.1960.0020.

Albert Farre and Tim Rapley, "The New Old (and Old New) Medical Model: Four Decades Navigating the Biomedical and Psychosocial Understandings of Health and Illness," *Healthcare* 5, no. 4 (November 18, 2017): 88, https://doi.org/10.3390/healthcare5040088.

Patrick L. Hill, "Chronic Pain: A Consequence of Dysregulated Protective Action," *British Journal of Pain* 13, no. 1 (September 10. 2018): 13–21, https://doi.org/10.1177/2049463718799784.

Harold G. Koenig, "Religion, Spirituality, and Health: The Research and Clinical Implications," *ISRN Psychiatry* (December 16, 2012): 1–33, https://pubmed.ncbi.nlm.nih.gov/23762764/.

Hari Kusnanto, Dwi Agustian, and Dany Hilmanto, "Biopsychosocial Model of Illnesses in Primary Care: A Hermeneutic Literature Review," *Journal of Family Medicine and Primary Care* 7, no. 3 (May–June, 2018): 497–500, https://doi.org/10.4103/jfmpc.jfmpc_145_17.

Lisa A. Miller et al., "Neuroanatomical Correlates of Religiosity and Spirituality," *JAMA Psychiatry* 71, no. 2 (February 1, 2014): 128, https://doi.org/10.1001/jamapsychiatry.2013.3067.

Marcelo Saad, Roberta De Medeiros, and Amanda Cristina Mosini, "Are We Ready for a True Biopsychosocial-Spiritual Model? The Many Meanings of 'Spiritual,'" *Medicines* 4, no. 4 (October 31, 2017): 79, https://doi.org/10.3390/medicines4040079.

Jessica Van Denend et al., "The Body, the Mind, and the Spirit: Including the Spiritual Domain in Mental Health Care," *Journal of Religion & Health* 61, no. 5 (July 19, 2022): 3571–88, https://doi.org/10.1007/s10943-022-01609-2.

Tyler J. VanderWeele et al., "Association Between Religious Service Attendance and Lower Suicide Rates Among US Women," *JAMA Psychiatry* 73, no. 8 (August 1, 2016): 845–851, https://doi.org/10.1001/jamapsychiatry.2016.1243.

Chapter 3: The Sensitive Nervous System: Its Role in Your Path to Healing

Bianca P. Acevedo et al., "The Highly Sensitive Brain: An fMRI Study of Sensory Processing Sensitivity and Response to Others' Emotions," *Brain and Behavior* 4, no. 4 (June 23, 2014): 580–94, https://doi.org/10.1002/brb3.242.

Bianca P. Acevedo, *The Highly Sensitive Brain: Research, Assessment, and Treatment of Sensory Processing Sensitivity* (Cambridge, MA: Academic Press, 2020).

Elaine N. Aron and Arthur Aron, "Sensory-Processing Sensitivity and Its Relation to Introversion and Emotionality," *Journal of Personality and Social Psychology* 73, no. 2 (August 1, 1997): 345–68, https://pubmed.ncbi.nlm.nih.gov/9248053/.

Elaine N. Aron, Arthur Aron, and Jadzia Jagiellowicz, "Sensory Processing Sensitivity: A Review in the Light of the Evolution of Biological Responsivity," *Personality and Social Psychology Review* 16, no. 3 (January 30, 2012): 262–82, https://doi.org/10.1177/1088868311434213.

Taraneh Attary and Ali Ghazizadeh, "Localizing Sensory Processing Sensitivity and Its Subdomains within Its Relevant Trait Space: A Data-Driven Approach," *Scientific Reports* 11, no. 20343 (October 13, 2021), https://doi.org/10.1038/s41598-021-99686-y.

A. J. Ayres, "The Development of Perceptual-Motor Abilities: A Theoretical Basis for Treatment of Dysfunction," *American Journal of Occupational Therapy* 17 (November-December 1963): 221–25, https://pubmed.ncbi.nlm.nih.gov/14072429.

Sharell Bas et al., "Experiences of Adults High in the Personality Trait Sensory Processing Sensitivity: A Qualitative Study," *Journal of Clinical Medicine* 10, no. 21 (October 24, 2021): 4912, https://doi.org/10.3390/jcm10214912.

Jay Belsky and Michael Pluess, "Beyond Diathesis Stress: Differential Susceptibility to Environmental Influences," *Psychological Bulletin* 135, no. 6 (November 1, 2009): 885–908, https://www.hsperson.com/pdf/Belsky_and_Pluess_2009_Beyond_Diathesis_Stress_-_%20Differential_Susceptibility_to_Environmental_Influences.pdf.

W. Thomas Boyce and Bruce J. Ellis, "Biological Sensitivity to Context: I. An Evolutionary-Developmental Theory of the Origins and Functions of Stress Reactivity," *Development and Psychopathology* 17, no. 2 (May 12, 2005), https://doi.org/10.1017/s0954579405050145.

Kristjana Cameron, John S. Ogrodniczuk, and George Hadjipavlou, "Changes in Alexithymia Following Psychological Intervention," *Harvard Review of Psychiatry* 22, no. 3 (May–June, 2014): 162–78, https://journals.lww.com/hrpjournal/Abstract/2014/05000/Changes_in_Alexithymia_Following_Psychological.3.aspx.

Caroline M. Coppens, Sietse F. de Boer, and Jaap M. Koolhaas, "Coping Styles and Behavioural Flexibility: Towards Underlying Mechanisms," *Philosophical Transactions of the Royal Society B* 365, no. 1560 (December 27, 2010): 4021–28, https://doi.org/10.1098/rstb.2010.0217.

Véronique De Gucht, Dion H A Woestenburg, and Tom F. Wilderjans, "The Different Faces of (High) Sensitivity, Toward a More Comprehensive Measurement Instrument. Development and Validation of the Sensory Processing Sensitivity Questionnaire (SPSQ)," *Journal of Personality Assessment* 104, no. 6 (February 17, 2022): 784–99, https://doi.org/10.1080/00223891.2022.2032101.

Bernadette de Villiers, Francesca Lionetti, and Michael Pluess, "Vantage Sensitivity: A Framework for Individual Differences in Response to Psychological Intervention," *Social Psychiatry and Psychiatric Epidemiology* 53, no. 6 (January 4, 2018): 545–54, https://doi.org/10.1007/s00127-017-1471-0.

Winnie Dunn, "Supporting Children to Participate Successfully in Everyday Life by Using Sensory Processing Knowledge," *Infants and Young Children* 20, no. 2 (April 1, 2007): 84–101, https://journals.lww.com/iycjournal/fulltext/2007/04000/supporting_children_to_participate_successfully_in.2.aspx.

Bruce J. Ellis et al., "Differential Susceptibility to the Environment: An Evolutionary–Neurodevelopmental Theory," *Development and Psychopathology* 23, no. 1 (February 1, 2011): 7–28, https://doi.org/10.1017/s0954579410000611.

Julie Ermer and Winnie Dunn, "The Sensory Profile: A Discriminant Analysis of Children with and without Disabilities," *American Journal of Occupational Therapy* 52, no. 4 (April 1, 1998): 283–90, https://research.aota.org/ajot/article-abstract/52/4/283/4192/The-Sensory-Profile-A-Discriminant-Analysis-of?redirectedFrom=fulltext.

Corina U. Greven et al., "Sensory Processing Sensitivity in the Context of Environmental Sensitivity: A Critical Review and Development of Research Agenda," *Neuroscience & Biobehavioral Reviews* 98 (March 1, 2019): 287–305, https://doi.org/10.1016/j.neubiorev.2019.01.009.

Hadas Grouper et al., "Increased Functional Connectivity between Limbic Brain Areas in Healthy Individuals with High versus Low Sensitivity to Cold Pain: A Resting State fMRI Study," *PLOS One* 17, no. 4 (April 20, 2022): e0267170, https://doi.org/10.1371/journal.pone.0267170.

Laura Harrison et al., "The Importance of Sensory Processing in Mental Health: A Proposed Addition to the Research Domain Criteria (RDoC) and Suggestions for RDoC 2.0," *Frontiers in Psychology* 10 (February 5, 2019), https://doi.org/10.3389/fpsyg.2019.00103.

Manfred J. C. Hessing et al., "Individual Behavioral and Physiological Strategies in Pigs," *Physiology & Behavior* 55, no. 1 (January 1, 1994): 39–46, https://www.sciencedirect.com/science/article/abs/pii/0031938494900078?via%3Dihub.

Shuhei Iimura, "Sensory-Processing Sensitivity and COVID-19 Stress in a Young Population: The Mediating Role of Resilience," *Personality and Individual Differences* 184 (January 1, 2022): 111183, https://doi.org/10.1016/j.paid.2021.111183.

Jadzia Jagiellowicz, Arthur Aron, and Elaine N. Aron, "Relationship Between the Temperament Trait of Sensory Processing Sensitivity and Emotional Reactivity," *Social Behavior and Personality* 44, no. 2 (January 1, 2016): 185–99, https://doi.org/10.2224/sbp.2016.44.2.185.

Lorna S. Jakobson and Sarah N. Rigby, "Alexithymia and Sensory Processing Sensitivity: Areas of Overlap and Links to Sensory Processing Styles," *Frontiers in Psychology* 12 (May 24, 2021), https://www.sciencedirect.com/science/article/abs/pii/0031938494900078?via%3Dihub.

Chieko Kibe et al., "Sensory Processing Sensitivity and Culturally Modified Resilience Education: Differential Susceptibility in Japanese Adolescents," *PLOS One* 15, no. 9 (September 14, 2020): e0239002, https://doi.org/10.1371/journal.pone.0239002.

Shelly J. Lane et al., "Neural Foundations of Ayres Sensory Integration®," *Brain Sciences* 9, no. 7 (June 28, 2019): 153, https://doi.org/10.3390/brainsci9070153.

Francesca Lionetti et al., "Dandelions, Tulips and Orchids: Evidence for the Existence of Low-Sensitive, Medium-Sensitive and High-Sensitive Individuals," *Translational Psychiatry* 8, no. 24 (January 22, 2018), https://doi.org/10.1038/s41398-017-0090-6.

Francesca Lionetti et al., "Sensory Processing Sensitivity and Its Association with Personality Traits and Affect: A Meta-Analysis," *Journal of Research in Personality* 81 (August 1, 2019): 138–52, https://www.sciencedirect.com/science/article/abs/pii/S0092656619300583?via%3Dihub.

Olivier Luminet, Kristy A. Nielson, and Nathan Ridout, "Cognitive-Emotional Processing in Alexithymia: An Integrative Review," *Cognition and Emotion* 35, no. 3 (March 31, 2021): 449–87, https://doi.org/10.1080/02699931.2021.1908231.

David Lyons, Edward Price, and Gary P. Moberg, "Social Modulation of Pituitary-Adrenal Responsiveness and Individual Differences in Behavior of Young Domestic Goats," *Physiology & Behavior* 43, no. 4 (January 1, 1988): 451–58, https://www.sciencedirect.com/science/article/abs/pii/0031938488901199?via%3Dihub.

Klara Malinakova et al., "Sensory Processing Sensitivity Questionnaire: A Psychometric Evaluation and Associations with Experiencing the COVID-19 Pandemic," *International Journal of Environmental Research and Public Health* 18, no. 24 (December 8, 2021): 12962, https://doi.org/10.3390/ijerph182412962.

Aino K. Mattila et al., "Taxometric Analysis of Alexithymia in a General Population Sample from Finland," *Personality and Individual Differences* 49, no. 3 (August 1, 2010): 216–21, https://doi.org/10.1016/j.paid.2010.03.038.

Amanda M. McQuarrie, Stephen D. Smith, and Lorna S. Jakobson, "Alexithymia and Sensory Processing Sensitivity Account for Unique Variance in the Prediction of Emotional Contagion and Empathy," *Frontiers in Psychology* 14 (April 20, 2023), https://doi.org/10.3389/fpsyg.2023.1072783.

Alexia E. Metz et al., "Dunn's Model of Sensory Processing: An Investigation of the Axes of the Four-Quadrant Model in Healthy Adults," *Brain Sciences* 9, no. 2 (February 7, 2019): 35, https://doi.org/10.3390/brainsci9020035.

Joseph Meyerson et al., "Burnout and Professional Quality of Life among Israeli Dentists: The Role of Sensory Processing Sensitivity," *International Dental Journal* 70, no. 1 (February 1, 2020): 29–37, https://doi.org/10.1111/idj.12523.

Michael Pluess et al., "Environmental Sensitivity in Children: Development of the Highly Sensitive Child Scale and Identification of Sensitivity Groups," *Developmental Psychology* 54, no. 1 (January 1, 2018): 51–70, https://doi.org/10.1037/dev0000406.

Michael Pluess and Ilona Boniwell, "Sensory-Processing Sensitivity Predicts Treatment Response to a School-Based Depression Prevention Program: Evidence of Vantage Sensitivity," *Personality and Individual Differences* 82 (August 1, 2015): 40–45, https://doi.org/10.1016/j.paid.2015.03.011.

Jessie Poquérusse et al., "Alexithymia and Autism Spectrum Disorder: A Complex Relationship," *Frontiers in Psychology* 9 (July 17, 2018), https://doi.org/10.3389/fpsyg.2018.01196.

Lucia Ricciardi et al., "Alexithymia in Neurological Disease: A Review," *Journal of Neuropsychiatry and Clinical Neurosciences* 27, no. 3 (February 6, 2015): 179–87, https://doi.org/10.1176/appi.neuropsych.14070169.

Joachim Schjolden and Svante Winberg, "Genetically Determined Variation in Stress Responsiveness in Rainbow Trout: Behavior and Neurobiology," *Brain Behavior and Evolution* 70, no. 4 (September 1, 2007): 227–38, https://doi.org/10.1159/000105486.

Andrew Sih, Alison M. Bell, and Jeffrey C. Johnson, "Behavioral Syndromes: An Ecological and Evolutionary Overview," *Trends in Ecology and Evolution* 19, no. 7 (July 1, 2004): 372–78, https://doi.org/10.1016/j.tree.2004.04.009.

Kathy Smolewska, Scott McCabe, and Erik Z. Woody, "A Psychometric Evaluation of the Highly Sensitive Person Scale: The Components of Sensory-Processing Sensitivity and Their Relation to the BIS/BAS and 'Big Five,'" *Personality and Individual Differences* 40, no. 6 (April 1, 2006): 1269–79, https://doi.org/10.1016/j.paid.2005.09.022.

Amanda L. Stone and Anna C. Wilson, "Transmission of Risk from Parents with Chronic Pain to Offspring: An Integrative Conceptual Model," *Journal of the International Association for the Study of Pain* 157, no. 12 (December 2016): 2628–39, https://doi.org/10.1097/j.pain.0000000000000637.

Stephen J. Suomi, "Risk, Resilience, and Gene x Environment Interactions in Rhesus Monkeys," *Annals of the New York Academy of Sciences* 1094, no. 1 (December 1, 2006): 52–62, https://doi.org/10.1196/annals.1376.006.

Yaara Turjeman-Levi and Avraham N. Kluger, "Sensory-Processing Sensitivity versus the Sensory-Processing Theory: Convergence and Divergence," *Frontiers in Psychology* 13 (December 1, 2022), https://doi.org/10.3389/fpsyg.2022.1010836.

Yuta Ujiie and Kohske Takahashi, "Subjective Sensitivity to Exteroceptive and Interoceptive Processing in Highly Sensitive Person," *Psychological Reports*, August 12, 2022, https://doi.org/10.1177/00332941221119403.

Frank Van Den Boogert et al., "Sensory Processing, Perceived Stress and Burnout Symptoms in a Working Population during the COVID-19 Crisis," *International Journal of Environmental Research and Public Health* 19, no. 4 (February 11, 2022): 2043, https://doi.org/10.3390/ijerph19042043.

Chapter 4: The Tipping Point: How Stress and Fear Lead to a Dysregulated Nervous System

Bianca P. Acevedo et al., "The Functional Highly Sensitive Brain: A Review of the Brain Circuits Underlying Sensory Processing Sensitivity and Seemingly Related Disorders," *Philosophical Transactions of the Royal Society B* 373, no. 1744 (April 19, 2018): 20170161, https://doi.org/10.1098/rstb.2017.0161.

Ghazi I. Al Jowf et al., "The Molecular Biology of Susceptibility to Post-Traumatic Stress Disorder: Highlights of Epigenetics and Epigenomics," *International Journal of Molecular Sciences* 22, no. 19 (October 4, 2021): 10743, https://doi.org/10.3390/ijms221910743.

Ghazi I. Al Jowf et al., "A Public Health Perspective of Post-Traumatic Stress Disorder," *International Journal of Environmental Research and Public Health* 19, no. 11 (May 26, 2022): 6474, https://www.mdpi.com/1660-4601/19/11/6474.

Rodrigo G. Arzate-Mejía and Isabelle M. Mansuy, "Epigenetic Inheritance: Impact for Biology and Society—Recent Progress, Current Questions and Future Challenges," *Environmental Epigenetics* 8, no. 1 (November 5, 2022), https://doi.org/10.1093/eep/dvac021.

Yann Auxéméry, "L'état de Stress Post-Traumatique Comme Conséquence de l'interaction Entre Une Susceptibilité Génétique Individuelle, Un Évènement Traumatogène et Un Contexte Social," *L'Encéphale* 38, no. 5 (October 1, 2012): 373–80, https://doi.org/10.1016/j.encep.2011.12.003.

J. Douglas Bremner et al., "Diet, Stress and Mental Health," *Nutrients* 12, no. 8 (August 13, 2020): 2428, https://doi.org/10.3390/nu12082428.

J. Douglas Bremner and Matthew T. Wittbrodt, "Chapter One— Stress, the Brain, and Trauma Spectrum Disorders," in *International Review of Neurobiology* 152 (2020), 1–22, https://www.sciencedirect.com/science/article/abs/pii/S0074774220300040?via%3Dihub.

Center for Substance Abuse Treatment (US), "Exhibit 1.3-4, DSM-5 Diagnostic Criteria for PTSD—Trauma-Informed Care in Behavioral Health Services—NCBI Bookshelf," n.d., https://www.ncbi.nlm.nih.gov/books/NBK207191/box/part1_ch3.box16.

Jacquelyn S. Christensen et al., "Diverse Autonomic Nervous System Stress Response Patterns in Childhood Sensory Modulation," *Frontiers in Integrative Neuroscience* 14 (February 18, 2020),https://www.frontiersin.org/articles/10.3389/fnint.2020.00006/full.

Kevin J. Clancy et al., "Intrinsic Sensory Disinhibition Contributes to Intrusive Re-Experiencing in Combat Veterans," *Scientific Reports* 10, no. 936 (January 22, 2020), https://doi.org/10.1038/s41598-020-57963-2.

Marco Del Giudice, "Attachment in Middle Childhood: An Evolutionary-Developmental Perspective," *New Directions for Child and Adolescent Development* 2015, no. 148 (June 18, 2015): 15–30, https://doi.org/10.1002/cad.20101.

Marco Del Giudice, "Differential Susceptibility to the Environment: Are Developmental Models Compatible with the Evidence from Twin Studies?" *Developmental Psychology* 52, no. 8 (June 16, 2016): 1330–39, https://doi.org/10.1037/dev0000153.

Marco Del Giudice, Bruce J. Ellis, and Elizabeth A. Shirtcliff, "The Adaptive Calibration Model of Stress Responsivity," *Neuroscience & Biobehavioral Reviews* 35, no. 7 (June 1, 2011): https://www.sciencedirect.com/science/article/abs/pii/S014976341000196X?via%3Dihub.

Jonathan DePierro et al., "Beyond PTSD: Client Presentations of Developmental Trauma Disorder from a National Survey of Clinicians," *Psychological Trauma: Theory, Research, Practice, and Policy* 14, no. 7 (December 19, 2019): 1167–74, https://doi.org/10.1037/tra0000532.

Pelin Karaca-Dinç, Seda Oktay, and Ayşegül Durak Batıgün, "Mediation Role of Alexithymia, Sensory Processing Sensitivity and Emotional-Mental Processes between Childhood Trauma and Adult Psychopathology: A Self-Report Study," *BMC Psychiatry* 21, no. 508 (October 15, 2021), https://doi.org/10.1186/s12888-021-03532-4.

Todd M. Everson et al., "Epigenetic Differences in Stress Response Gene *FKBP5* among Children with Abusive vs Accidental Injuries," *Pediatric Research* 94 (January 9, 2023): 193–9 https://doi.org/10.1038/s41390-022-02441-w.

Robyn Fivush et al., "The Making of Autobiographical Memory: Intersections of Culture, Narratives and Identity," *International Journal of Psychology* 46, no. 5 (October 6, 2011): 321–45, https://doi.org/10.1080/00207594.2011.596541.

Julian D. Ford et al., "Can Developmental Trauma Disorder Be Distinguished from Posttraumatic Stress Disorder? A Symptom-Level Person-Centred Empirical Approach," *European Journal of Psychotraumatology* 13, no. 2 (November 2, 2022), https://doi.org/10.1080/20008066.2022.2133488.

Christine Gimpel et al., "Changes and Interactions of Flourishing, Mindfulness, Sense of Coherence, and Quality of Life in Patients of a Mind-Body Medicine Outpatient Clinic," *Complementary Medicine Research* 21, no. 3 (June 18, 2014): 154–62, https://doi.org/10.1159/000363784.

Julia Anna Glombiewski et al., "Do Patients with Chronic Pain Show Autonomic Arousal When Confronted with Feared Movements? An Experimental Investigation of the Fear–Avoidance Model," *Journal of the International Association for the Study of Pain* 156, no. 3 (March 1, 2015): 547–54, https://doi.org/10.1097/01.j.pain.0000460329.48633.ce.

Lisa Hancock and Richard A. Bryant, "Posttraumatic Stress, Stressor Controllability, and Avoidance," *Behaviour Research and Therapy* 128 (February 19, 2020): 103591 https://doi.org/10.1016/j.brat.2020.103591.

Georgia E. Hodes and C. Neill Epperson, "Sex Differences in Vulnerability and Resilience to Stress Across the Life-span," *Biological Psychiatry* 86, no. 6 (September 15, 2019): 421–32, https://www.biologicalpsychiatryjournal.com/article/S0006-3223(19)31325-3/fulltext.

Caitlyn O. Hood and Christal L. Badour, "The Effects of Posttraumatic Stress and Trauma-Focused Disclosure on Experimental Pain Sensitivity Among Trauma-Exposed Women," *Journal of Traumatic Stress* 33, no. 6 (August 13, 2020): 1071–81, https://doi.org/10.1002/jts.22571.

Emily R. Hunt et al., "Using Massage to Combat Fear-Avoidance and the Pain Tension Cycle," *International Journal of Athletic Therapy and Training* 24, no. 5 (September 1, 2019): 198-201 https://doi.org/10.1123/ijatt.2018-0097.

Ali Jawaid, Katherina-Lynn Jehle, and Isabelle M. Mansuy, "Impact of Parental Exposure on Offspring Health in Humans," *Trends in Genetics* 37, no. 4 (April 1, 2021): 373–88, https://doi.org/10.1016/j.tig.2020.10.006.

Payton J. Jones et al., "Exposure to Descriptions of Traumatic Events Narrows One's Concept of Trauma," *Journal of Experimental Psychology: Applied* 29, no. 1 (March 2022): 179–87, https://pubmed.ncbi.nlm.nih.gov/35025575/.

Payton J. Jones and Richard J. McNally, "Does Broadening One's Concept of Trauma Undermine Resilience?" *Psychological Trauma: Theory, Research, Practice, and Policy* 14, no. S1 (April 1, 2022): S131–39, https://pubmed.ncbi.nlm.nih.gov/34197173/.

Ned H. Kalin, "Trauma, Resilience, Anxiety Disorders, and PTSD," *American Journal of Psychiatry* 178, no. 2 (February 1, 2021): 103–5, https://doi.org/10.1176/appi.ajp.2020.20121738.

David C. Knight, "Neurocognitive Profiles Predict Susceptibility and Resilience to Posttraumatic Stress," *American Journal of Psychiatry* 178, no. 11 (November 4, 2021): 991–93, https://ajp.psychiatryonline.org/doi/10.1176/appi.ajp.2021.21090890.

Franziska Köhler-Dauner et al., "Maternal Sensitivity Modulates Child's Parasympathetic Mode and Buffers Sympathetic Activity in a Free Play Situation," *Frontiers in Psychology* 13 (April 19, 2022), https://doi.org/10.3389/fpsyg.2022.868848.

Mirko Lehmann et al., "Insights into the Molecular Genetic Basis of Individual Differences in Metacognition," *Physiology & Behavior* 264 (May 15, 2023): 114139, https://doi.org/10.1016/j.physbeh.2023.114139.

Eleonora Marzilli et al., "Internet Addiction among Young Adult University Students during the COVID-19 Pandemic: The Role of Peritraumatic Distress, Attachment, and Alexithymia," *International Journal of Environmental Research and Public Health* 19, no. 23 (November 24, 2022): 15582, https://doi.org/10.3390/ijerph192315582.

Vasiliki Michopoulos et al., "Inflammation in Fear- and Anxiety-Based Disorders: PTSD, GAD, and Beyond," *Neuropsychopharmacology* 42, no. 1 (January 1, 2017): 254–70, https://doi.org/10.1038/npp.2016.146.

Gavin E. Morris et al., "Mitigating Contemporary Trauma Impacts Using Ancient Applications," *Frontiers in Psychology* 13 (August 2, 2022), https://doi.org/10.3389/fpsyg.2022.645397.

Caroline M. Nievergelt et al., "International Meta-Analysis of PTSD Genome-Wide Association Studies Identifies Sex- and Ancestry-Specific Genetic Risk Loci," *Nature Communications* 10, no. 1 (October 8, 2019), https://doi.org/10.1038/s41467-019-12576-w.

Carol S. North et al., "The Evolution of PTSD Criteria across Editions of DSM," *Annuals of Clinical Psychiatry* 28, no. 3 (August 1, 2016): 197-208, https://pubmed.ncbi.nlm.nih.gov/27490836.

Michael Notaras and Maarten van den Buuse, "Neurobiology of BDNF in Fear Memory, Sensitivity to Stress, and Stress-Related Disorders," *Molecular Psychiatry* 25, no. 10 (January 3, 2020): 2251–74, https://pubmed.ncbi.nlm.nih.gov/31900428/.

Andrea L. Roberts et al., "The Stressor Criterion for Posttraumatic Stress Disorder : Does It Matter?," *Journal of Clinical Psychiatry* 73, no. 2 (February 15, 2012): e264–70, https://pubmed.ncbi.nlm.nih.gov/22401487/.

Judith R. Schore and Allan N. Schore, "Modern Attachment Theory: The Central Role of Affect Regulation in Development and Treatment," *Clinical Social Work Journal* 36, no. 1 (March 1, 2008): 9–20, https://link.springer.com/article/10.1007/s10615-007-0111-7#citeas.

Khushbu Shah et al., "Mind-Body Treatments of Irritable Bowel Syndrome Symptoms: An Updated Meta-Analysis," *Behaviour Research and Therapy* 128 (May 1, 2020): 103462, https://www.sciencedirect.com/science/article/abs/pii/S0005796719301482?via%3Dihub.

Joseph Spinazzola, Bessel A. van der Kolk, and Julian D. Ford, "Developmental Trauma Disorder: A Legacy of Attachment Trauma in Victimized Children," *Journal of Traumatic Stress* 34, no. 4 (May 28, 2021): 711–20, https://doi.org/10.1002/jts.22697.

Jennifer S. Stevens et al., "Brain-Based Biotypes of Psychiatric Vulnerability in the Acute Aftermath of Trauma," *American Journal of Psychiatry* 178, no. 11 (October 14, 2021): 1037–49, https://ajp.psychiatryonline.org/doi/10.1176/appi.ajp.2021.20101526.

Kristina M. Thumfart et al., "Epigenetics of Childhood Trauma: Long Term Sequelae and Potential for Treatment," *Neuroscience & Biobehavioral Reviews* 132 (January 1, 2022): 1049–66, https://www.sciencedirect.com/science/article/pii/S014976342100484X?via%3Dihub.

Lisa J. M. van den Berg et al., "A New Perspective on PTSD Symptoms after Traumatic vs Stressful Life Events and the Role of Gender," *European Journal of Psychotraumatology* 8, no. 1 (November 13, 2017), https://doi.org/10.1080/20008198.2017.1380470.

Bessel A. van der Kolk, "Trauma and Memory," *Psychiatry and Clinical Neurosciences* 52, no. S1 (September 1, 1998): S52-64, https://doi.org/10.1046/j.1440-1819.1998.0520s5s97.x.

Christiaan H. Vinkers et al., "An Integrated Approach to Understand Biological Stress System Dysregulation across Depressive and Anxiety Disorders," *Journal of Affective Disorders* 283 (March 15, 2021): 139–46, https://doi.org/10.1016/j.jad.2021.01.051.

Marielle Wathelet et al., "Posttraumatic Stress Disorder in Time of COVID-19: Trauma or Not Trauma, Is That the Question?" *Acta Psychiatrica Scandinavica* 144, no. 3 (June 9, 2021): 310–11, https://doi.org/10.1111/acps.13336.

Martin C. S. Wong et al., "Resilience Level and Its Association with Maladaptive Coping Behaviours in the COVID-19 Pandemic: A Global Survey of the General Populations," *Globalization and Health* 19, no. 1 (January 3, 2023), https://doi.org/10.1186/s12992-022-00903-8.

Samantha A. Wong et al., "Internal Capsule Microstructure Mediates the Relationship between Childhood Maltreatment and PTSD Following Adulthood Trauma Exposure," *Molecular Psychiatry* (March 17, 2023), https://doi.org/10.1038/s41380-023-02012-3.

Anthony S. Zannas et al., "Epigenetic Aging and PTSD Outcomes in the Immediate Aftermath of Trauma," *Psychological Medicine* (March 23, 2023): 1–10, https://doi.org/10.1017/S0033291723000636.

Chapter 5: The 5-Stage Plan to Reverse Nervous System Dysregulation

Aliya Alimujiang et al., "Association Between Life Purpose and Mortality Among US Adults Older Than 50 Years," *JAMA Network Open* 2, no. 5 (May 24, 2019): e194270, https://doi.org/10.1001/jamanetworkopen.2019.4270.

Manoj K. Bhasin et al., "Relaxation Response Induces Temporal Transcriptome Changes in Energy Metabolism, Insulin Secretion and Inflammatory Pathways," *PLOS One* 12, no. 25 (May 1, 2013): e0172873, https://journals.plos.org/plosone/article?id=10.1371/journal.pone.0062817.

Manoj K. Bhasin et al., "Specific Transcriptome Changes Associated with Blood Pressure Reduction in Hypertensive Patients After Relaxation Response Training," *Journal of Alternative and Complementary Medicine* 24, no. 5 (May 1, 2018): 486–504, https://doi.org/10.1089/acm.2017.0053.

Randy Cohen, Chirag Bavishi, and Alan Rozanski, "Purpose in Life and Its Relationship to All-Cause Mortality and Cardiovascular Events, A Meta Analysis" *Psychosomatic Medicine* 78, no. 2 (February–March, 2016): 122–33, https://journals.lww.com/psychosomaticmedicine/abstract/2016/02000/purpose_in_life_and_its_relationship_to_all_cause.2.aspx.

Jeffery A. Dusek et al., "Genomic Counter-Stress Changes Induced by the Relaxation Response," *PLOS One* 3, no. 7 (July 2, 2008): e2576, https://doi.org/10.1371/journal.pone.0002576.

Donald C. Goff et al., "Tardive Dyskinesia and Substrates of Energy Metabolism in CSF," *American Journal of Psychiatry* 152, no. 12 (December 1, 1995): 1730–36, https://doi.org/10.1176/ajp.152.12.1730.

Jeffrey J. Goldberger et al., "Autonomic Nervous System Dysfunction: A JACC Focus Seminar," *Journal of the American College of Cardiology* 73, no. 10 (March 19, 2019): 1189–1206, https://doi.org/10.1016/j.jacc.2018. 12.064.

Minmin Hu et al., "Resveratrol Prevents Haloperidol-Induced Mitochondria Dysfunction through the Induction of Autophagy in SH-SY5Y Cells," *NeuroToxicology* 87 (October 22, 2021): 231–42, https://doi.org/10.1016/j.neuro.2021.10.007.

Braden Kuo et al., "Genomic and Clinical Effects Associated with a Relaxation Response Mind-Body Intervention in Patients with Irritable Bowel Syndrome and Inflammatory Bowel Disease," *PLOS One* 10, no. 4 (April 30, 2015): e0123861, https://doi.org/10.1371/journal.pone.0123861.

Ian W. Listopad et al., "Bio-Psycho-Socio-Spirito-Cultural Factors of Burnout: A Systematic Narrative Review of the Literature," *Frontiers in Psychology* 12 (December 1, 2021), https://doi.org/10.3389/fpsyg.2021.722862.

Lisa A. Miller et al., "Neuroanatomical Correlates of Religiosity and Spirituality: A Study in Adults at High and Low Familial Risk for Depression," *JAMA Psychiatry* 71, no. 2 (February 1, 2014): 135, https://doi.org/10.1001/jamapsychiatry.2013.3067.

Juan C. Sánchez-Manso et al., *Autonomic Dysfunction* (Treasure Island, FL: StatPearls Publishing, 2022), https://pubmed.ncbi.nlm.nih.gov/28613638.

Chapter 6: A Structure to Support Your Nervous System

Walid Kamal Abdelbasset et al., "Therapeutic Effects of Proprioceptive Exercise on Functional Capacity, Anxiety, and Depression in Patients with Diabetic Neuropathy: A 2-Month Prospective Study," *Clinical Rheumatology* 39, no. 10 (April 16, 2020): 3091–97, https://doi.org/10.1007/s10067-020-05086-4.

Victoria A. Acosta-Rodríguez et al., "Circadian Alignment of Early Onset Caloric Restriction Promotes Longevity in Male C57BL/6J Mice," *Science* 376, no. 6598 (May 5, 2022): 1192–1202, https://doi.org/10.1126/science.abk0297.

Kirsten Berding et al., "Feed Your Microbes to Deal with Stress: A Psychobiotic Diet Impacts Microbial Stability and Perceived Stress in a Healthy Adult Population," *Molecular Psychiatry* 28, no. 2 (October 27, 2022): 601-10, https://doi.org/10.1038/s41380-022-01817-y.

Fivos Borbolis, Eirini Mytilinaiou, and Konstantinos Palikaras, "The Crosstalk between Microbiome and Mitochondrial Homeostasis in Neurodegeneration," *Cells* 12, no. 3 (January 28, 2023): 429, https://www.mdpi.com/2073-4409/12/3/429.

"Brain Basics: Understanding Sleep," National Institute of Neurological Disorders and Stroke (March 17, 2023), https://www.ninds.nih.gov/health-information/public-education/brain-basics/brain-basics-understanding-sleep.

Jiezhong Chen and Luis Vitetta, "Mitochondria Could Be a Potential Key Mediator Linking the Intestinal Microbiota to Depression," *Journal of Cellular Biochemistry* 121, no. 1 (January 1, 2020): 17–24, https://onlinelibrary.wiley.com/doi/10.1002/jcb.29311.

Teris Cheung et al., "The Effectiveness of Electrical Vestibular Stimulation (VeNS) on Symptoms of Anxiety: Study Protocol of a Randomized, Double-Blinded, Sham-Controlled Trial," *International Journal of Environmental Research and Public Health* 20, no. 5 (February 27, 2023): 4218, https://doi.org/10.3390/ijerph20054218.

Agata Chudzik et al., "Probiotics, Prebiotics and Postbiotics on Mitigation of Depression Symptoms: Modulation of the Brain–Gut–Microbiome Axis," *Biomolecules* 11, no. 7 (July 7, 2021): 1000, https://www.mdpi.com/2218-273X/11/7/1000.

Alejandro Déniz-García et al., "Impact of Anxiety, Depression and Disease-Related Distress on Long-Term Glycaemic Variability among Subjects with Type 1 Diabetes Mellitus," *BMC Endocrine Disorders* 22, no. 122 (May 11, 2022), https://doi.org/10.1186/s12902-022-01013-7.

Laura R. Dowling et al., "Enteric Nervous System and Intestinal Epithelial Regulation of the Gut-Brain Axis," *Journal of Allergy and Clinical Immunology* 150, no. 3 (September 1, 2022): 513–22, https://doi.org/10.1016/j.jaci.2022.07.015.

Joseph R. Ferrari and Catherine A. Roster, "Delaying Disposing: Examining the Relationship between Procrastination and Clutter across Generations," *Current Psychology* 37, no. 2 (June 1, 2018): 426–31, https://doi.org/10.1007/s12144-017-9679-4.

Jane A. Foster, Glen B. Baker, and Serdar M. Dursun, "The Relationship Between the Gut Microbiome-Immune System-Brain Axis and Major Depressive Disorder," *Frontiers in Neurology* 12 (September 28, 2021), https://doi.org/10.3389/fneur.2021.721126.

Pengfei Han et al., "Sensitivity to Sweetness Correlates to Elevated Reward Brain Responses to Sweet and High-Fat Food Odors in Young Healthy Volunteers," *NeuroImage* 208 (March 1, 2020): 116413, https://www.sciencedirect.com/science/article/pii/S1053811919310043?via%3Dihub.

Lauren E. Hartstein et al., "High Sensitivity of Melatonin Suppression Response to Evening Light in Preschool-Aged Children," *Journal of Pineal Research* 72, no. 2 (January 8, 2022): e12780, https://onlinelibrary.wiley.com/doi/10.1111/jpi.12780.

Anja Hilbert et al., "Meta-Analysis on the Long_Term Effectiveness of Psychological and Medical Treatments for Binge-Eating Disorder," *International Journal of Eating Disorders* 53, no. 9 (June 25, 2020): 1353–76, https://doi.org/10.1002/eat.23297.

Roman Holzer, Wilhelm Bloch, and Christian Brinkmann, "Continuous Glucose Monitoring in Healthy Adults—Possible Applications in Health Care, Wellness, and Sports," *Sensors* 22, no. 5 (March 5, 2022): 2030, https://doi.org/10.3390/s22052030.

Andrew Huberman, "Dr. Satchin Panda: Intermittent Fasting to Improve Health, Cognition, & Longevity," *Huberman Lab* (March 18, 2023), https://hubermanlab.com/dr-satchin-panda-intermittent-fasting-to-improve-health-cognition-and-longevity/.

Gaspard Kerner, Jeremy Choin, and Lluis Quintana-Murci, "Ancient DNA as a Tool for Medical Research," *Nature Medicine* 29 (March 15, 2023): 1048–51, https://doi.org/10.1038/s41591-023-02244-4.

Annelise Madison and Janice K. Kiecolt-Glaser, "Stress, Depression, Diet, and the Gut Microbiota: Human–Bacteria Interactions at the Core of Psychoneuroimmunology and Nutrition," *Current Opinion in Behavioral Sciences* 28 (March 25, 2019): 105–10, https://doi.org/10.1016/j.cobeha.2019.01.011.

Sai Sailesh Kumar Goothy et al., "Effect of Selected Vestibular Exercises on Depression, Anxiety and Stress in Elderly Women with Type 2 Diabetes," *International Journal of Biochemistry & Physiology* (November 20, 2019), https://doi.org/10.23880/ijbp-16000169.

Hiroshi Kunugi, "Gut Microbiota and Pathophysiology of Depressive Disorder," *Annals of Nutrition and Metabolism* 77, no. Suppl. 2 (January 1, 2021): 11–20, https://doi.org/10.1159/000518274.

Atsukazu Kuwahara et al., "Microbiota-Gut-Brain Axis: Enteroendocrine Cells and the Enteric Nervous System Form an Interface between the Microbiota and the Central Nervous System," *Biomedical Research* 41, no. 5 (October 16, 2020): 199–216, https://doi.org/10.2220/biomedres.41.199.

Sarah A. McCormick, Kirby Deater-Deckard, and Claire Hughes, "Household Clutter and Crowding Constrain Associations between Maternal Sensitivity and Child Theory of Mind," *British Journal of Developmental Psychology* 40, no. 2 (February 17, 2022): 271–86, https://doi.org/10.1111/bjdp.12406.

Elisa Menardo et al., "Nature and Mindfulness to Cope with Work-Related Stress: A Narrative Review," *International Journal of Environmental Research and Public Health* 19, no. 10 (May 13, 2022): 5948, https://www.mdpi.com/1660-4601/19/10/5948.

Katja Oomen-Welke et al., "Spending Time in the Forest or the Field: Investigations on Stress Perception and Psychological Well-Being—A Randomized Cross-Over Trial in Highly Sensitive Persons," *International Journal of Environmental Research and Public Health* 19, no. 22 (November 19, 2022): 15322, https://www.mdpi.com/1660-4601/19/22/15322.

Andrew J. K. Phillips et al., "High Sensitivity and Interindividual Variability in the Response of the Human Circadian System to Evening Light," *Proceedings of the National Academy of Sciences of the United States of America* 116, no. 24 (May 28, 2019): 12019–24, https://doi.org/10.1073/pnas.1901824116.

Joseph R. Rausch, "Measures of Glycemic Variability and Links with Psychological Functioning," *Current Diabetes Reports* 10, no. 6 (October 5, 2010): 415–21, https://doi.org/10.1007/s11892-010-0152-0.

Sujana Reddy et al., *Physiology, Circadian Rhythm* (Treasure Island, FL: StatPearls Publishing, 2022), https://www.ncbi.nlm.nih.gov/books/NBK519507.

Catia Scassellati et al., "The Complex Molecular Picture of Gut and Oral Microbiota–Brain-Depression System: What We Know and What We Need to Know," *Frontiers in Psychiatry* 12 (November 2, 2021), https://doi.org/10.3389/fpsyt.2021.722335.

Katherine Semenkovich et al., "Depression in Type 2 Diabetes Mellitus: Prevalence, Impact, and Treatment," *Drugs* 75, no. 6 (April 8, 2015): 577–87, https://doi.org/10.1007/s40265-015-0347-4.

Sik Yu So and Tor C. Savidge, "Gut Feelings: The Microbiota-Gut-Brain Axis on Steroids," *American Journal of Physiology-Gastrointestinal and Liver Physiology* 322, no. 1 (December 16, 2021): G1–20, https://journals.physiology.org/doi/full/10.1152/ajpgi.00294.2021.

Chao Song et al., "The Influence of Occupational Therapy on College Students' Home Physical Exercise Behavior and Mental Health Status under the Artificial Intelligence Technology," *Occupational Therapy International* 2022 , no..20 (September 9, 2022): 1–13, https://doaj.org/article/7cfcd5e1932c4b8e9b9c594721ca8fe7.

Ellen R. Stothard et al., "Circadian Entrainment to the Natural Light-Dark Cycle across Seasons and the Weekend," *Current Biology* 27, no. 4 (February 20, 2017): 508–13, https://doi.org/10.1016/j.cub.2016.12.041.

Garen V. Vartanian et al., "Melatonin Suppression by Light in Humans Is More Sensitive Than Previously Reported," *Journal of Biological Rhythms* 30, no. 4 (May 27, 2015): 351–54, https://doi.org/10.1177/0748730415585413.

Kathleen T. Watson et al., "Incident Major Depressive Disorder Predicted by Three Measures of Insulin Resistance: A Dutch Cohort Study," *American Journal of Psychiatry* 178, no. 10 (September 23, 2021): 914–20, https://doi.org/10.1176/appi.ajp.2021.20101479.

Marsha C. Wibowo et al., "Reconstruction of Ancient Microbial Genomes from the Human Gut," *Nature* 594, no. 7862 (May 12, 2021): 234–39, https://doi.org/10.1038/s41586-021-03532-0.

Christian Franz Josef Woll and Felix D. Schönbrodt, "A Series of Meta-Analytic Tests of the Efficacy of Long-Term Psychoanalytic Psychotherapy," *European Psychologist* 25, no. 1 (January 1, 2020): 51–72, https://econtent.hogrefe.com/doi/10.1027/1016-9040/a000385.

Hidenori Yoshii et al., "The Importance of Continuous Glucose Monitoring-Derived Metrics Beyond HbA1c for Optimal Individualized Glycemic Control," *Journal of Clinical Endocrinology and Metabolism* 107, no. 10 (July 31, 2022): e3990–4003, https://doi.org/10.1210/clinem/dgac459.

Jing Zhang and Natasha Slesnick, "The Effects of a Family Systems Intervention on Co-Occurring Internalizing and Externalizing Behaviors of Children with Substance Abusing Mothers: A Latent Transition Analysis," *Journal of Marital and Family Therapy* 44, no. 4 (October 3, 2017): 687–701, https://doi.org/10.1111/jmft.12277.

Chapter 7: Stage 1: Awareness—Recognizing Your Nervous System Patterns

Kaitlyn Bakker and Richard Moulding, "Sensory-Processing Sensitivity, Dispositional Mindfulness and Negative Psychological Symptoms," *Personality and Individual Differences* 53, no. 3 (August 1, 2012): 341–46, https://doi.org/10.1016/j.paid.2012.04.006.

J. De Jonckheere et al., "Heart Rate Variability Analysis as an Index of Emotion Regulation Processes: Interest of the Analgesia Nociception Index (ANI)," *2012 Annual International Conference of the IEEE Engineering in Medicine and Biology Society* (2012), https://doi.org/10.1109/embc.2012.6346703.

Hani M. Elwafi et al., "Mindfulness Training for Smoking Cessation: Moderation of the Relationship between Craving and Cigarette Use," *Drug and Alcohol Dependence* 130, nos. 1–3 (June 1, 2013): 222–29, https://www.sciencedirect.com/science/article/abs/pii/S0376871612004565?via%3Dihub.

Kieran C. R. Fox et al., "Functional Neuroanatomy of Meditation: A Review and Meta-Analysis of 78 Functional Neuroimaging Investigations," *Neuroscience & Biobehavioral Reviews* 65 (June 1, 2016): 208–28, https://doi.org/10.1016/j.neubiorev.2016.03.021.

Kieran C. R. Fox et al., "Is Meditation Associated with Altered Brain Structure? A Systematic Review and Meta-Analysis of Morphometric Neuroimaging in Meditation Practitioners," *Neuroscience & Biobehavioral Reviews* 43 (June 1, 2014): 48–73, https://doi.org/10.1016/j.neubiorev.2014.03.016.

Roberto Guidotti et al., "Neuroplasticity within and between Functional Brain Networks in Mental Training Based on Long-Term Meditation," *Brain Sciences* 11, no. 8 (August 18, 2021): 1086, https://www.mdpi.com/2076-3425/11/8/1086.

Sean Dae Houlihan and Judson A. Brewer, "The Emerging Science of Mindfulness as a Treatment for Addiction," *Advances in Mental Health and Addiction* (New York: Springer, 2016), 191–210, https://link.springer.com/chapter/10.1007/978-3-319-22255-4_9.

Mara Mather and Julian F. Thayer, "How Heart Rate Variability Affects Emotion Regulation Brain Networks," *Current Opinion in Behavioral Sciences* 19 (February 1, 2018): 98–104, https://www.sciencedirect.com/science/article/abs/pii/S2352154617300621?via%3Dihub.

Peter Sedlmeier et al., "The Psychological Effects of Meditation: A Meta-Analysis," *Psychological Bulletin* 138, no. 6 (May 14, 2012): 1139–71, https://doi.org/10.1037/a0028168.

Toru Takahashi et al., "Dispositional Mindfulness Mediates the Relationship Between Sensory-Processing Sensitivity and Trait Anxiety, Well-Being, and Psychosomatic Symptoms," *Psychological Reports* 123, no. 4 (August 1, 2020): 1083–98, https://doi.org/10.1177/0033294119841848.

Chapter 8: Stage 2: Regulation—Building Agency through Embodied Safety

Marta Alda et al., "Zen Meditation, Length of Telomeres, and the Role of Experiential Avoidance and Compassion," *Mindfulness* 7, (February 22, 2016): 651–59, https://doi.org/10.1007/s12671-016-0500-5.

Melis Yilmaz Balban et al., "Brief Structured Respiration Practices Enhance Mood and Reduce Physiological Arousal," *Cell Reports Medicine* 4, no. 1 (January 17, 2023): 100895, https://doi.org/10.1016/j.xcrm.2022.100895.

Lisa Feldman Barrett. 2017. *How Emotions Are Made: The Secret Life of the Brain.* London, England: Macmillan.

Esther T. Beierl et al., "Cognitive Paths from Trauma to Posttraumatic Stress Disorder: A Prospective Study of Ehlers and Clark's Model in Survivors of Assaults or Road Traffic Collisions," *Psychological Medicine* 50, no. 13 (September 11, 2019): 2172–81, https://doi.org/10.1017/s0033291719002253.

Natalia Bobba-Alves, Robert-Paul Juster, and Martin Picard, "The Energetic Cost of Allostasis and Allostatic Load," *Psychoneuroendocrinology* 146 (December 1, 2022): 105951, https://doi.org/10.1016/j.psyneuen.2022.105951.

Elissa S. Epel et al., "Meditation and Vacation Effects Have an Impact on Disease-Associated Molecular Phenotypes," *Translational Psychiatry* (August 30, 2016): e880, https://doi.org/10.1038/tp.2016.164.

Brian Hsueh et al., "Cardiogenic Control of Affective Behavioural State," *Nature* 615, no. 7951 (March 1, 2023): 292–99, https://doi.org/10.1038/s41586-023-05748-8.

Andrew Huberman, "Dr. David Spiegel: Using Hypnosis to Enhance Mental & Physical Health & Performance," *Huberman Lab* (July 17, 2022), https://hubermanlab.com/dr-david-spiegel-using-hypnosis-to-enhance-mental-and-physical-health-and-performance/.

Andrew Huberman, "Dr. Elissa Epel: Control Stress for Healthy Eating, Metabolism & Aging," *Huberman Lab* (April 4, 2023), https://hubermanlab.com/dr-elissa-epel-control-stress-for-healthy-eating-metabolism-and-aging.

Breanne E. Kearney and Ruth A. Lanius, "The Brain-Body Disconnect: A Somatic Sensory Basis for Trauma-Related Disorders," *Frontiers in Neuroscience* 16 (November 21, 2022), https://www.frontiersin.org/articles/10.3389/fnins.2022.1015749/full.

Ning-Cen Li et al., "The Anti-Inflammatory Actions and Mechanisms of Acupuncture from Acupoint to Target Organs via Neuro-Immune Regulation," *Journal of Inflammation Research* 2021, no. 14 (December 21, 2021): 7191–224, https://doi.org/10.2147/jir.s341581.

Qiufu Ma, "Somato-Autonomic Reflexes of Acupuncture," *Medical Acupuncture* 32, no. 6 (December 16, 2020): 362–66, https://doi.org/10.1089/acu.2020.1488.

Francie Moehring et al., "Uncovering the Cells and Circuits of Touch in Normal and Pathological Settings," *Neuron* 100, no. 2 (October 24, 2018): 349–60, https://doi.org/10.1016/j.neuron.2018.10.019.

Mount Sinai Health System, "Systems Biology Research Study Reveals Benefits of Vacation and Meditation," (August 30, 2016), https://www.mountsinai.org/about/newsroom/2016/systems-biology-research-study-reveals-benefits-of-vacation-and-meditation.

Martin Picard et al., "A Mitochondrial Health Index Sensitive to Mood and Caregiving Stress," *Biological Psychiatry* 84, no. 1 (July 1, 2018): 9–17, https://doi.org/10.1016/j.biopsych.2018.01.012.

Carolyn M. Schmitt and Sarah A. Schoen, "Interoception: A Multi-Sensory Foundation of Participation in Daily Life," *Frontiers in Neuroscience* 16 (June 9, 2022), https://doi.org/10.3389/fnins.2022.875200.

Chapter 9: Stage 3: Restoration—Rebuilding Nervous System Flexibility

Jay Belsky and Michael Pluess, "Beyond Diathesis Stress: Differential Susceptibility to Environmental Influences," *Psychological Bulletin* 135, no. 6 (November 1, 2009): 885–908, https://doi.org/10.1037/a0017376.

George A. Bonanno, *The End of Trauma: How the New Science of Resilience Is Changing How We Think About PTSD* (London: Hachette UK, 2021).

Daniel P. Brown and David S. Elliot, *Attachment Disturbances in Adults: Treatment for Comprehensive Repair* (New York: W. W. Norton and Company, 2016).

Richard A. Bryant and Rachael Foord, "Activating Attachments Reduces Memories of Traumatic Images," *PLOS One* 11, no. 9 (September 15, 2016): e0162550, https://doi.org/10.1371/journal.pone.0162550.

Jude Cassidy, Jason D. Jones, and Phillip R. Shaver, "Contributions of Attachment Theory and Research: A Framework for Future Research, Translation, and Policy," *Development and Psychopathology* 25, no. 4, pt. 2 (December 17,, 2013): 1415–34, https://doi.org/10.1017/s0954579413000692.

Jessica E. Cooke et al., "Parent–Child Attachment and Children's Experience and Regulation of Emotion: A Meta-Analytic Review," *Emotion* 19, no. 6 (September 1, 2019): 1103–26, https://doi.org/10.1037/emo0000504.

Louis F. Damis, "The Role of Implicit Memory in the Development and Recovery from Trauma-Related Disorders," *NeuroSci* 3, no. 1 (January 18, 2022): 63–88, https://doi.org/10.3390/neurosci3010005

Echo, "Echo Training," May 15, 2023, https://www.echotraining.org.

R.M. Pasco Fearon and Glenn I. Roisman, "Attachment Theory: Progress and Future Directions," *Current Opinion in Psychology* 15 (June 1, 2017): 131–36, https://doi.org/10.1016/j.copsyc.2017.03.002.

R. Chris Fraley, Niels G. Waller, and Kelly Brennan, "An Item Response Theory Analysis of Self-Report Measures of Adult Attachment," *Journal of Personality and Social Psychology* 78, no. 2 (January 1, 2000): 350–65, https://doi.org/10.1037/0022-3514.78.2.350.

Isaac R. Galatzer-Levy, Sandy H. Huang, and George A. Bonanno, "Trajectories of Resilience and Dysfunction Following Potential Trauma: A Review and Statistical Evaluation," *Clinical Psychology Review* 63 (July 1, 2018): 41–55, https://doi.org/10.1016/j.cpr.2018.05.008.

Sarah N. Garfinkel et al., "Knowing Your Own Heart: Distinguishing Interoceptive Accuracy from Interoceptive Awareness," *Biological Psychology* 104 (January 1, 2015): 65–74, https://doi.org/10.1016/j.biopsycho.2014.11.004.

Sahib S. Khalsa et al., "Interoception and Mental Health: A Roadmap," *Biological Psychiatry: Cognitive Neuroscience and Neuroimaging* 3, no. 6 (June 1, 2018): 501–13, https://doi.org/10.1016/j.bpsc.2017.12.004.

Lachlan J. Kerley, Pamela J. Meredith, and Paul H. Harnett, "The Relationship Between Sensory Processing and Attachment Patterns: A Scoping Review," *Canadian Journal of Occupational Therapy* 90, no. 1 (May 24, 2022): 79–91, https://doi.org/10.1177/00084174221102726.

Anne Kever et al., "Interoceptive Sensitivity Facilitates Both Antecedent- and Response-Focused Emotion Regulation Strategies," *Personality and Individual Differences* 87 (December 1, 2015): 20–23, https://www.sciencedirect.com/science/article/abs/pii/S0191886915004584?via%3Dihub.

Mariska Klein Velderman et al., "Effects of Attachment-Based Interventions on Maternal Sensitivity and Infant Attachment: Differential Susceptibility of Highly Reactive Infants," *Journal of Family Psychology* 20, no. 2 (June 29, 2005): 266–74, https://doi.org/10.1037/0893-3200.20.2.266.

Anthony Wing Kosner, "The Mind at Work: Lisa Feldman Barrett on the Metabolism of Emotion," *The Mind at Work* (February 10, 2021), https://blog.dropbox.com/topics/work-culture/the-mind-at-work--lisa-feldman-barrett-on-the-metabolism-of-emot.

F.H. Norris, "Epidemiology of Trauma: Frequency and Impact of Different Potentially Traumatic Events on Different Demographic Groups," *Journal of Consulting and Clinical Psychology* 60, no. 3 (June 1, 1992): 409–18, https://doi.org/10.1037/0022-006x.60.3.409.

Susanna Pallini et al., "Attachment and Attention Problems: A Meta-Analysis," *Clinical Psychology Review* 74 (October 31, 2019): 101772, https://doi.org/10.1016/j.cpr.2019.101772.

Susanna Pallini et al., "The Relation of Attachment Security Status to Effortful Self-Regulation: A Meta-Analysis," *Psychological Bulletin* 144, no. 5 (March 8, 2018): 501–31, https://doi.org/10.1037/bul0000134.

Federico Parra et al., "Ideal Parent Figure Method in the Treatment of Complex Posttraumatic Stress Disorder Related to Childhood Trauma: A Pilot Study," *European Journal of Psychotraumatology* 8, no. 1 (November 16, 2017), https://doi.org/10.1080/20008198.2017.1400879.

Olga Pollatos, Ellen Matthias, and Johannes Keller, "When Interoception Helps to Overcome Negative Feelings Caused by Social Exclusion," *Frontiers in Psychology* 6 (June 15, 2015), https://www.frontiersin.org/articles/10.3389/fpsyg.2015.00786/full.

Holly G. Prigerson et al., "Enhancing & Mobilizing the POtential for Wellness & Emotional Resilience (EMPOWER) among Surrogate Decision-Makers of ICU Patients: Study Protocol for a Randomized Controlled Trial," *Trials* 20, no. 1 (July 9, 2019): 408, https://doi.org/10.1186/s13063-019-3515-0.

Lisa Quadt et al., "Interoceptive Training to Target Anxiety in Autistic Adults (ADIE): A Single-Center, Superiority Randomized Controlled Trial," *EClinicalMedicine* 39 (September 1, 2021): 101042, https://www.thelancet.com/journals/eclinm/article/PIIS2589-5370(21)00322-9/fulltext.

Pernille Darling Rasmussen et al., "Attachment as a Core Feature of Resilience: A Systematic Review and Meta-Analysis," *Psychological Reports* 122, no. 4 (August 1, 2019): 1259–96, https://doi.org/10.1177/0033294118785577.

G. I. Roismanet et al., "The Adult Attachment Interview and Self-Reports of Attachment Style: An Empirical Rapprochement," *Journal of Personality and Social Psychology* 92, no. 4 (April 2007): 678–97 https://pubmed.ncbi.nlm.nih.gov/17469952/.

Myeong-Gu Seo and Lisa Feldman Barrett, "Being Emotional During Decision Making—Good or Bad? An Empirical Investigation," *Academy of Management Journal* 50, no. 4 (August 1, 2007): 923–40, https://journals.aom.org/doi/10.5465/amj.2007.26279217.

Clay Skipper, "Your Brain Doesn't Work the Way You Think It Does," GQ, (November 30, 2020), https://www.gq.com/story/lisa-feldman-barrett-interview.

"Trauma-Informed Care and Practice," in *Trauma-Informed Toolkit*, 2nd ed. (Winnipeg: Klinic Community Health Centre, 2013), 15–21, https://makingsenseoftrauma.com/wp-content/uploads/2016/01/Trauma-Informed-Care-and-Practice.pdf.

Everett Waters, Brian E. Vaughn, and Harriet S. Waters, *Measuring Attachment: Developmental Assessment across the Lifespan* (New York: Guilford Press, 2021), https://www.guilford.com/books/Measuring-Attachment/Waters-Vaughn-Waters/9781462546473.

Thomas L. Webb, Eleanor Miles, and Paschal Sheeran, "Dealing with Feeling: A Meta-Analysis of the Effectiveness of Strategies Derived from the Process Model of Emotion Regulation," *Psychological Bulletin* 138, no. 4 (May 14, 2012): 775–808, https://doi.org/10.1037/a0027600.

Sarah Woodhouse, Susan Ayers, and Andy P. Field, "The Relationship between Adult Attachment Style and Post-Traumatic Stress Symptoms: A Meta-Analysis," *Journal of Anxiety Disorders* 35 (October 1, 2015): 103–17, https://doi.org/10.1016/j.janxdis.2015.07.002.

Susan S. Woodhouse et al., "Secure Base Provision: A New Approach to Examining Links Between Maternal Caregiving and Infant Attachment," *Child Development* 91, no. 1 (January–February, 2020), https://srcd.onlinelibrary.wiley.com/doi/10.1111/cdev.13224.

Chapter 10: Stage 4: Connection—Repairing Bonds and Cultivating Kinship

Kilian Abellaneda-Pérez et al., "Purpose in Life Promotes Resilience to Age-Related Brain Burden in Middle-Aged Adults," *Alzheimer's Research & Therapy* 15, no. 1 (March 8, 2023), https://www.frontiersin.org/articles/10.3389/fpsyt.2023.1134865/full.

Minhal Ahmed et al., "Breaking the Vicious Cycle: The Interplay between Loneliness, Metabolic Illness, and Mental Health," *Frontiers in Psychiatry* 14 (March 8, 2023), https://doi.org/10.3389/fpsyt.2023.1134865.

Kaho Akimoto et al., "Effect of 528 Hz Music on the Endocrine System and Autonomic Nervous System," *Health* 10, no. 9 (January 1, 2018): 1159–70, https://doi.org/10.4236/health.2018.109088.

Aliya Alimujiang et al., "Association Between Life Purpose and Mortality Among US Adults Older Than 50 Years," *JAMA Network Open* 2, no. 5 (May 24, 2019): e194270, https://jamanetwork.com/journals/jamanetworkopen/fullarticle/2734064.

Megan E. Beerse et al., "Biobehavioral Utility of Mindfulness-Based Art Therapy: Neurobiological Underpinnings and Mental Health Impacts," *Experimental Biology and Medicine* 245, no. 2 (October 21, 2019): 122–30, https://doi.org/10.1177/1535370219883634.

Julia F. Christensen et al., "Dance Expertise Modulates Behavioral and Psychophysiological Responses to Affective Body Movement," *Journal of Experimental Psychology: Human Perception and Performance* 42, no. 8 (August 1, 2016): 1139–47, https://doi.org/10.1037/xhp0000176.

Julia F. Christensen, Ruben T. Azevedo, and Manos Tsakiris, "Emotion Matters: Different Psychophysiological Responses to Expressive and Non-Expressive Full-Body Movements," *Acta Psychologica* 212 (January 1, 2021): 103215, https://doi.org/10.1016/j.actpsy.2020.103215.

T. Babayi Daylari et al., "Influence of Various Intensities of 528 Hz Sound-Wave in Production of Testosterone in Rat's Brain and Analysis of Behavioral Changes," *Genes & Genomics* 41, no. 2 (November 9, 2018): 201-11, https://doi.org/10.1007/s13258-018-0753-6.

Robin I. M. Dunbar, "Coevolution of Neocortical Size, Group Size and Language in Humans," *Behavioral and Brain Sciences* 16, no. 4 (December 1, 1993): 681–94, https://doi.org/10.1017/s0140525x00032325.

Robin I. M. Dunbar, *Friends: Understanding the Power of Our Most Important Relationships* (New York: Little, Brown Book Group, (2021).

Robin Dunbar, "Why Drink Is the Secret to Humanity's Success," *Financial Times* (August 10, 2018), https://www.ft.com/content/c5ce0834-9a64-11e8-9702-5946bae86e6d.

Robert A. Emmons, *The Psychology of Ultimate Concerns: Motivation and Spirituality in Personality* (New York: Guilford Press, 1999).

Evren Erzen and Özkan Çikrikci, "The Effect of Loneliness on Depression: A Meta-Analysis," *International Journal of Social Psychiatry* 64, no. 5 (May 23, 2018): 427–35, https://doi.org/10.1177/0020764018776349.

Elizabeth Finnis, "Canticle of the Creatures: Francis of Assisi—Praised Be You My Lord, with All Your Creatures," FranciscanSeculars.com (February 28, 2019), http://franciscanseculars.com/the-canticle-of-the-creatures.

David A. Fryburg, "Kindness as a Stress Reduction–Health Promotion Intervention: A Review of the Psychobiology of Caring," *American Journal of Lifestyle Medicine* 16, no. 1 (January 29, 2021): 89–100, https://doi.org/10.1177/1559827620988268.

Ellen Galinsky, "PBS's 'This Emotional Life': The Magic of Relationships," *HuffPost* (November 17, 2011), https://www.huffpost.com/entry/pbss-this-emotional-life_b_568178.

Robyn Gobbel, "What to Do After We Mess Up," RobynGobbel.com (May 17, 2022), https://robyngobbel.com/rupturerepair.

Jason G. Goldman, "Ed Tronick and the 'Still Face Experiment,'" *Scientific American Blog Network* (October 18, 2010), https://blogs.scientificamerican.com/thoughtful-animal/ed-tronick-and-the-8220-still-face-experiment-8221.

Margaret M. Hansen, Reo J. F. Jones, and Kirsten Tocchini, "Shinrin-Yoku (Forest Bathing) and Nature Therapy: A State-of-the-Art Review," *International Journal of Environmental Research and Public Health* 14, no. 8 (July 28, 2017): 851, https://doi.org/10.3390/ijerph14080851.

Lyanda Lynn Haupt, *Rooted: Life at the Crossroads of Science, Nature, and Spirit* (New York: Little, Brown Spark, 2021).

Louise C. Hawkley and John T. Cacioppo, "Loneliness Matters: A Theoretical and Empirical Review of Consequences and Mechanisms," *Annals of Behavioral Medicine* 40, no. 2 (October 1, 2010): 218–27, https://doi.org/10.1007/s12160-010-9210-8.

Julianne Holt-Lunstad et al., "Loneliness and Social Isolation as Risk Factors for Mortality," *Perspectives on Psychological Science* 10, no. 2 (March 11, 2015): 227–37, https://doi.org/10.1177/1745691614568352.

Julianne Holt-Lunstad, "Loneliness and Social Isolation as Risk Factors: The Power of Social Connection in Prevention," *American Journal of Lifestyle Medicine* 15, no. 5 (May 6, 2021): 567–73, https://doi.org/10.1177/15598276211009454.

Julianne Holt-Lunstad, Timothy B. Smith, and J. Bradley Layton, "Social Relationships and Mortality Risk: A Meta-Analytic Review," *PLOS Medicine* 7, no. 7 (July 27, 2010): e1000316, https://journals.plos.org/plosmedicine/article?id=10.1371/journal.pmed.1000316.

Girija Kaimal et al., "Functional Near-Infrared Spectroscopy Assessment of Reward Perception Based on Visual Self-Expression: Coloring, Doodling, and Free Drawing," *Arts in Psychotherapy* 55 (September 1, 2017): 85–92, https://doi.org/10.1016/j.aip.2017.05.004.

Girija Kaimal, Kendra Ray, and Juan Muniz, "Reduction of Cortisol Levels and Participants' Responses Following Art Making," *Art Therapy* 33, no. 2 (May 23, 2016): 74–80, https://doi.org/10.1080/07421656.2016.1166832.

Victor Kaufman et al., "Unique Ways in Which the Quality of Friendships Matter for Life Satisfaction," *Journal of Happiness Studies* 23, no. 6 (March 5, 2022): 2563–80, https://doi.org/10.1007/s10902-022-00502-9.

Malcolm Koo, Hsuan-Pin Chen, and Yueh-Chiao Yeh, "Coloring Activities for Anxiety Reduction and Mood Improvement in Taiwanese Community-Dwelling Older Adults: A Randomized Controlled Study," *Evidence-Based Complementary and Alternative Medicine* 2020 (January 21, 2020): https://pubmed.ncbi.nlm.nih.gov/32063986/.

Patrik Lindenfors, Andreas Wartel, and Johan Lind, "'Dunbar's Number' Deconstructed," *Biology Letters* 17, no. 5 (May 5, 2021), https://doi.org/10.1098/rsbl.2021.0158.

Melissa Madeson, "Logotherapy: Viktor Frankl's Theory of Meaning," PositivePsychology.com (August 30, 2023), https://positivepsychology.com/viktor-frankl-logotherapy.

Christopher M. Masi et al., "A Meta-Analysis of Interventions to Reduce Loneliness," *Personality and Social Psychology Review* 15, no. 3 (August 17, 2011): 219–66, https://doi.org/10.1177/1088868310377394.

F. Stephan Mayer and Cynthia McPherson Frantz, "The Connectedness to Nature Scale: A Measure of Individuals' Feeling in Community with Nature," *Journal of Environmental Psychology* 24, no. 4 (December 1, 2004): 503–15, https://doi.org/10.1016/j.jenvp.2004.10.001.

James W. Pennebaker, "Expressive Writing in Psychological Science," *Perspectives on Psychological Science* 13, no. 2 (October 9, 2017): 226–29, https://doi.org/10.1177/1745691617707315.

Homa Pourriyahi et al., "Loneliness: An Immunometabolic Syndrome," *International Journal of Environmental Research and Public Health* 18, no. 22 (November 19, 2021): 12162, https://doi.org/10.3390/ijerph182212162.

Alison E. Pritchard et al., "The Relationship Between Nature Connectedness and Eudaimonic Well-Being: A Meta-Analysis," *Journal of Happiness Studies* 21, no. 3 (April 30, 20190): 1145–67, https://doi.org/10.1007/s10902-019-00118-6.

Laura Alejandra Rico-Uribe et al., "Association of Loneliness with All-Cause Mortality: A Meta-Analysis," *PLOS One* 13, no. 1 (January 4, 2018): e0190033, https://doi.org/10.1371/journal.pone.0190033.

Tania Singer and Olga Klimecki, "Empathy and Compassion," *Current Biology* 24, no. 18 (September 22, 2014): PR875–78, https://doi.org/10.1016/j.cub.2014.06.054.

Toshimasa Sone et al., "Sense of Life Worth Living (Ikigai) and Mortality in Japan: Ohsaki Study," *Psychosomatic Medicine* 70, no. 6 (July 1, 2008): 709–15, https://doi.org/10.1097/psy.0b013e31817e7e64.

Annette W. M. Spithoven et al., "Genetic Contributions to Loneliness and Their Relevance to the Evolutionary Theory of Loneliness," *Perspectives on Psychological Science* 14, no. 3 (March 7, 2019): https://journals.sagepub.com/doi/10.1177/1745691618812684.

Siri Jakobsson Støre and Niklas Jakobsson, "The Effect of Mandala Coloring on State Anxiety: A Systematic Review and Meta-Analysis," *Art Therapy* 39, no. 4 (January 4, 2022): 173–81, https://www.tandfonline.com/doi/full/10.1080/07421656.2021.2003144.

Clara Strauss et al., "What Is Compassion and How Can We Measure It? A Review of Definitions and Measures," *Clinical Psychology Review* 47 (July 1, 2016): 15–27, https://doi.org/10.1016/j.cpr.2016.05.004.

Barna Konkolÿ Thege, Róbert Urbán, and Mária S Kopp, "Four-Year Prospective Evaluation of the Relationship between Meaning in Life and Smoking Status," *Substance Abuse Treatment, Prevention, and Policy* 8, no. 8 (2013): 89–100, https://doi.org/10.1186/1747-597X-8-8.

E. Tronick, L. B. Adamson, and T. B. Brazelton, "Infant Emotions in Normal and Pertubated Interactions," paper presented at the biennial meeting of the Society for Research in Child Development, Denver, CO, April 1975.

Ed Tronick and Marjorie Beeghly, "Infants' Meaning-Making and the Development of Mental Health Problems," *American Psychologist* 66, no. 2 (February–March, 2011): 107–19, https://doi.org/10.1037/a0021631.

Caoimhe Twohig-Bennett and Andy Jones, "The Health Benefits of the Great Outdoors: A Systematic Review and Meta-Analysis of Greenspace Exposure and Health Outcomes," *Environmental Research* 166 (October 1, 2018): 628–37, https://doi.org/10.1016/j.envres.2018.06.030.

Roger S. Ulrich et al., "A Review of the Research Literature on Evidence-Based Healthcare Design," *HERD: Health Environments Research & Design Journal* 1, no. 3 (April 1, 2008): 61–125, https://doi.org/10.1177/193758670800100306.

Roger S. Ulrich, "View Through a Window May Influence Recovery from Surgery," *Science* 224, no. 4647 (April 27, 1984): 420–21, https://doi.org/10.1126/science.6143402.

Janneke E. P. van Leeuwen et al., "More Than Meets the Eye: Art Engages the Social Brain," *Frontiers in Neuroscience* 16 (February 25, 2022), https://doi.org/10.3389/fnins.2022.738865.

Awel Vaughan-Evans et al., "Implicit Detection of Poetic Harmony by the Naïve Brain," *Frontiers in Psychology* 7 (November 25, 2016), https://doi.org/10.3389/fpsyg.2016.01859.

Bronnie Ware, *Top Five Regrets of the Dying: A Life Transformed by the Dearly Departing* (Carlsbad, CA: Hay House, 2019).

Wenfei Yao et al., "Impact of Exposure to Natural and Built Environments on Positive and Negative Affect: A Systematic Review and Meta-Analysis," *Frontiers in Public Health* 9 (November 25, 2021), https://doi.org/10.3389/fpubh.2021.758457.

Yongju Yu, "Thwarted Belongingness Hindered Successful Aging in Chinese Older Adults: Roles of Positive Mental Health and Meaning in Life," *Frontiers in Psychology* 13 (February 24, 2022), https://www.frontiersin.org/articles/10.3389/fpsyg.2022.839125/full.

David D. Zhang et al., "Earliest Parietal Art: Hominin Hand and Foot Traces from the Middle Pleistocene of Tibet," *Science Bulletin* 66, no. 24 (December 30, 2021): 2506–15, https://doi.org/10.1016/j.scib.2021.09.001.

Xiaofeng Zhang et al., "A Systematic Review of the Anxiety-Alleviation Benefits of Exposure to the Natural Environment," *Reviews on Environmental Health* 38, no. 2 (March 24, 2022): 281–93, https://www.degruyter.com/document/doi/10.1515/reveh-2021-0157/html.

Chapter 11: Stage 5: Expansion—Growing Your Capacity

Aliya Alimujiang et al., "Association Between Life Purpose and Mortality Among US Adults Older Than 50 Years," *JAMA Network Open* 2, no. 5 (May 24, 2019): e194270, https://jamanetwork.com/journals/jamanetworkopen/fullarticle/2734064.

Summer Allen, "The Science of Awe," *The Greater Good Science Center* Berkeley.edu (September 2018), https://ggsc.berkeley.edu/images/uploads/GGSC-JTF_White_Paper-Awe_FINAL.pdf.

Muhammed Mustafa Atakan, Şükran Nazan Koşar, and Hüseyin Hüsrev Turnagöl, "Six Sessions of Low-Volume High-Intensity Interval Exercise Improves Resting Fat Oxidation," *International Journal of Sports Medicine* 43, no. 14 (September 23, 2022): 1206–13, https://doi.org/10.1055/a-1905-7985.

Ruth Ann Atchley, David L. Strayer, and Paul Atchley, "Creativity in the Wild: Improving Creative Reasoning through Immersion in Natural Settings," *PLOS One* 7, no. 12 (December 12, 2012): e51474, https://doi.org/10.1371/journal.pone.0051474.

Melis Yilmaz Balban et al., "Brief Structured Respiration Practices Enhance Mood and Reduce Physiological Arousal," *Cell Reports Medicine* 4, no. 1 (January 17, 2023): 100895, https://doi.org/10.1016/j.xcrm.2022.100895.

Roy F. Baumeister et al., "Some Key Differences between a Happy Life and a Meaningful Life," *The Journal of Positive Psychology* 8, no. 6 (August 22, 2013): 505–16, https://doi.org/10.1080/17439760.2013.830764.

Megan E. Beerse et al., "Biobehavioral Utility of Mindfulness-Based Art Therapy: Neurobiological Underpinnings and Mental Health Impacts," *Experimental Biology and Medicine* 245, no. 2 (October 21, 2019): 122–30, https://doi.org/10.1177/1535370219883634.

P. Blardi et al., "Stimulation of Endogenous Adenosine Release by Oral Administration of Quercetin and Resveratrol in Man," *Drugs Under Experimental and Clinical Research* 25, nos. 2–3 (1999): 105–10, https://pubmed.ncbi.nlm.nih.gov/10370871.

Patricia A. Boyle et al., "Purpose in Life Is Associated with Mortality Among Community-Dwelling Older Persons," *Psychosomatic Medicine* 71, no. 5 (June 2009): 574–79, https://journals.lww.com/psychosomaticmedicine/abstract/2009/06000/purpose_in_life_is_associated_with_mortality_among.13.aspx.

Annie Britton and Martin J. Shipley, "Bored to Death?" *International Journal of Epidemiology* 39, no. 2 (February 1, 2010): 370–71, https://doi.org/10.1093/ije/dyp404.

Emilia Bunea, "'Grace Under Pressure': How CEOs Use Serious Leisure to Cope with the Demands of Their Job," *Frontiers in Psychology* 11 (July 3, 2020), https://doi.org/10.3389/fpsyg.2020.01453.

"The Burden of Stress in America," Robert Wood Johnson Foundation (July 7, 2014), https://www.rwjf.org/en/insights/our-research/2014/07/the-burden-of-stress-in-america.html.

Colin A. Capaldi, Raelyne L. Dopko, and John M. Zelenski, "The Relationship between Nature Connectedness and Happiness: A Meta-Analysis," *Frontiers in Psychology* 5 (September 8, 2014), https://www.frontiersin.org/articles/10.3389/fpsyg.2014.00976/full.

Anne Cleary et al., "Exploring Potential Mechanisms Involved in the Relationship between Eudaimonic Wellbeing and Nature Connection," *Landscape and Urban Planning* 158 (February 1, 2017): 119–28, https://doi.org/10.1016/j.landurbplan.2016.10.003.

Geoffrey L. Cohen and David K. Sherman, "The Psychology of Change: Self-Affirmation and Social Psychological Intervention," *Annual Review of Psychology* 65, no. 1 (January 3, 2014): 333–71, https://doi.org/10.1146/annurev-psych-010213-115137.

Alessia Costa et al., "Doing Nothing? An Ethnography of Patients' (In)Activity on an Acute Stroke Unit," *Health* 26, no. 4 (January 9, 2021): 457–74, https://doi.org/10.1177/1363459320969784.

Alia J. Crum, Jeremy P. Jamieson, and Modupe Akinola, "Optimizing Stress: An Integrated Intervention for Regulating Stress Responses," *Emotion* 20, no. 1 (February 1, 2020): 120–25, https://doi.org/10.1037/emo0000670.

Alia J. Crum, Peter Salovey, and Shawn Achor, "Rethinking Stress: The Role of Mindsets in Determining the Stress Response," *Journal of Personality and Social Psychology* 104, no. 4 (February 25, 2013): 716–33, https://psycnet.apa.org/doiLanding?doi=10.1037%2Femo0000670.

Christina Daskalopoulou et al., "Physical Activity and Healthy Ageing: A Systematic Review and Meta-Analysis of Longitudinal Cohort Studies," *Ageing Research Reviews* 38 (June 23, 2017): 6–17, https://doi.org/10.1016/j.arr.2017.06.003.

Jennifer Daubenmier et al., "Changes in Stress, Eating, and Metabolic Factors Are Related to Changes in Telomerase Activity in a Randomized Mindfulness Intervention Pilot Study," *Psychoneuroendocrinology* 37, no. 7 (July 1, 2012): 917–28, https://doi.org/10.1016/j.psyneuen.2011.10.008.

Elissa S. Epel et al., "Can Meditation Slow Rate of Cellular Aging? Cognitive Stress, Mindfulness, and Telomeres," *Annals of the New York Academy of Sciences* 1172, no. 1 (August 28, 2009): 34–53, https://doi.org/10.1111/j.1749-6632.2009.04414.x.

Elissa S. Epel et al., "Effects of a Mindfulness-Based Intervention on Distress, Weight Gain, and Glucose Control for Pregnant Low-Income Women: A Quasi-Experimental Trial Using the ORBIT Model," *International Journal of Behavioral Medicine* 26, no. 5 (October 1, 2019): 461–73, https://doi.org/10.1007/s12529-019-09779-2.

Elissa S. Epel, "The Geroscience Agenda: Toxic Stress, Hormetic Stress, and the Rate of Aging," *Ageing Research Reviews* 63 (September 28, 2020): 101167, https://doi.org/10.1016/j.arr.2020.101167.

Elissa S. Epel, *The Stress Prescription: Seven Days to More Joy and Ease* (New York: Penguin Life, 2022).

Elissa S. Epel, Bruce S. McEwen, and Jeannette R. Ickovics, "Embodying Psychological Thriving: Physical Thriving in Response to Stress," *Journal of Social Issues* 54, no. 2 (April 9, 2010): 301–22, https://spssi.onlinelibrary.wiley.com/doi/10.1111/j.1540-4560.1998.tb01220.x/

Omid Fotuhi, "Implicit Processes in Smoking Interventions," UWSpace.com (September 19, 2013), https://www.uwspace.uwaterloo.ca/handle/10012/7885?show=full.

Astrid T. Groot and Marcel Dicke, "Insect-Resistant Transgenic Plants in a Multi-Trophic Context," *Plant Journal* 31, no. 4 (August 16, 2002): 387–406, https://doi.org/10.1046/j.1365-313x.2002.01366.x.

Margaret M. Hansen, Reo J. F. Jones, and Kirsten Tocchini, "Shinrin-Yoku (Forest Bathing) and Nature Therapy: A State-of-the-Art Review," *International Journal of Environmental Research and Public Health* 14, no. 8 (July 28, 2017): 851, https://doi.org/10.3390/ijerph14080851.

David Heber, "Vegetables, Fruits and Phytoestrogens in the Prevention of Diseases," *Journal of Postgraduate Medicine* 5, no. 2 (April–June 2004): 145–49, https://www.jpgmonline.com/text.asp?2004/50/2/145/8259

Konrad T. Howitz et al., "Small Molecule Activators of Sirtuins Extend *Saccharomyces Cerevisiae* Lifespan," *Nature* 425, no. 6954 (August 24, 2003): 191–96, https://doi.org/10.1038/nature01960.

Andrew Huberman, "Dr. Alia Crum: Science of Mindsets for Health & Performance," *Huberman Lab* (April 22, 2023), https://hubermanlab.com/dr-alia-crum-science-of-mindsets-for-health-performance.

Andrew Huberman, "Dr. Elissa Epel: Control Stress for Healthy Eating, Metabolism & Aging," *Huberman Lab* (April 4, 2023), https://hubermanlab.com/dr-elissa-epel-control-stress-for-healthy-eating-metabolism-and-aging.

Gabriel Sahlgren, "Work Longer, Live Healthier: The Relationship between Economic Activity, Health and Government Policy," Institute of Economic Affairs (May 16, 2013), https://iea.org.uk/publications/research/work-longer-live-healthier-the-relationship-between-economic-activity-health-a.

Dacher Keltner and Jonathan Haidt, "Approaching Awe, a Moral, Spiritual, and Aesthetic Emotion," *Cognition and Emotion* 17, no. 2 (March 1, 2003): 297–314, https://doi.org/10.1080/02699930302297.

Matthijs Kox et al., "Voluntary Activation of the Sympathetic Nervous System and Attenuation of the Innate Immune Response in Humans," *Proceedings of the National Academy of Sciences* 111, no. 20 (May 20, 2014): 7379–84, https://doi.org/10.1073/pnas.1322174111.

Jun Lin and Elissa S. Epel, "Stress and Telomere Shortening: Insights from Cellular Mechanisms," *Ageing Research Reviews* 73 (January 1, 2022): 101507, https://doi.org/10.1016/j.arr.2021.101507.

Mark P. Mattson, "Hormesis and Disease Resistance: Activation of Cellular Stress Response Pathways," *Human & Experimental Toxicology* 27, no. 2 (February 1, 2008): 155–62, https://doi.org/10.1177/0960327107083417.

Kelly McGonigal, *The Upside of Stress: Why Stress Is Good for You (and How to Get Good at It)* (New York: Avery, 2016).

Maria Monroy and Dacher Keltner, "Awe as a Pathway to Mental and Physical Health," *Perspectives on Psychological Science* 18, no. 2 (August 22, 2022): 309–20, https://doi.org/10.1177/17456916221094856.

Rhonda P. Patrick and Teresa L. Johnson, "Sauna Use as a Lifestyle Practice to Extend Healthspan," *Experimental Gerontology* 154 (October 15, 2021): 111509, https://doi.org/10.1016/j.exger.2021.111509.

Joshua D. Perlin and Leon Li, "Why Does Awe Have Prosocial Effects? New Perspectives on Awe and the Small Self," *Perspectives on Psychological Science* 15, no. 2 (January 13, 2020): 291–308, https://doi.org/10.1177/1745691619886006.

Martin Picard et al., "A Mitochondrial Health Index Sensitive to Mood and Caregiving Stress," *Biological Psychiatry* 84, no. 1 (July 1, 2018): 9–17, https://doi.org/10.1016/j.biopsych.2018.01.012.

Leo Pruimboom et al., "Influence of a 10-Day Mimic of Our Ancient Lifestyle on Anthropometrics and Parameters of Metabolism and Inflammation: The 'Study of Origin,'" *BioMed Research International* 2016, no. 6935123 (June 6, 2016): 1–9, https://doi.org/10.1155/2016/6935123.

Stefan E. Schulenberg, "Empirical Research and Logotherapy," *Psychological Reports* 93, no. 1 (August 1, 2003): 307–19, https://doi.org/10.2466/pr0.2003.93.1.307.

Ekin Secinti et al., "The Relationship between Acceptance of Cancer and Distress: A Meta-Analytic Review," *Clinical Psychology Review* 71 (July 1, 2019): 27–38, https://doi.org/10.1016/j.cpr.2019.05.001.

M. N. Shiota, D. Keltner, and O. P. John, " Positive Emotion Dispositions Differentially Associated with Big Five Personality and Attachment Style," *Journal of Positive Psychology* 1, no. 2 (February 18, 2007): 61–71, https://doi.org/10.1080/17439760500510833.

Toshimasa Sone et al., "Sense of Life Worth Living (Ikigai) and Mortality in Japan: Ohsaki Study," *Psychosomatic Medicine* 70, no. 6 (July 1, 2008): 709–15, https://doi.org/10.1097/psy.0b013e31817e7e64.

P. Šrámek et al., "Human Physiological Responses to Immersion into Water of Different Temperatures," *European Journal of Applied Physiology* 81, no. 5 (March 1, 2000): 436–42, https://link.springer.com/article/10.1007/s004210050065.

Ekaterina R. Stepanova, Denise Quesnel, and Bernhard E. Riecke, "Understanding AWE: Can a Virtual Journey, Inspired by the Overview Effect, Lead to an Increased Sense of Interconnectedness?" *Frontiers in Digital Humanities* 6 (May 22, 2019), https://doi.org/10.3389/fdigh.2019.00009.

Cassandra Vieten et al., "The Mindful Moms Training: Development of a Mindfulness-Based Intervention to Reduce Stress and Overeating during Pregnancy," *BMC Pregnancy and Childbirth* 18, no. 1 (June 1, 2018): 201, https://doi.org/10.1186/s12884-018-1757-6.

Gregory M. Walton et al., "Two Brief Interventions to Mitigate a 'Chilly Climate' Transform Women's Experience, Relationships, and Achievement in Engineering," *Journal of Educational Psychology* 107, no. 2 (May 1, 2014): 468–85, https://doi.org/10.1037/a0037461.

Florence Williams, *The Nature Fix: Why Nature Makes Us Happier, Healthier, and More Creative* (New York: W. W. Norton & Company, 2017).

Ala Yankouskaya et al., "Short-Term Head-Out Whole-Body Cold-Water Immersion Facilitates Positive Affect and Increases Interaction between Large-Scale Brain Networks," *Biology* 12, no. 2 (January 29, 2023): 211, https://doi.org/10.3390/biology12020211.

John M. Zelenski and Elizabeth K. Nisbet, "Happiness and Feeling Connected: The Distinct Role of Nature Relatedness," *Environment and Behavior* 46, no. 1 (January 1, 2014): 3–23, https://doi.org/10.1177/0013916512451901.

David D. Zhang et al., "Earliest Parietal Art: Hominin Hand and Foot Traces from the Middle Pleistocene of Tibet," *Science Bulletin* 66, no. 24 (December 30, 2021): 2506–15, https://doi.org/10.1016/j.scib.2021.09.001.

Chapter 12: Connecting the Dots: The Ongoing Practice of Building a Coherent Life Narrative

Rebecca L. Cann, Mark Stoneking, and Allan C. Wilson, "Mitochondrial DNA and Human Evolution," *Nature* 325, no. 6099 (January 1, 1987): 31–36, https://www.nature.com/articles/325031a0.

Jasmine R. Connell et al., "Evaluating the Suitability of Current Mitochondrial DNA Interpretation Guidelines for Multigenerational Whole Mitochondrial Genome Comparisons," *Journal of Forensic Sciences* 67, no. 5 (September 2022): 1766–75, https://pubmed.ncbi.nlm.nih.gov/35855536.

Richard Dawkins, *River Out of Eden: A Darwinian View of Life* (New York: Basic Books, 1996).

Ann Gibbons, "Mitochondrial Eve: Wounded, But Not Dead Yet," *Science* 257, no. 5072 (August 14. 1992): 873–75, https://www.science.org/doi/10.1126/science.1502551.

Michael F. Hammer, "A Recent Common Ancestry for Human Y Chromosomes," *Nature* 378, no. 6555 (November 23, 1995): 376–78, https://www.nature.com/articles/378376a0.

Ingebor Stiefel, Poppy Harris, and Andreas W. F. Zollman, "Family Constellation—A Therapy Beyond Words," *Australian & New Zealand Journal of Family Therapy* 23, no. 1 (March 2002): 38–44, https://onlinelibrary.wiley.com/doi/10.1002/j.1467-8438.2002.tb00484.x.

Barna Konkolÿ Thege, Carla Petroll, Carlos Rivas, and Salome Scholtens. "The Effectiveness of Family Constellation Therapy in Improving Mental Health: A Systematic Review," *Family Process* 60, no. 2 (February 2, 2021): 409–23, https://pubmed.ncbi.nlm.nih.gov/33528854.

Chapter 13: Flourishing Like the Fern: Adapting Amid Challenges and Inspiring Others

Bailey Burns, "Thin Blue Line Stories," A Space Story, https://aspacestory.com/thin-blue-line-stories.

Alice Chirico et al., "'Standing Up for Earth Rights': Awe-Inspiring Virtual Nature for Promoting Pro-Environmental Behaviors," *Cyberpsychology, Behavior, and Social Networking* 26, no. 4 (April 4, 2023), https://doi.org/10.1089/cyber.2022.0260.

Lyanda Lynn Haupt, *Rooted: Life at the Crossroads of Science, Nature, and Spirit* (New York: Little, Brown Spark, 2021).

Amy Isham, Patrick Elf, and Tim Jackson, "Self-Transcendent Experiences as Promoters of Ecological Wellbeing? Exploration of the Evidence and Hypotheses to Be Tested," *Frontiers in Psychology* 13 (November 14, 2022), https://doi.org/10.3389/fpsyg.2022.1051478.

William R. Miller, "The Phenomenon of Quantum Change," *Journal of Clinical Psychology* 60, no. 5 (May 1, 2004): 453–60, https://doi.org/10.1002/jclp.20000.

Karen O'Brien, *You Matter More Than You Think: Quantum Social Change for a Thriving World* (Oslo: cCHANGE press, 2021).

Rebecca Solnit and Thelma Young Lutunatabua, *Not Too Late: Changing the Climate Story from Despair to Possibility* (Chicago: Haymarket Books, 2023).

John M. Zelenski and Jessica E. Desrochers, "Can Positive and Self-Transcendent Emotions Promote Pro-Environmental Behavior?" *Current Opinion in Psychology* 42 (March 4, 2021): 31–35, https://doi.org/10.1016/j.copsyc.2021.02.009.

Index